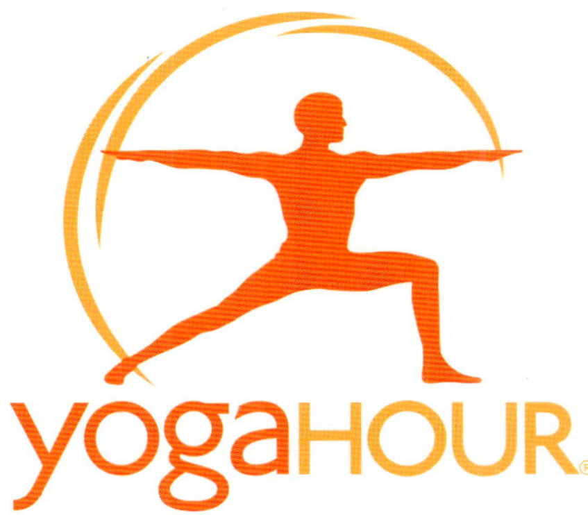

Inform Your Flow

Shape, Safety, and Refinement Instructions
for over 200 poses in the yogahour® syllabus

Darren Rhodes

ISBN 978-0-9979103-0-8
Third Edition.
© Darren Rhodes, Yogahour 2014, 2015, 2016

All rights reserved. The contents of this book may not be reproduced in any form, without written permission. Your purchase is for personal use only. Please respect the copyright of this product and do not copy, distribute, or sell any of the contents. For more information please visit yogahour.com

Inform Your Flow Credits:
Content: Darren Rhodes
Cover and Graphic Design: Mackie Osborne
Photography: Jade Beall
Editors: Joanne Miller, Shawn Asplundh, Bre Downing, Christine Reitmayr, Neda Honarvar, and Teagan Schweitzer
Printed in China by Prolong Press Limited

LIMIT OF LIABILITY: THE EXERCISE AND SEQUENCES CONTAINED HEREIN MAY NOT BE SUITABLE FOR EVERY INDIVIDUAL. NEITHER THE PUBLISHER NOR THE AUTHOR SHALL BE LIABLE FOR ANY LOSS OF PROFIT OR ANY OTHER COMMERCIAL DAMAGES, INCLUDING BUT NOT LIMITED TO SPECIAL, INCIDENTAL, CONSEQUENTIAL, OR OTHER DAMAGES. CONSULTATION WITH A PHYSICIAN IS SUGGESTED BEFORE COMMENCING ANY EXERCISE PROGRAM. PERSONS USING THESE SEQUENCES DO SO ENTIRELY AT THEIR OWN RISK.

Foreward

In the same way that the banks of a river channel the flow of water and direct its course, biomechanical alignment in asana provides a structure through which the flow of one's awareness and energy can be directed with clarity and focus. Alignment and flow exist on every level of our being– from our subtle intentions and heart-felt feelings to intellectual understanding and knowledge, all the way to our breath-based movement and sustained physical action. As we bend, stretch, breathe, stabilize and open our bodies through persistent postural practice, we invoke a transformational process aimed at the alignment with, and integration of, who we most truly are. We are engaging a process that shows us the deepest flows of our being and the structures through which we might bring that spiritual essence to life.

Whether you prefer a flowing, movement-oriented expression of asana or you enjoy a more static practice with a form-based emphasis, this book, with its captivating photographs, succinct descriptions and pithy alignment cues will help you. New and experienced students will gain access to the rich insights of Darren Rhodes' masterful synthesis and teachers will find a never-ending source of inspiration for their class planning and implementation. Truly, there is something in this book for every sincere asana practitioner.

Don't be fooled by the seeming simplicity in the presentation of the following material. Finding depth in the basics is a journey of the most profound order and the ability to convey sophisticated concepts in a simple manner speaks volumes about the understanding that lives in the foundation of this offering. Darren Rhodes has brought together a lifetime of study, practice and teaching in this manual. Please enjoy the work required to integrate his insights into your own experience and know that in doing so, you are standing on the shoulders of giants.

May all that is good, true and loving bless you on your path of yoga.

Christina Sell
Author, *Yoga From the Inside Out: Making Peace with Your Body through Yoga* and *My Body is a Temple: Yoga as a Path to Wholeness*

Welcome to Yogahour®

Yogahour is an accessible, affordable, expertly taught flow/form class that offers clear and specific alignment instructions. Yogahour aims to be the most doable yet difficult one-hour flow/form class offered anywhere.

Yogahour originated in Tucson Arizona by founder, Darren Rhodes. One of the central aims of yogahour is to support and sustain the local studio and the longevity of practice.

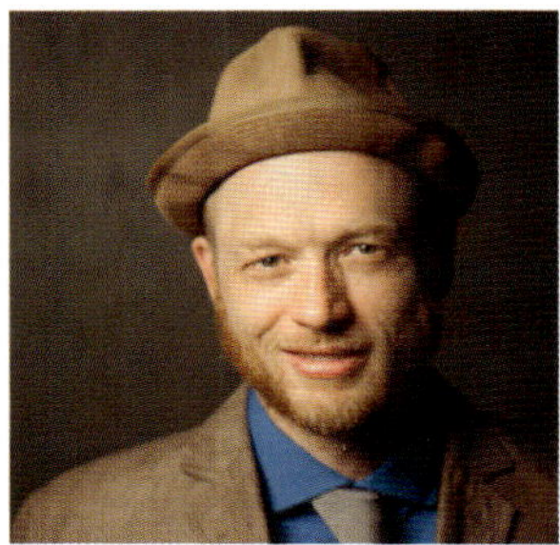 Darren Rhodes is the owner of YogaOasis and the founder of yogahour.
He lives in Tucson with his wife and two children.

Introduction

In early 2006, YogaOasis (YO) studios faced a financial challenge. Our financial advisor summed up our situation this way: "You are like a ship that is slowly sinking. You have about three months to turn this situation around." At the time, failure seemed more likely than survival, let alone success. We learned the hard way that challenge can promote positive change. When failure seems inevitable but you refuse to give up, pivotal and lasting transformations can, and often do, take place. Without the pressing possibility of failure, what would push us to discover our true capacity?

Around that time, one of our students gave me a card with this quote: "What would you do if you knew you couldn't fail?" An even more interesting question to me is: "What would you do anyway, even if failure seemed inevitable?" Armed with determination, intention, and creativity, a small group of us decided to fight the good fight for YO, no matter what. It was during these weekly meetings that the concept of yogahour® was born.

This was all happening during a period of economic turmoil around the globe. We realized that people needed a way to relieve stress and strengthen their bodies without breaking the bank. We decided that this was an opportunity to create a new type of yoga class experience. Our goal was to remove as many of the obstacles as possible for people who wanted to practice yoga. The classes needed to be both accessible to new students and engaging for longtime practitioners. We would need to offer expert alignment instruction while drawing from a difficult-but-doable palette of poses for our flow oriented sequences. Lastly, the classes needed to be affordable.

The yogahour class itself started with just four slots per week on the YO schedule. Two years later we had built up to 25 classes. By our third year, many of the yogahour classes became so popular we had to offer overflow classes. Standby teachers taught the overflow students in an adjacent room to avoid turning students away. When even the overflow classes started to overflow, we decided to open an additional studio on the east side of Tucson, YO | east. On January 22, 2010, we opened our third studio, YO | downtown.

Yogahour was thriving at YO studios in Tucson, but we had a growing number of out of state practitioners who wanted access to the practice on the go and in their hometowns. During this time, my longtime friend and collaborator Milo (Michael Longstaff) came up with the idea of creating a yogahour App and gave me the task of creating a yogahour set sequence and a class script as the basis of it. At first, second, and third I protested because I didn't think I had what it took to articulate alignment cues effectively. Milo said, "Do it anyway."

The first draft of the script for this one hour class took me nearly two hours to recite! Necessity, as they say, is the mother of invention– and I realized that sutra-like vernacular was the only option. Creating this sequence (yogahour set sequence 1) and writing the sutra-style script that went along with it set the foundation for what yogahour is today. Both the sutra-style vernacular used in yogahour and the 33 set sequences we have today were modeled after this initial project. The yogahour vision would never have become what it is today if it wasn't for the talents that Milo brought to the table.

Another indelible offering from Milo is the brand identity of yogahour, which gave it a professional feel. He then passed the baton to Mackie Osborne, who has since kept the essence of Milo's design, while adding her own signature flare so roar and rare.

In 2012, several studios around the country started offering official yogahour classes. This was sparked by a week-long yoga training intensive I was teaching with Christina Sell. We had yogahour classes directly following these training sessions. Brigette Finley, now yogahour director, took note of how big these classes were (often 52 students). She and her husband Alexis, who together owned a local studio in St. Louis, MO, took me to coffee to tell me two things:
1. Yogahour was worthy of becoming a distinct style of Hatha yoga.
2. She and her husband wanted to start offering yogahour at their local studio.

Within less than a year, yogahour became the most popular class at their studio. This has become the story of many local studios around the world. This points to the very purpose of yogahour: to support and help sustain the local studio and longevity of practice. Yogahour will only ever be as big as the local studio. As you may well know, there is nothing like the community connection born out of the local studio. The "it takes a village" concept applies to yogahour. Since its inception, many others have evolved yogahour way beyond my initial expression of it. For that I offer you my Namaste, please stay, Pranams.

~ Darren Rhodes

How Shape, Safety, and Refinement Instructions Inform Flow

Shape
Shape instructions efficiently and effectively get students into and out of the basic form of each pose.

Safety (strength)
Safety instructions create stability and reduce risk of injury.

Refinement (stretch)
Refinement instructions stretch the pose, enhance awareness, and add nuance.

Prep/Pose
Prep is part and parcel to each pose. Knowing where each pose starts and stops promotes clarity, safety, and sets the practitioner up for success.

Sutra-like vernacular
A sutra is a concentrated teaching presented in the most succinct statement possible. To maximize accessibility, yogahour uses sutra-like vernacular.

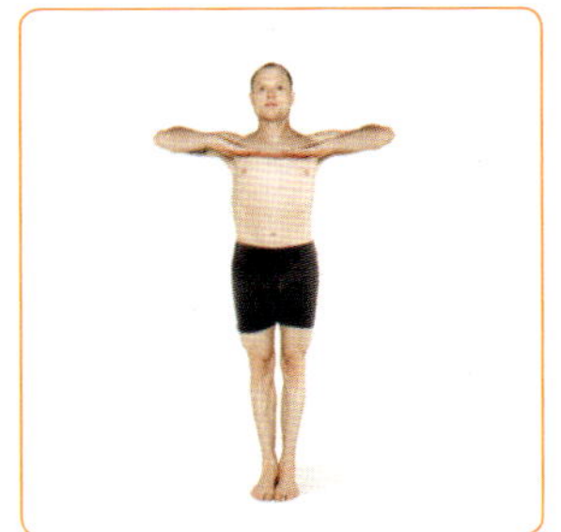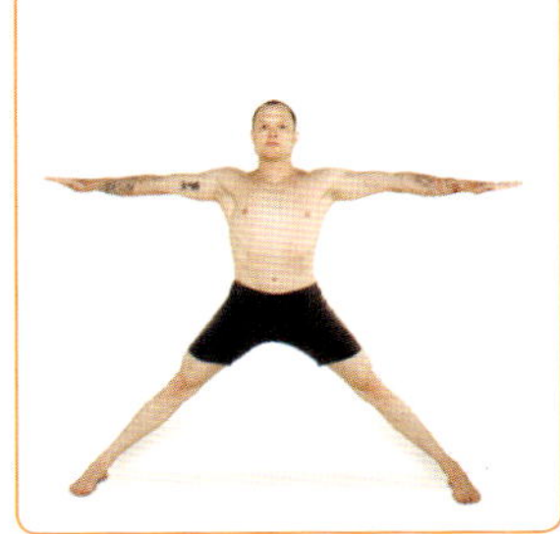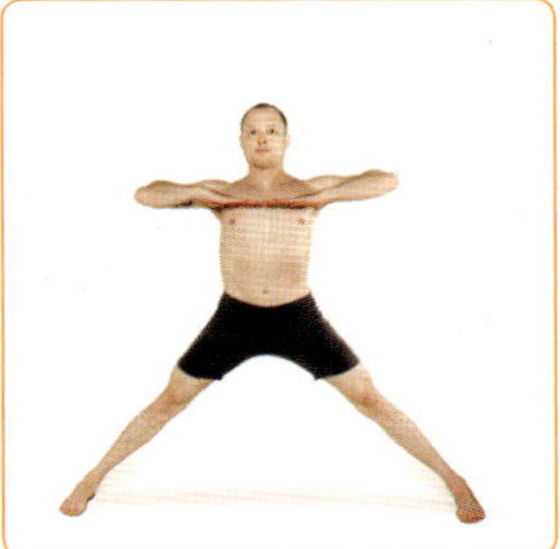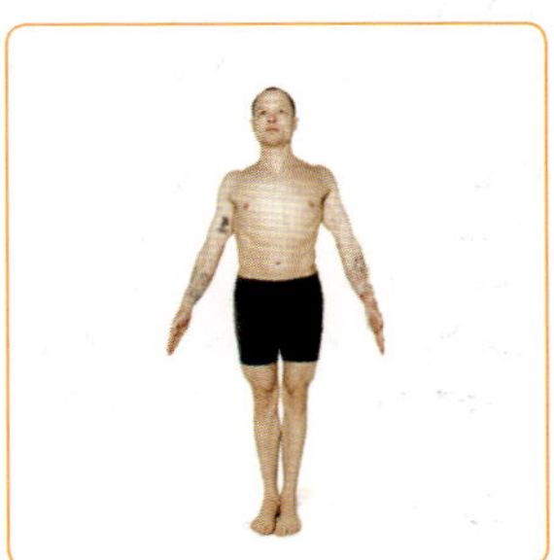

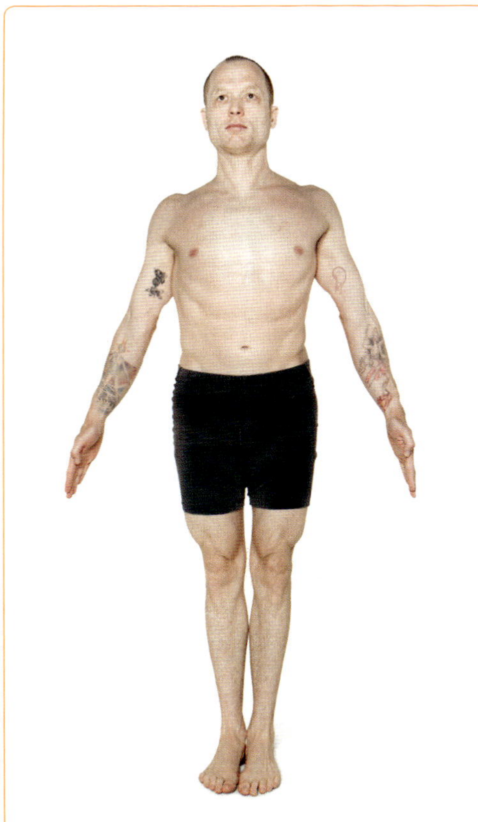

mountain
tadasana

shape prep
- Bring inner edges of feet together.

shape pose
- Bring arms by sides. Close fingers, point palms in.
- Straighten arms, legs.
- Lift chin slightly, look straight ahead.

safety (strength) pose
- Distribute weight evenly on feet. Do not lean forward, back, or to the side.
- Press big toes down, flare toes.
- Tone thighs, tighten kneecaps, firm hamstrings.
- Squeeze feet/legs together.
- Tighten glutes, press tailbone down, tone abdomen.

refinement (stretch) pose
- Lift chest, stretch spine. Extend arms down.
- Soften eyes, jaw. Notice breath.
- Mountain pose promotes poise, focus, pith.

Mountain is a pose, not a pause between poses. It's a chance to come to center and get that much more centered. I discovered mountain as a pose during Barefoot Boot Camp out of pure necessity. In that moment I experienced the truth of David Williams' words, "Before you've practiced, the theory is useless. After you've practiced, the theory is obvious."

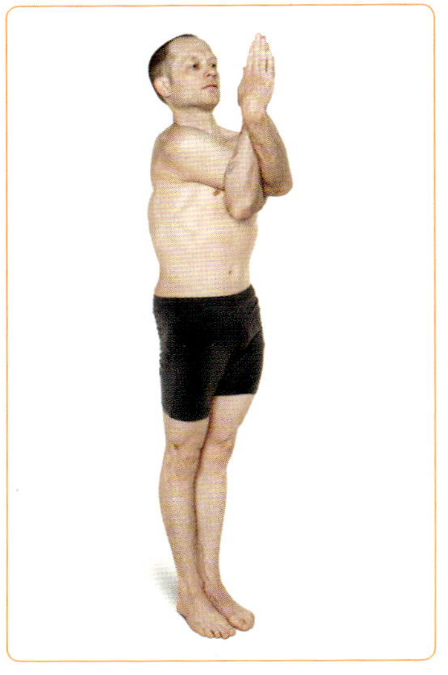

summit

shape pose (from mountain)
- Interlace fingers, lift arms overhead, point palms up.
- Straighten arms.
- Lift chin slightly, look straight ahead.

safety (strength) pose
- Press big toes down, flare toes.
- Tone thighs, tighten kneecaps, firm hamstrings.
- Squeeze legs together.
- Tighten glutes, press tailbone down, tone abdomen.
- Move ribs back.
- Squeeze elbows in.

refinement (stretch) pose
- Lift chest. Stretch spine. Extend arms up, back.
- Soften eyes, jaw. Notice breath.

Parvatasana warms up the shoulders. It works well prior to indudalasana, vrksasana, surya namaskar, and adho mukha vrksasana.

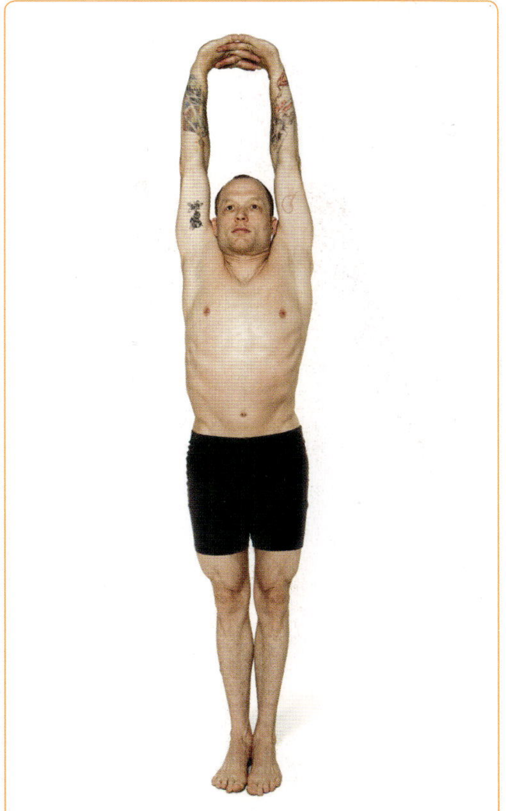

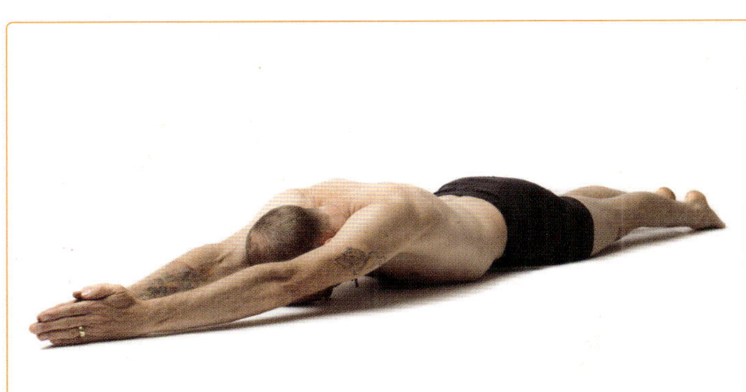

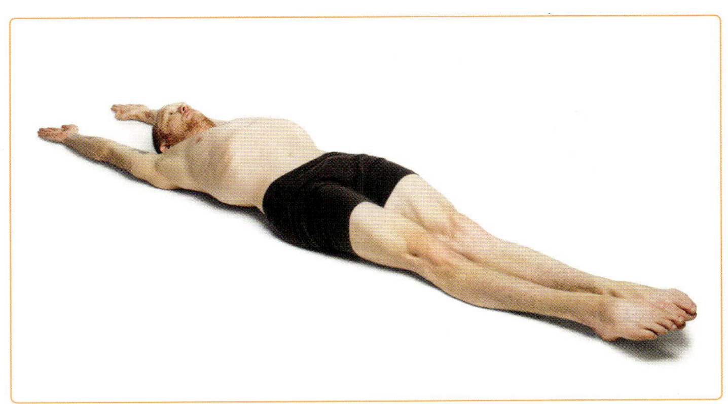

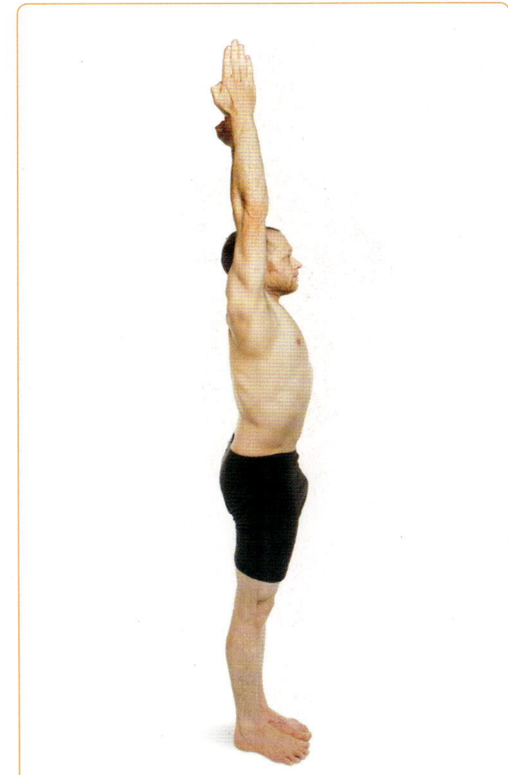

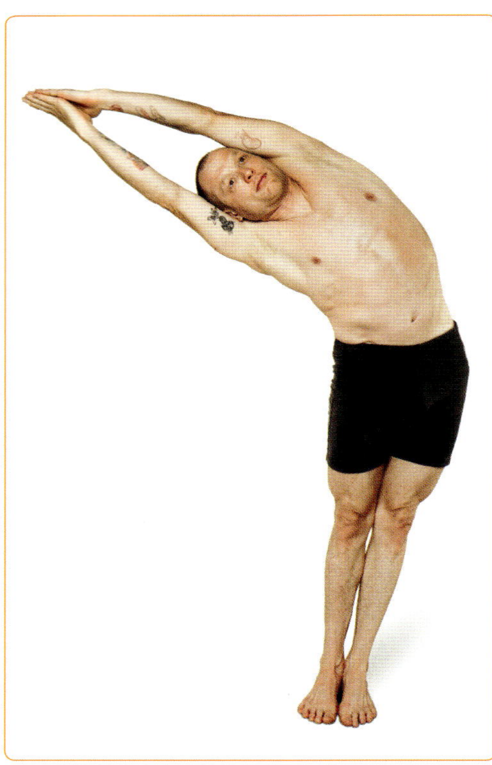

crescent
indudalasana

shape prep (from mountain)
- Lift arms overhead.
- Place palms together, cross thumbs.
- Straighten arms.

shape pose
- Sway hips to left, torso to right.
- Keep head placed evenly between arms.
- Look straight ahead.

safety (strength) pose
- Press big toes down, flare toes.
- Tone thighs, tighten kneecaps, firm hamstrings.
- Squeeze feet/legs together.
- Tighten glutes, press tailbone down, tone abdomen.
- Move ribs back.
- Move shoulders back.
- Squeeze elbows in.
- Do not overstretch or compress either side of the torso.

refinement (stretch) prep
- Lift chest, stretch spine.

refinement (stretch) pose
- Turn hips, torso slightly to left—move left hip, shoulder back.
- Press left foot down, stretch left hand out.

Repeat on the second side.

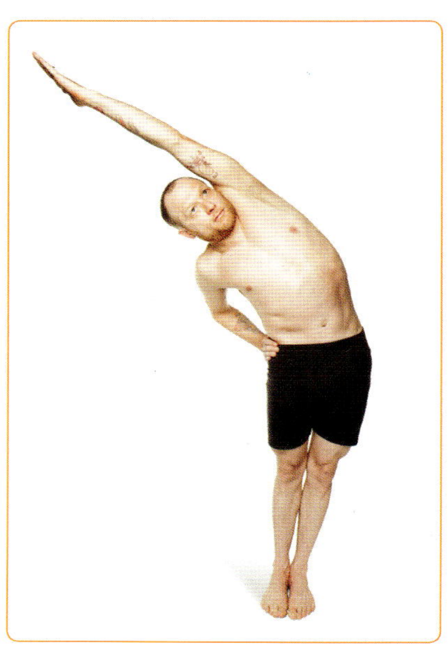

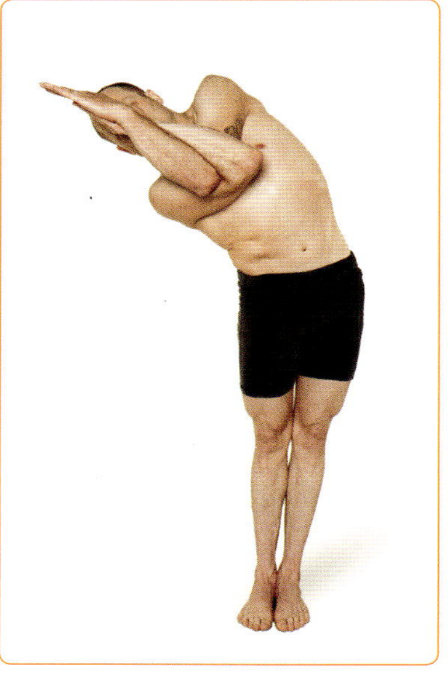

crescent 1 *wrist*
indudalasana

shape prep (from mountain)
- Lift arms overhead.
- Hold left wrist with right hand.
- Straighten arms.

shape pose
- Sway hips to left, torso to right.
- Keep head placed evenly between arms.
- Look straight ahead.

safety (strength) pose
- Press big toes down, flare toes.
- Tone thighs, tighten kneecaps, firm hamstrings.
- Squeeze feet/legs together.
- Tighten glutes, press tailbone down, tone abdomen.
- Move ribs back.
- Move shoulders back.
- Do not overstretch or compress either side of the torso.

refinement (stretch) prep
- Lift chest, stretch spine.

refinement (stretch) pose
- Turn hips, torso slightly to left.
- Press left foot down, stretch left hand out.
- Lift left wrist with right hand.

Repeat on the second side.

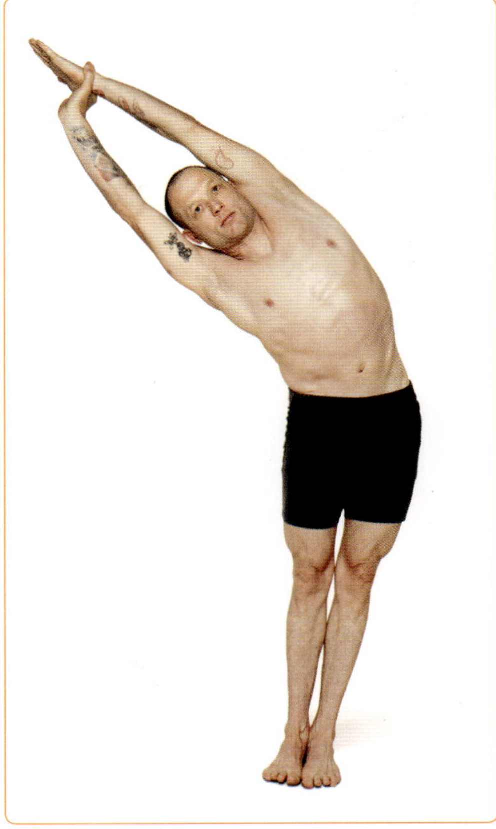

Few poses strengthen and stretch the obliques. I, therefore and thereafter, include crescent in one variation or another in almost every practice. It can be held for fifteen to thirty seconds, or you can move into and out of it with your breath. For example: exhale, indudalasana to the right. Inhale, come back to center. Exhale, indudalasana to the left and so on and so forth.

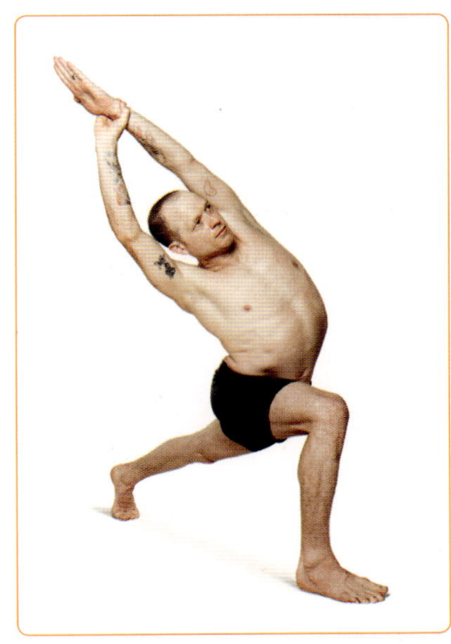

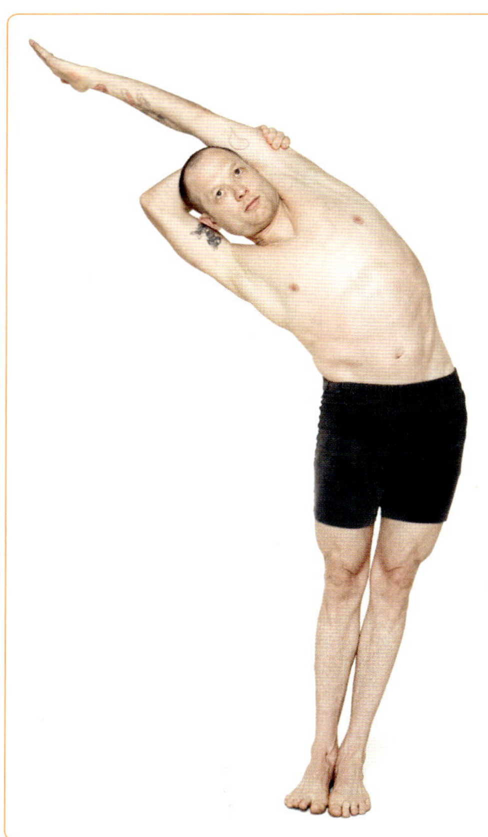

crescent 2 *triceps*
indudalasana

shape prep (from mountain)
- Lift arms overhead.
- Hold upper left triceps with right hand.

shape pose
- Sway hips to left, torso to right.
- Keep head placed evenly between arms.
- Look straight ahead.

safety (strength) pose
- Press big toes down, flare toes.
- Tone thighs, tighten kneecaps, firm hamstrings.
- Squeeze feet/legs together.
- Tighten glutes, press tailbone down, tone abdomen.
- Move ribs back.
- Move shoulders back.
- Press head into right forearm, forearm into head; move shoulders back.
- Press triceps, hand together.
- Do not overstretch or compress either side of the torso.

refinement (stretch) prep
- Lift chest, stretch spine.

refinement (stretch) pose
- Turn hips, torso slightly to left—move left hip, shoulder back.
- Press left foot down, stretch left hand out.
- Lift left arm with right hand.

Repeat on the second side.

crescent 3 *leg lifted*
indudalasana

shape prep (from mountain)
- Lift arms overhead.
- Place palms together, cross thumbs.
- Straighten arms.
- Sway hips to left, torso to right.

shape pose
- Lift right leg out to side.
- Keep head placed evenly between arms.
- Look straight ahead.

safety (strength) pose
- Tone thighs, tighten kneecaps, firm hamstrings.
- Press tailbone down, tone abdomen.
- Move ribs back.
- Move shoulders back.
- Squeeze elbows in.

refinement (stretch) prep
- Lift chest, stretch spine.

refinement (stretch) pose
- Extend feet down; arms up, back.

Repeat on the second side.

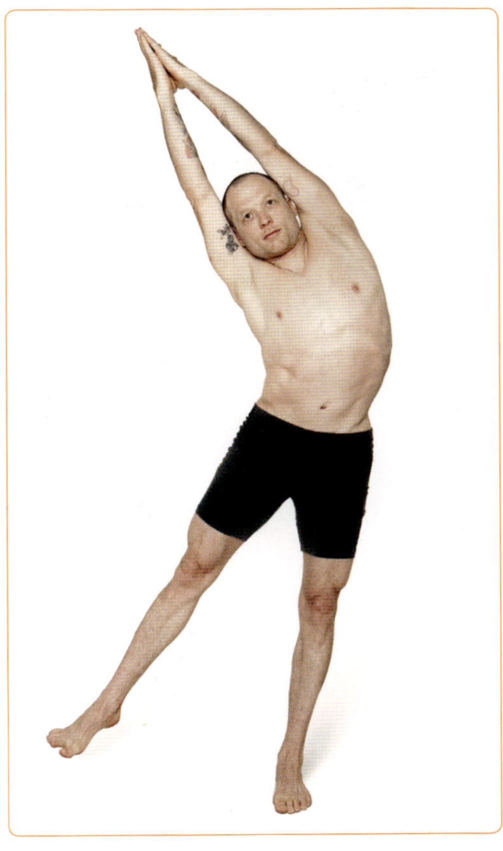

This pose warms up and works the glutes of the lifted leg. A key alignment instruction in yogahour: tighten glutes. This pose gives students an experience of that. A good teaching tool: "Notice how this pose tightens the glutes of your lifted leg." (passive instruction) Then, when teaching another pose in your sequence where that doesn't happen automatically, instruct: "Like you did in crescent, one leg lifted, tighten your glutes."

lunge

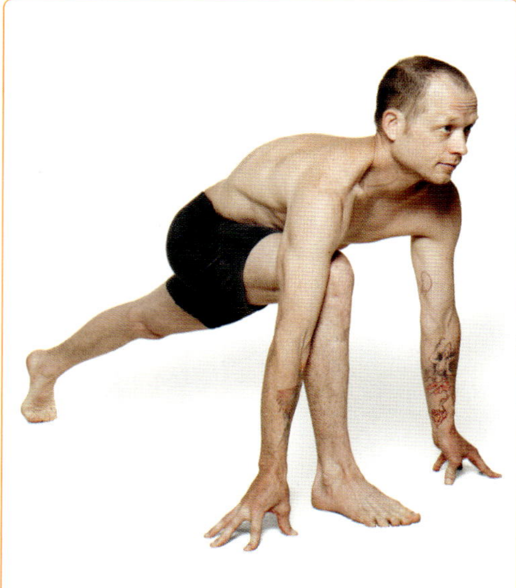

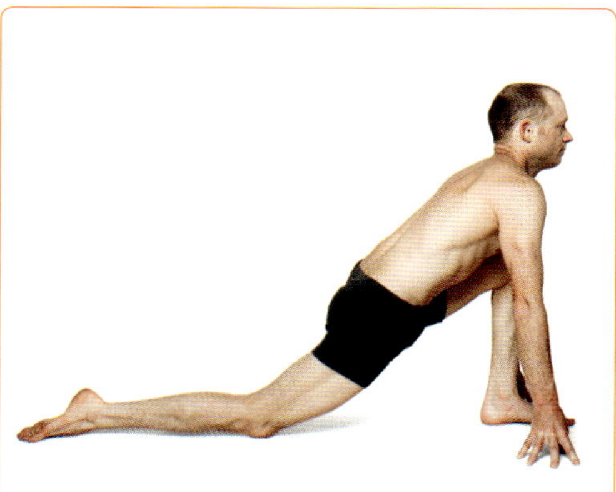

shape prep (from mountain)
■ Step left foot back, lower fingertips to floor under shoulders; straighten arms.

shape pose
■ Lunge pose is a back heel vertical, back leg straight, front thigh parallel, front shin vertical to the floor pose. (To accommodate tight hips/hip flexors shorten stance and lift hips higher than front knee.)
■ Move left hip forward, right hip back to square hips.
■ Round back evenly.
■ Lift chin slightly, look straight ahead.

safety (strength) pose
■ Squeeze feet toward each other.
■ Tighten glutes, press tailbone down, tone abdomen.
■ Lift back thigh.

refinement (stretch) pose
■ Press fingertips down.
■ Stretch spine.

Repeat on the second side.

A common technique: get into lunge from downward facing dog, warrior 1 prep from lunge. Equally as often, yogahour teachers get students into lunge and warrior 1 prep from mountain pose—front, middle, or back of mat.

One benefit of back heel vertical in lunge is the toes/sole of foot stretch.

down-dog lunge

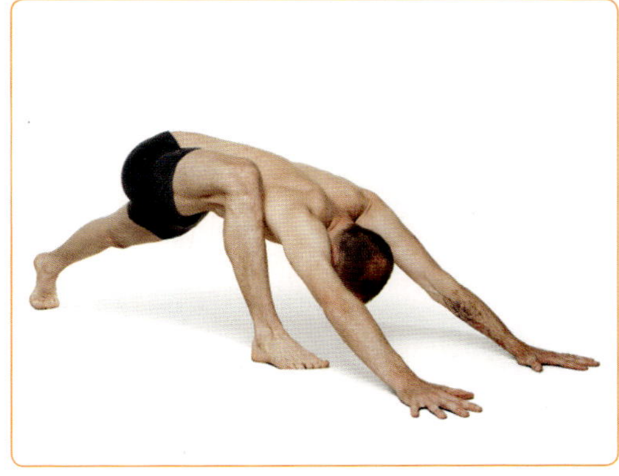

shape prep (from lunge)
- Fold torso inside front thigh.

shape pose
- Walk hands forward, straighten arms—right hand in front of right foot, hands shoulder-width apart; separate fingers evenly.
- Move back heel vertical, straighten back leg.
- Move front knee out (knee tends to move in).
- In down dog lunge, the lower body takes the shape of lunge, the upper body takes the shape of downward facing dog.

safety (strength) pose
- Press front big toe down, flare toes.
- Tighten glutes, press tailbone down, tone abdomen.
- Press hands down, lift shoulders up.
- Lift back thigh.

refinement (stretch) pose
- Press hands down, forward; feet down, back.
- Without changing shape, extend front knee, back heel apart.
- Relax neck.

Repeat on the second side.

Every pose can have a drishti—a point of visual focus. A benefit of drishti is the focus it promotes. A steady gaze on a single point or object can balance inward and outward attention. One name for that balanced attention is Shambhavi Mudra. (The great Siddha saint Bhagawan Nityananda was said to continually live in that practitioner-perfect-state.)

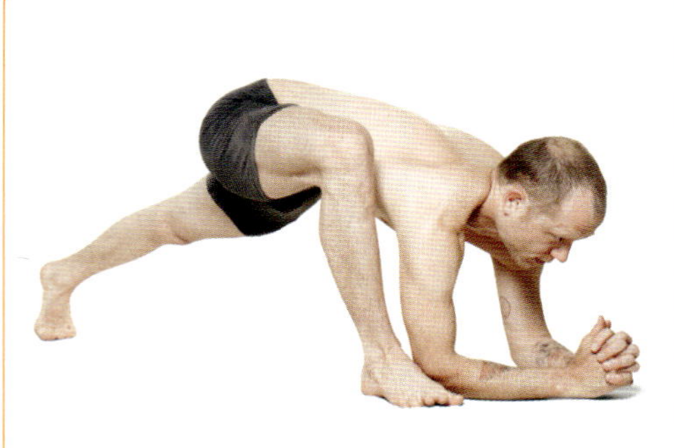

forearm lunge

shape pose (from lunge)
- Place forearms on floor inside front foot—elbow to arch of foot.
- Interlace fingers, place palms together.
- Separate elbows shoulder-width apart.
- Look down.
- Move back heel vertical; straighten back leg.
- Move front knee out (more doable: place hands under shoulders. Lower back knee to floor).
- Round back evenly.

safety (strength) pose
- Press front big toe down; flare toes.
- Tighten glutes, press tailbone down, tone abdomen.
- Lift back thigh.

refinement (stretch) pose
- Press forearms down, forward; feet down, back.
- Without changing shape, extend front knee, back heel apart.

Repeat on the second side.

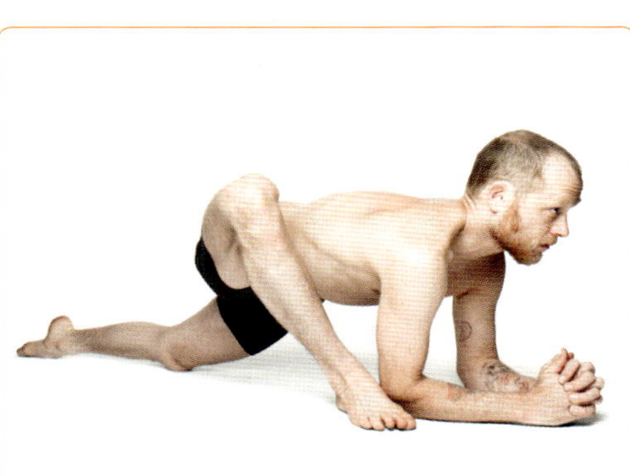

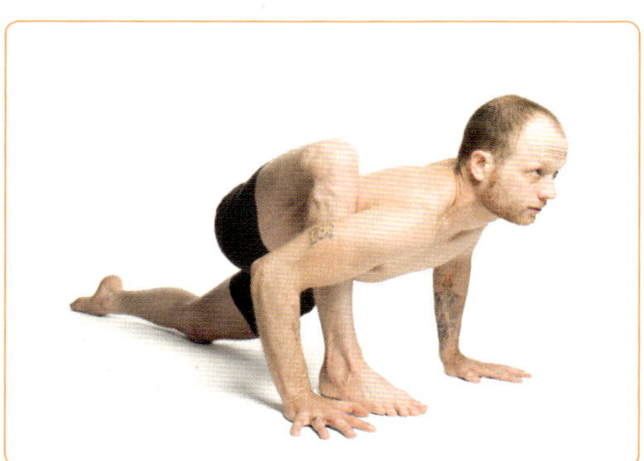

crouching monkey

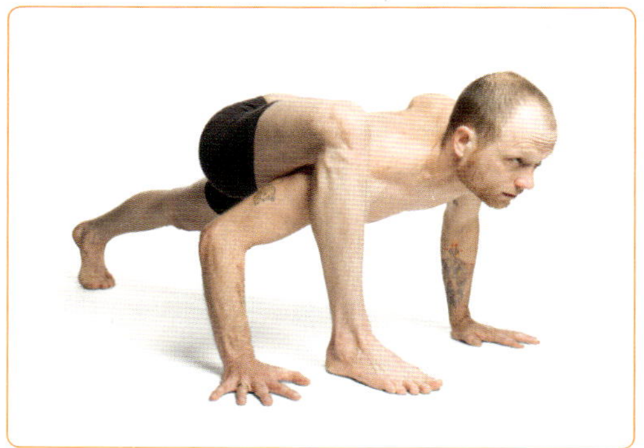

crouching warrior

revolved lunge

shape pose (from lunge)
- Twist to right, lift arm up vertical to floor.
- Stack shoulders.
- Look down, out, or up.
- Move back heel vertical; straighten back leg, arms.
- Line up head with hips.
- Line up bottom biceps with bottom hand.
- Point top palm out; close or open fingers. In either case stretch palm open and make hand flat.

safety (strength) pose
- Move front knee out.
- Tighten glutes, press tailbone down, tone low belly. Move ribs back.
- Lift back thigh.

refinement (stretch) pose
- Without changing shape, extend front knee, back heel apart.
- Lift chest, stretch spine.
- Stretch arms.

Repeat on the second side.

When the fingers are together, students tend to cup their palms. When the fingers are open, students tend to hyperextend their fingers. In either case, if a student put their top hand on the floor, their palm and fingertips should all touch the floor. Apply this across the board. That said, many yogahour teachers and studios teach "fingers together" exclusively. So although fingers together is not a hard and fast rule, it may be accurate to call it a principle shape of yogahour.

Done properly, twists compress, release, and remove toxins from the abdominal organs. They can also make for a strong and supple spine—a valuable asset.

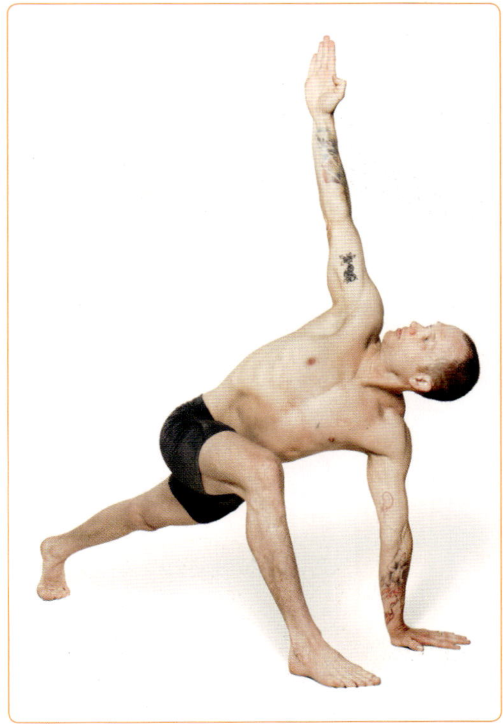

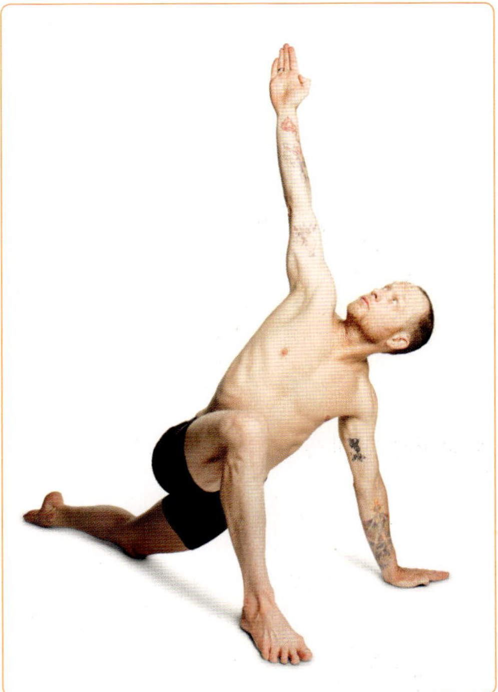

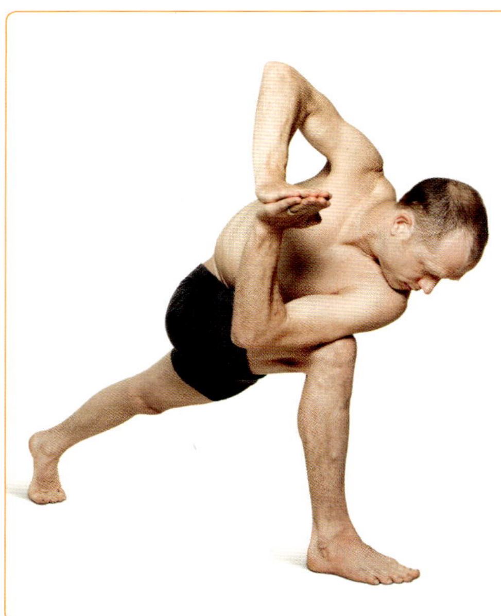

twisted lunge

shape prep (from lunge)
- Hold upper right thigh with right hand—thumb in, fingers out.
- Lift torso, left arm vertical.
- Twist to right, place left shoulder on right knee.

shape pose
- Press palms together—point right elbow up.
- Look down. Line up head with foot. Line up hips with head.
- Stack shoulders.
- Look down, out, or up.

safety (strength) pose
- Squeeze feet toward each other.
- Press palms, arm/leg together.
- Squeeze front hip, back thigh together.
- Tighten glutes, press tailbone down, tone/turn abdomen up, move ribs back.
- Move front knee out.
- Lift back thigh.

refinement (stretch) pose
- Without changing shape, extend front knee, back heel apart.
- Lift chest, stretch spine.
- Allow your breath to breathe itself.

Repeat on the second side.

forward fold *knees bent*
uttanasana prep

shape prep (from mountain)
- Bend knees slightly—knees in line with toes.
- Place torso against thighs.

shape pose
- Place palms on floor outside feet, slightly wider than shoulders.
- Straighten arms (which may require sliding hands behind feet).
- Bring face to shins.
- Round back evenly.

safety (strength) pose
- Squeeze legs together.
- Press hands down, forward; press feet down, back.
- Press tailbone down, tone abdomen.

refinement (stretch) pose
- Stretch spine.

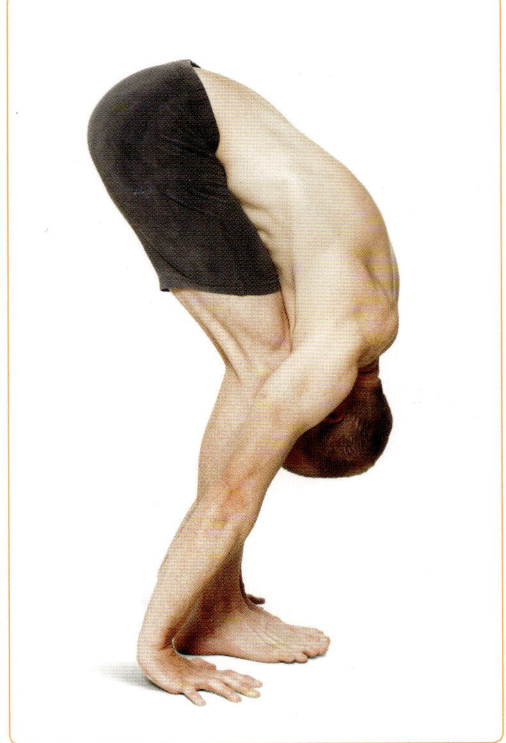

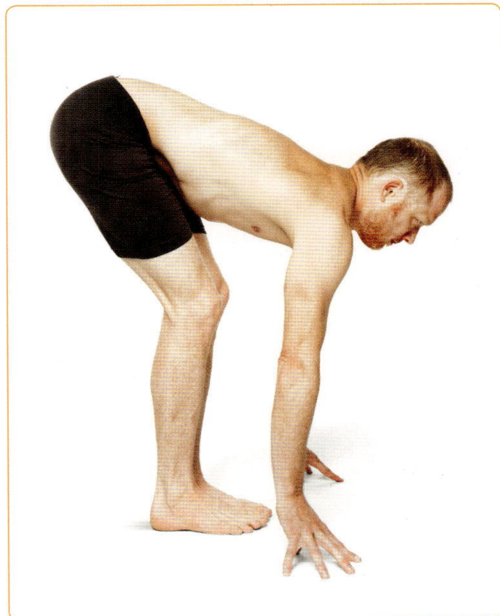

half forward fold *knees bent*

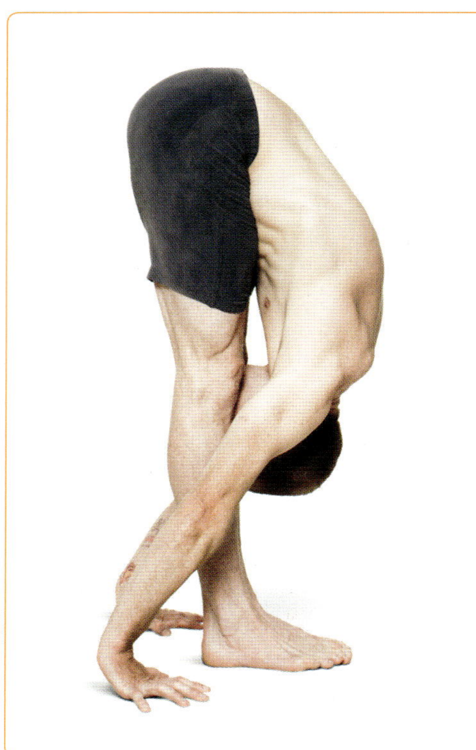

forward fold
uttanasana

shape prep (from mountain)
▥ Place palms on floor outside or behind feet—slightly wider than shoulders.
▥ Place torso against thighs.

shape pose
▥ Straighten legs, arms (more doable: bend knees slightly).
▥ Bring face to shins.
▥ Round back evenly.
▥ Lean forward slightly—hips directly above ankles.

safety (strength) pose
▥ Squeeze legs together.
▥ Press hands down, forward; press feet down, back.
▥ Press tailbone down, tone abdomen.

refinement (stretch) pose
▥ Stretch spine.

half forward fold
ardha uttanasana

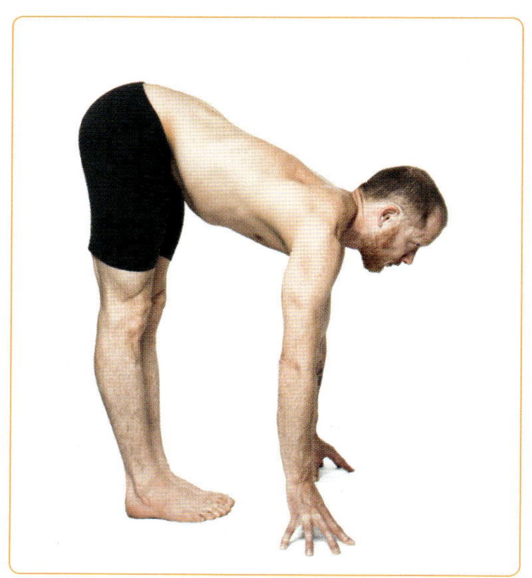

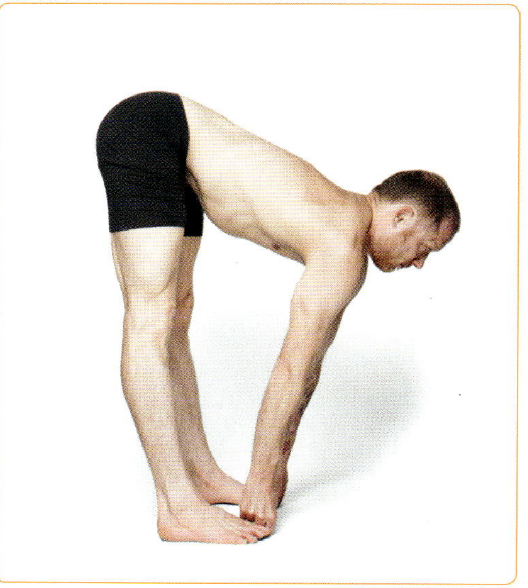

foot to hand pose
padahastasana

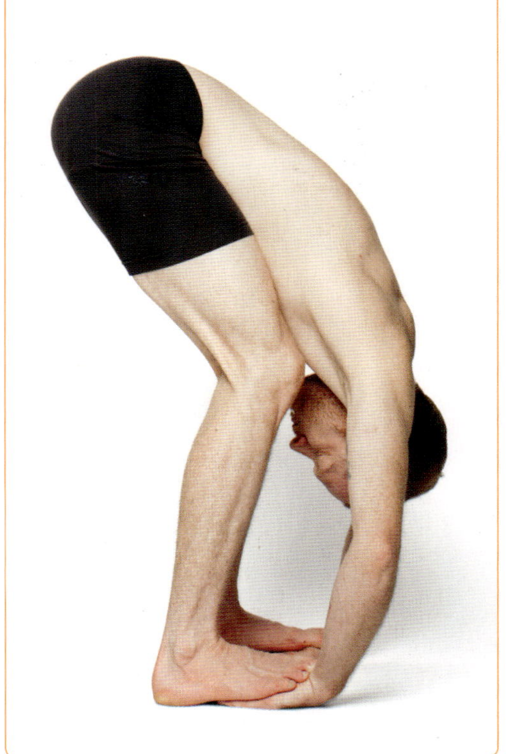

shape prep (from mountain)
- Separate feet outer hip-width apart.
- Bend knees slightly—knees in line with toes.

shape pose
- One at a time, place palms underneath feet, tips of toes against wrists.
- Bend and point elbows out.
- Keep knees bent or straighten legs.
- Lean forward slightly, hips directly above ankles.

safety (strength) prep
- Tone thighs, tighten kneecaps, firm hamstrings.

safety (strength) pose
- Press toes, tailbone down; tone abdomen.

refinement (stretch) pose
- Extend elbows out, shoulders down.
- Stretch spine.
- Relax neck.

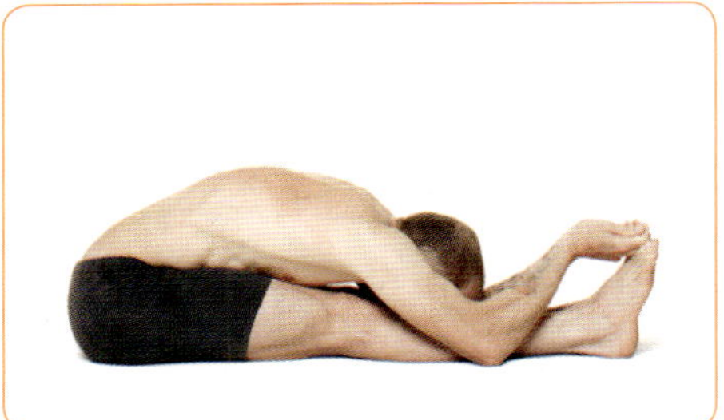

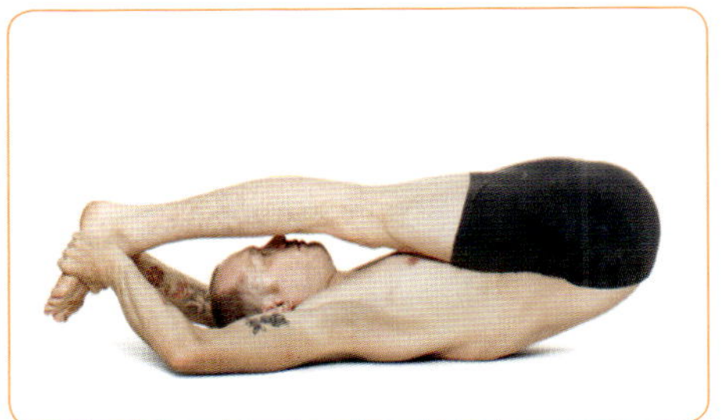

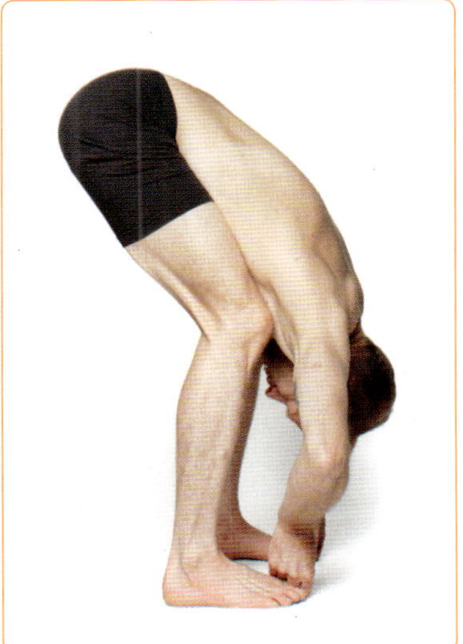

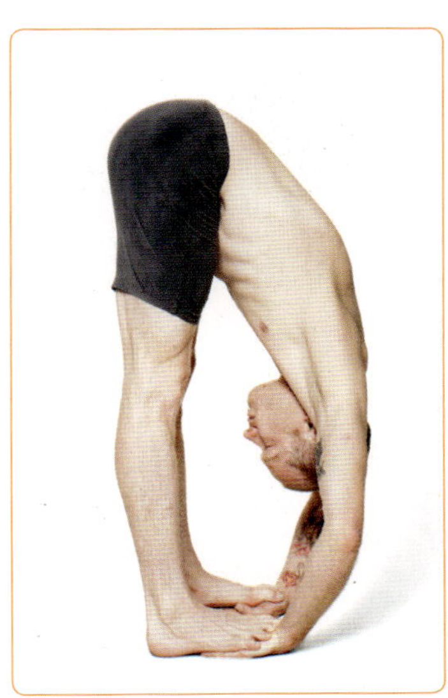

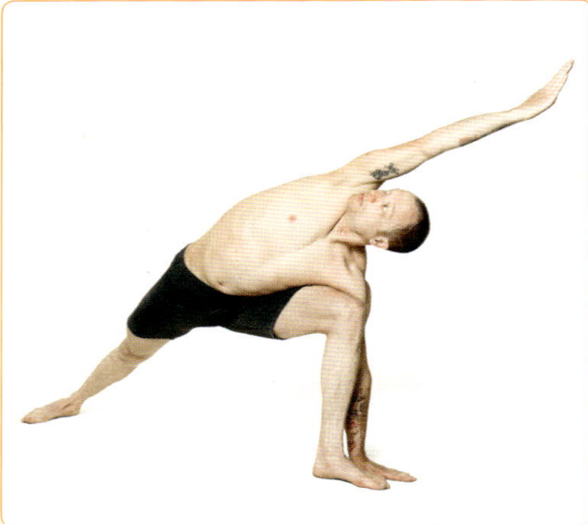

extended side angle
utthita parsvakonasana

shape prep
(from mountain middle of mat, facing long edge of mat)

- Take a wide stance—arms parallel to floor.
(wide stance = ankles directly under wrists. More doable: shorten stance slightly).
- Close fingers.
- Point big toes straight ahead. Make outer heels widest part of pose.
- Turn right foot out 90 degrees.
- Line up front heel to back center arch.
- Look past right fingertips.
- Bend right knee over heel.
- Place right hand on floor outside front foot (more doable: elbow to knee).

shape pose
- Bring left arm across face.
- Straighten arms. Point top palm down, bottom biceps forward.
- Look at top hand (more doable: look down or out).

safety (strength) pose
- Press back foot, front heel down; squeeze feet toward each other.
- Tighten back knee; move back thigh back.
- Press front knee into bottom arm.
- Move tailbone, abdomen in.
- Move top shoulder back, hollow out armpit.

refinement (stretch) pose
- Lift chest, stretch spine.
- Stretch arms.

Repeat on the second side.

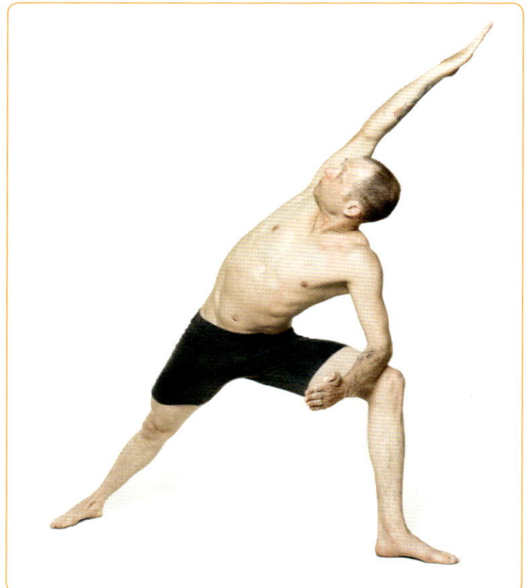

no-handed lunge
baddha hasta parsvakonasana

shape prep (from downward facing dog)
▨ Step right foot forward between hands, pivot back heel down. Make outer heel widest part of pose.
▨ Stand up, straighten front leg.
▨ Interlace fingers behind back with elbows slightly bent. Pull palms apart, straighten arms to capacity (more difficult: place palms together).

shape pose
▨ Bend front knee over heel, lower head to/toward ankle (more doable: place shoulder on knee or keep torso above front thigh).
▨ Lift arms toward or beyond vertical.
▨ Tilt front shin out slightly.
▨ Move right hip in line with back heel.

safety (strength) pose
▨ Press back foot down; lift abdomen.
▨ Squeeze shoulders together on back.

refinement (stretch) pose
▨ Extend shoulders away from head.
▨ Stretch hands up.

Repeat on the second side.

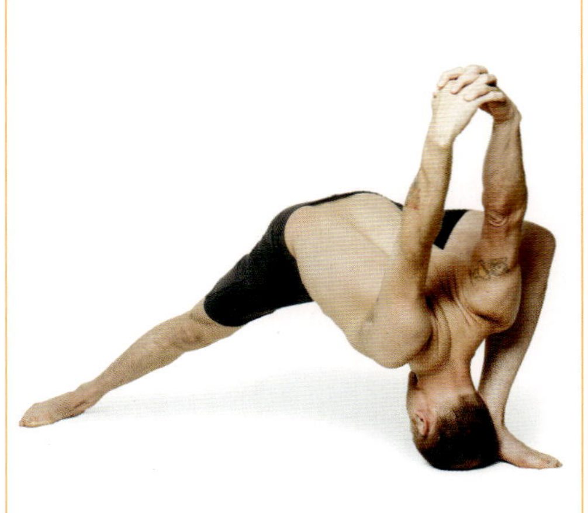

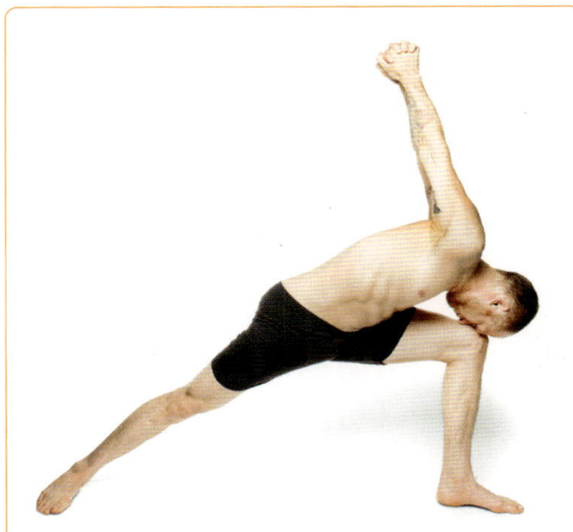

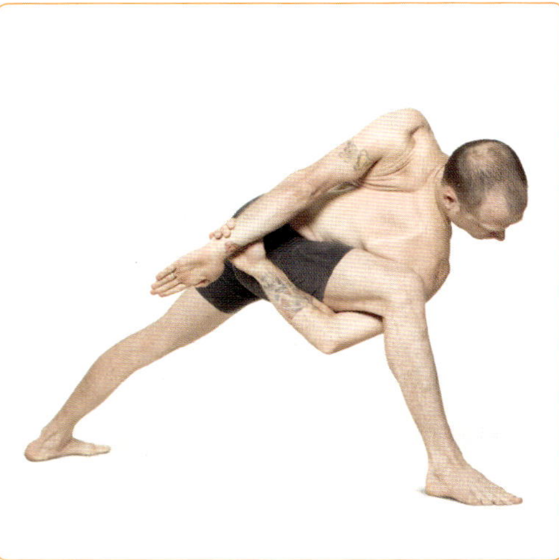

bound side angle

shape prep (from downward facing dog)
- Step right foot forward between hands, pivot back heel down. Make outer heel the widest part of the pose.
- Stand up, straighten front leg. Line up front heel with center of back arch.
- Bend front knee over heel.
- Bring right shoulder underneath right knee.
- Place right hand behind right hip (more doable: place hands on floor inside front leg).

shape pose
- Swing left arm onto low back, bind hands (more doable: use strap to bind).
- Stack shoulders, look up (more doable: bring shoulders equidistant to floor, look down or out).

safety (strength) pose
- Press back foot, front heel, down; lift abdomen.
- Move right hip under left hip.
- Move tailbone, abdomen in.
- Squeeze shoulders toward spine.

refinement (stretch) pose
- Lift chest, stretch spine.

Repeat on the second side.

What is interesting to me about this pose is I have never actually done it in a practice. The only time I've ever done it in my life is for the photo to be taken. So I will be practicing it soon to research its benefits. That is a practice I recommend: look through this book to find a pose you rarely or never practice. Mix it into your practice several times to see what it has to offer, and how it affects your practice and perspective." ~ Yoga Resource Practice Manual eBook

Wow, the yogahour set sequences and Barefoot Boot Camp certainly changed that! I now practice bound side angle on a regular basis.

wide-leg forward fold
prasarita padottanasana

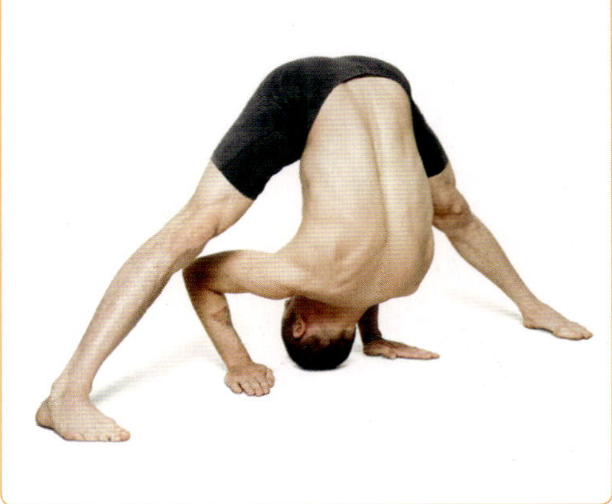

shape prep
(from mountain middle of mat, facing long edge of mat)
- Take a wide stance—arms parallel to floor, ankles under wrists.
- Point big toes straight ahead. Make outer heels widest part of pose or outer edge of feet parallel to short edge of mat.

shape pose
- Place hands on floor between feet—hands shoulder-width apart; round back evenly, place head between hands (more doable: place hands under shoulders, straighten arms, bend knees slightly).
- Lean forward slightly so legs are straight up and down.

safety (strength) prep
- Press inner edges of feet down; flare toes.
- Tone thighs, tighten kneecaps, firm hamstrings.

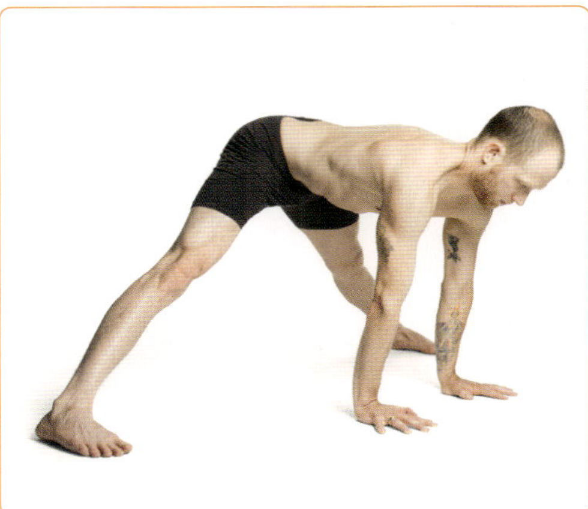

safety (strength) pose
- Press tailbone down, low belly in.
- Press hands down, forward—feet down, back.
- Minimize rounding in low back.
- Do not put any weight on head.

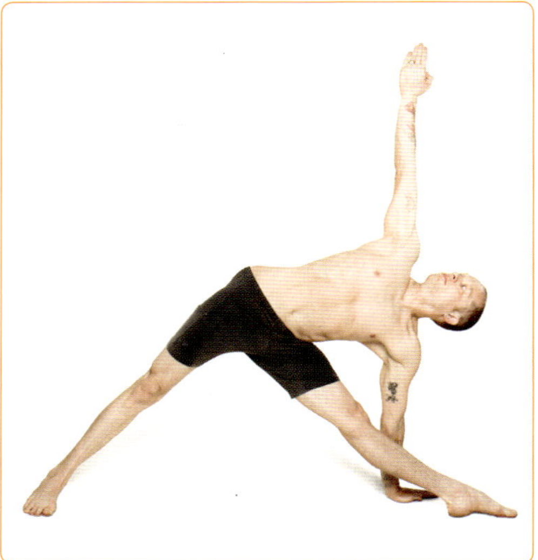

triangle
utthita trikonasana

shape prep
(from mountain middle of mat, facing long edge of mat)

■ Step or jump feet into a wide stance—arms parallel to the floor (wide stance = ankles directly under wrists. More doable: shorten stance slightly).

■ Point big toes straight ahead. Make outer heels the widest part of the pose.

■ Turn right foot out 90 degrees—make a straight line from front heel to middle of back arch.

■ Look past right fingertips.

shape pose

■ Hinge sideways at hips, place right hand on floor outside leg, under shoulder (more doable: bend front knee slightly or use a block).

■ Line up head, top hand, with front foot. Line up hips with head.

■ Look up (more doable: look out or down).

■ Stack shoulders.

■ Point biceps straight ahead; line up right kneecap with right foot.

safety (strength) prep

■ Tone thighs, tighten kneecaps, firm hamstrings. Tight kneecaps do not droop or wobble. Droopy kneecaps are like droopy eyelids: indications of sleepiness. Stay asana alert!

safety (strength) pose

■ Tighten glutes, press tailbone in, tone abdomen, move ribs back.

refinement (stretch) prep

■ Lift chest, stretch spine.

refinement (stretch) pose

■ Press feet down, apart.
■ Stretch arms.

Repeat on the second side.

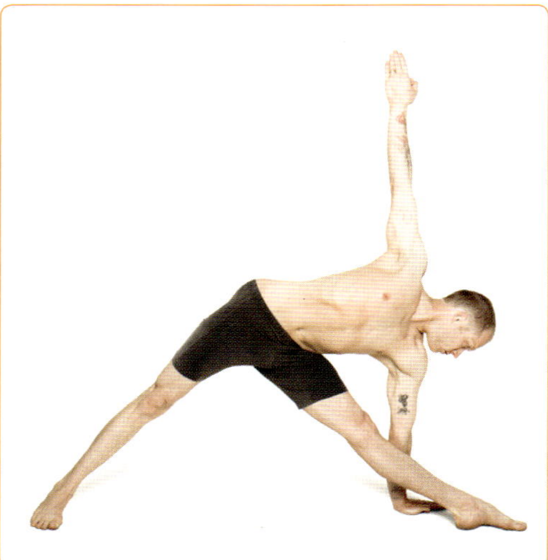

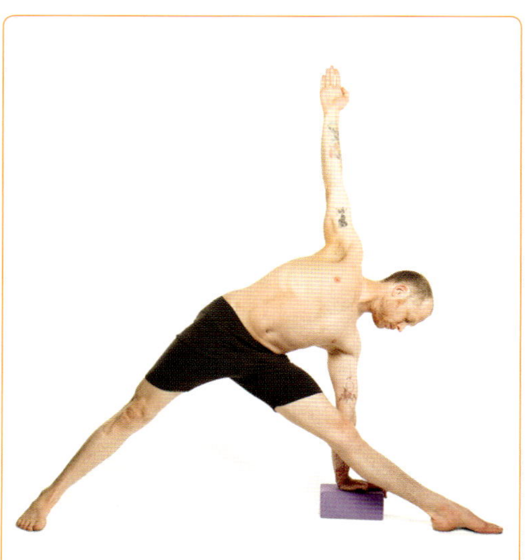

revolved triangle
parivrtta trikonasana

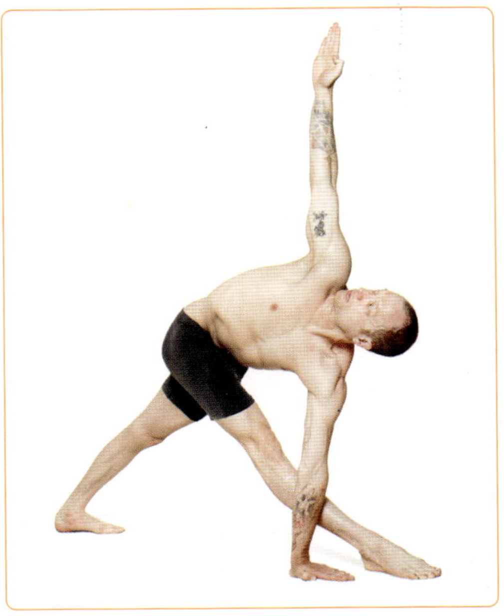

shape prep
(from mountain middle of mat, facing long edge of mat)
- Take a wide stance—arms parallel to floor (wide stance = ankles directly under wrists. More doable: shorten stance slightly).
- Point big toes straight ahead. Make outer heels widest part of pose.
- Pivot on heels—turn left foot in 60 degrees, right foot open 90 degrees.
- Square hips to right.
- Straighten legs.

shape pose
- Place left hand outside of right foot (more doable: place hand inside foot, under shoulder or use a block).
- Look down. Line up head, top hand, with front leg.
- Extend right hand up—arm vertical to floor.
- Close fingers.
- Look up, out, or continue to look down.

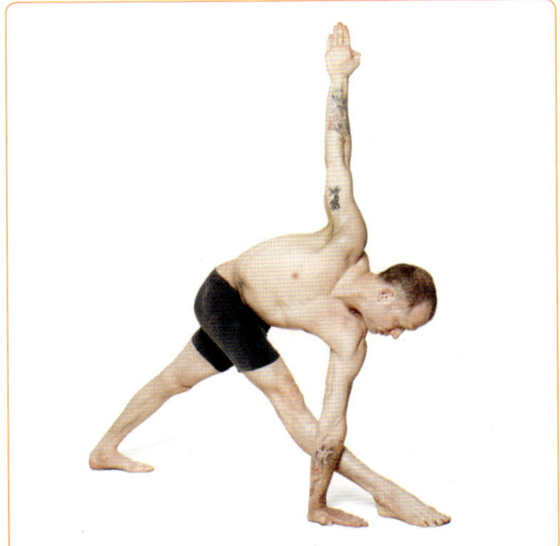

safety prep
- Press feet down.
- Tone thighs, tighten kneecaps, firm hamstrings.
- Squeeze inner thighs of both legs toward each other.

safety pose
- Tighten glutes, press tailbone down.
- Tone, turn abdomen up.
- Move ribs back.

refinement pose
- Stretch legs.
- Stretch spine.
- Stretch arms.

Repeat on the second side.

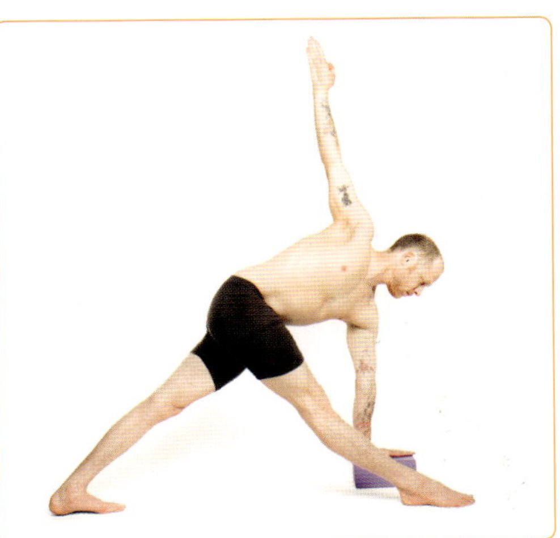

Keep hips steady and still. If the hips follow the twist, the shoulders will turn more but the spine will twist less; the twist must happen in the spine, not the hips.

Practice doesn't reverse problematic patterns. Practice is the opportunity to align with what is optimal time after time after time. Even seasoned practitioners often relax quads and slacken kneecaps as they go into the twisting aspect of this pose. A good "alerting adjustment" is to tap their quads with your fingertips and say "tone your quads."

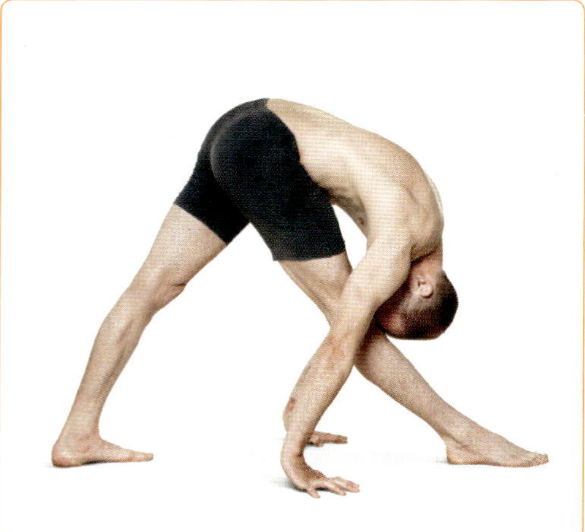

reverse mudra *hands on floor*
parsvottanasana

shape prep
(from mountain middle of mat, facing long edge of mat)
- Take a wide stance, place hands on hips.
- Point big toes straight ahead. Make outer heels widest part of pose.
- Shorten stance two inches.
- Pivot on heels—turn left foot in 60 degrees, right foot open 90 degrees.
- Square hips to right.
- Straighten legs.

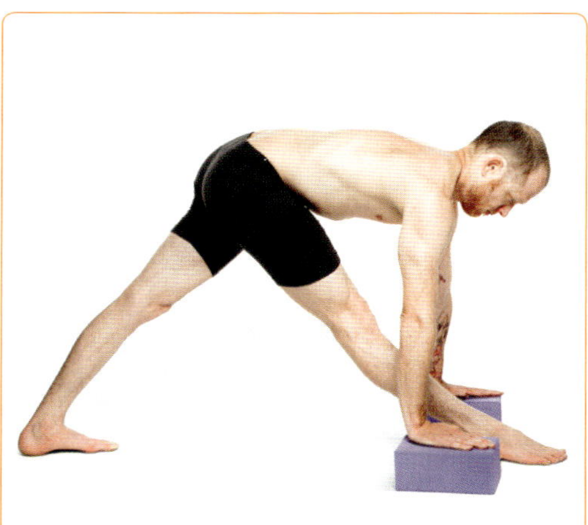

shape pose
- Fold forward, place hands on floor under shoulders (more doable: bend front knee slightly or use blocks).
- Stay here or slide hands back, place forehead on knee or chin to shin.
- Round back evenly.

safety (strength) prep
- Press feet down.
- Tone thighs, tighten kneecaps, firm hamstrings.
- Squeeze inner thighs toward each other.

safety (strength) pose
- Tighten glutes, press tailbone down.
- Tone and turn abdomen to right.

refinement (stretch) pose
- Press feet down, apart.
- Stretch spine.

Repeat on the second side.

The distance between your feet (the length of your stance) depends on your body type and range of motion. For the most part, the stance in reverse mudra is shorter than that of warrior 1. In both instances, what determines stance is one's ability to square hips, while keeping the back heel down. A shorter stance can accommodate tight hamstrings or calves, while a longer stance may be optimal for those with a short torso, long legs, or flexible hamstrings.

reverse mudra
parsvottanasana

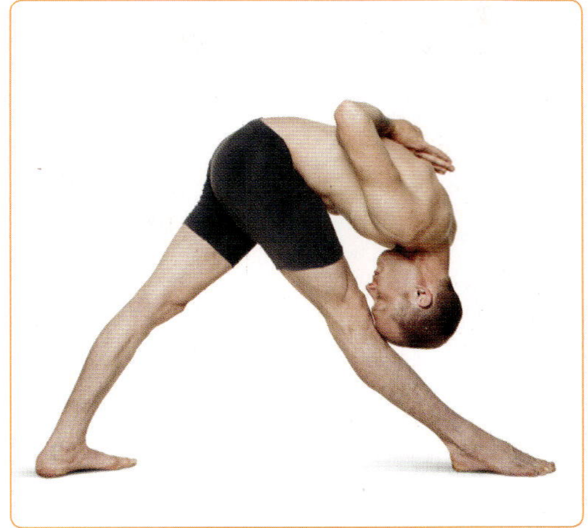

shape prep
(from mountain middle of mat, facing long edge of mat)
- Place palms together, behind upper back—point fingers up (more doable: clasp wrist with hand behind hips.) Slide wrists up back to, not beyond, capacity.
- Take a wide stance, then shorten stance 2 inches.
- Point big toes straight ahead. Make outer heels widest part of pose.
- Pivot on heels—turn left foot in 60 degrees, right foot open 90 degrees.
- Square hips to right.
- Straighten legs.

shape pose
- Place forehead on front knee or chin to shin (more doable: bend front knee slightly; more difficult: do a backbend before folding forward).
- Round back evenly.

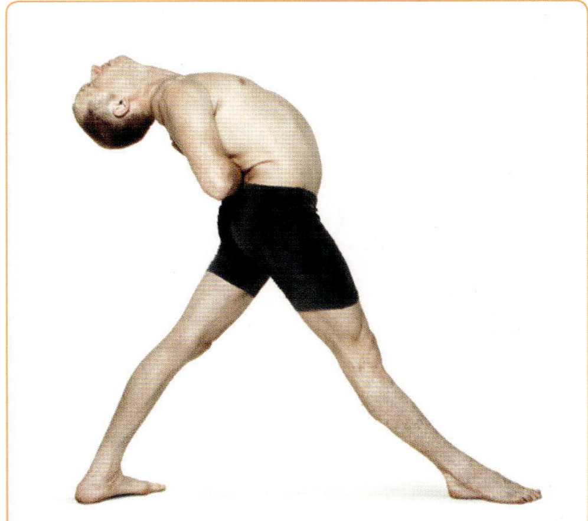

safety (strength) prep
- Press feet down.
- Tone quads, tighten kneecaps, firm hamstrings.
- Squeeze inner thighs toward each other.

safety (strength) pose
- Tighten glutes, press tailbone down.
- Tone and turn abdomen to right.
- Squeeze shoulders together on back.
- Do not overly round any part of spine.

refinement (stretch) pose
- Press feet down, apart. Stretch legs.
- Stretch spine.

Repeat on the second side.

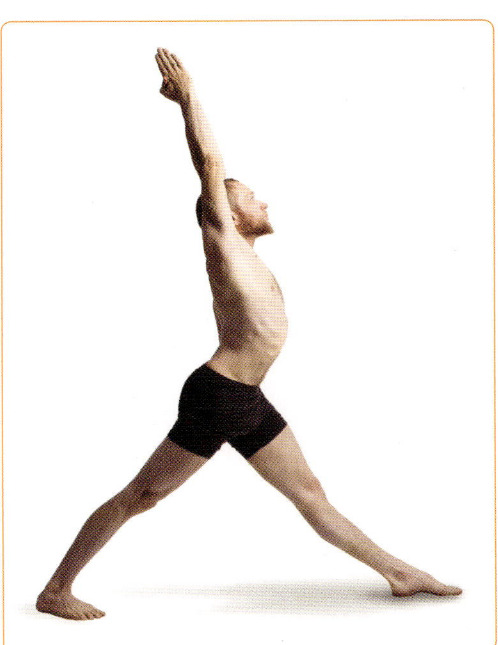

Modifications are often a must. The point of modifications is not to distance you from a given pose, but rather give deeper access to it. I recommend regarding the classical forms of these poses as guides not goals.

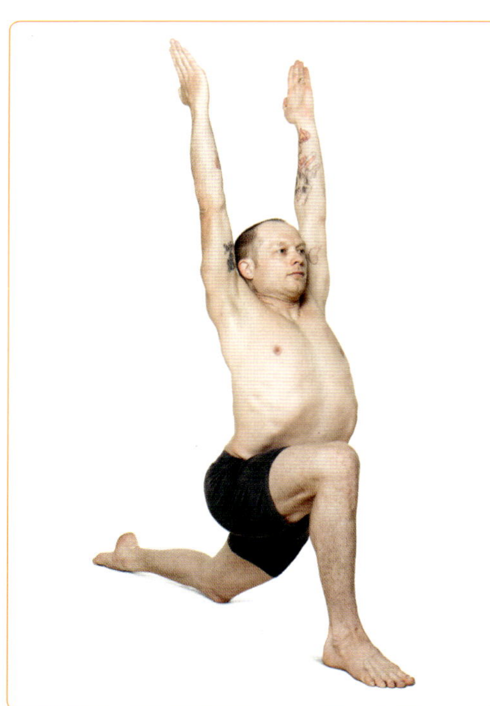

monkey lunge
anjaneyasana

shape prep (from lunge pose)
- Lower back knee, top of back foot to floor; point back foot—squeeze heel in.

shape pose
- Lift torso, arms upright. Straighten arms.
- Separate hands shoulder-width apart. Close fingers (more difficult: keeping arms straight, place palms together, cross thumbs).
- Lift chin slightly, look straight ahead or look down.

safety (strength) pose
- Squeeze front foot, back knee toward each other.
- Tighten glutes, press tailbone down, tone abdomen.

refinement (stretch) pose
- Lift chest, stretch spine.
- Extend arms up, back.

Repeat on the second side.

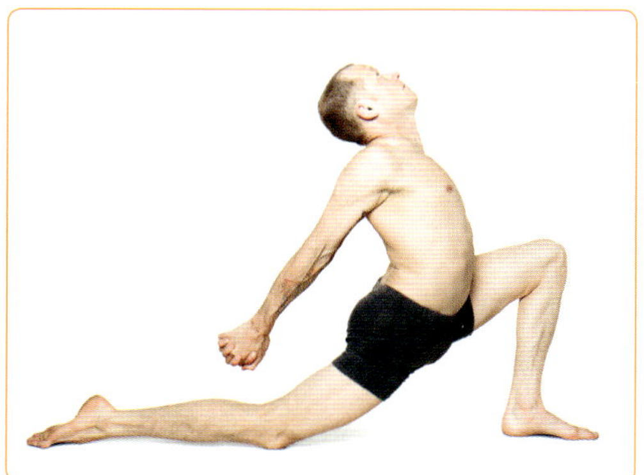

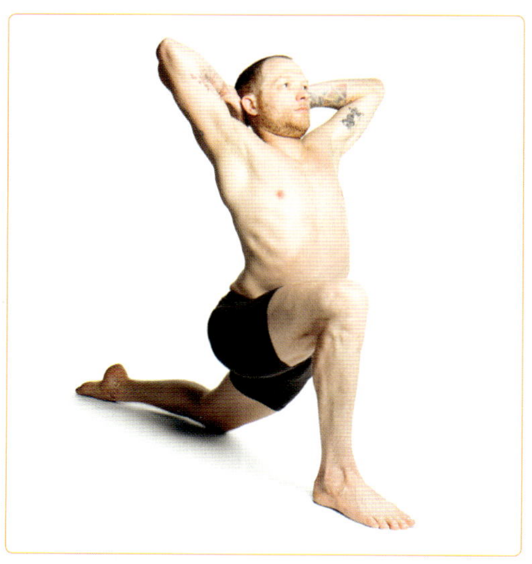

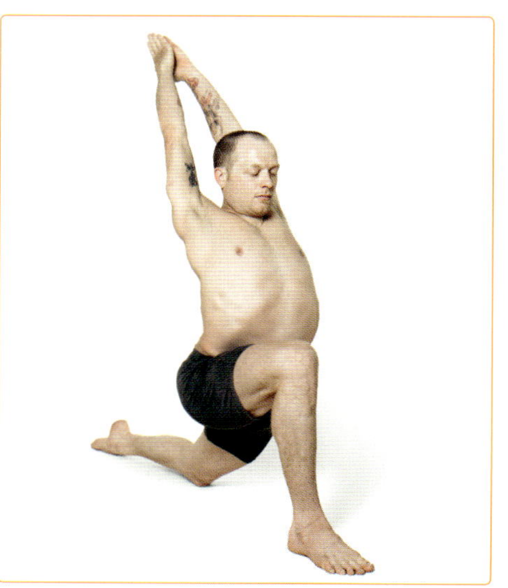

high lunge
virabhadrasana 1 prep

shape prep (from mountain back of mat)
- Step right foot forward toward front of mat.
- Lift arms overhead, hands shoulder-width apart.

shape pose
- Bend right knee directly above heel—shin vertical.
- Square hips somewhat.
- Lift chin slightly, look straight ahead (more difficult: look up).
- Move back heel vertical, heel directly above toe mounds.
- Straighten back leg.

safety (strength) pose
- Tighten glutes, press tailbone down, tone abdomen.
- Minimize backbend in low back.

refinement (stretch) pose
- Lift chest, stretch spine.
- Stretch arms up, back.

Repeat on the second side.

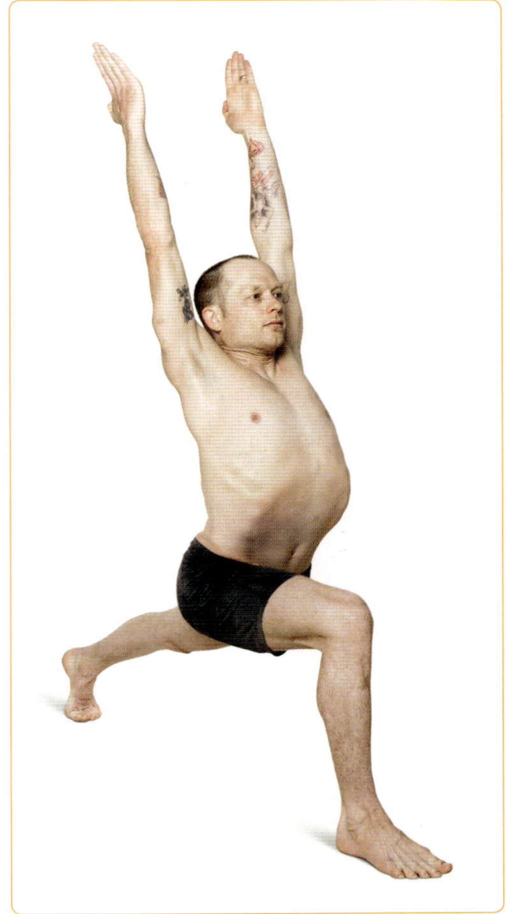

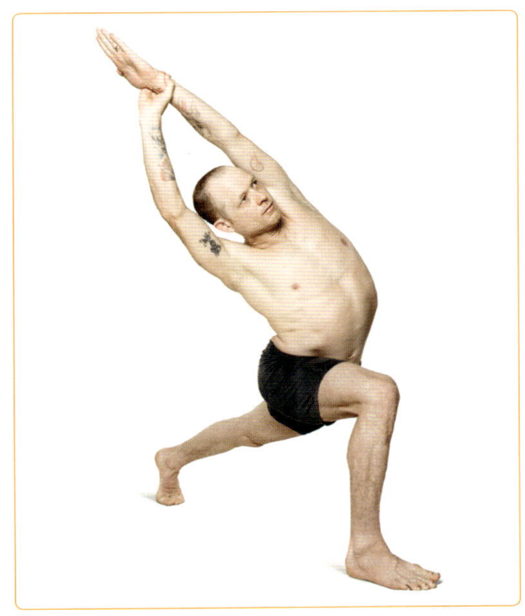

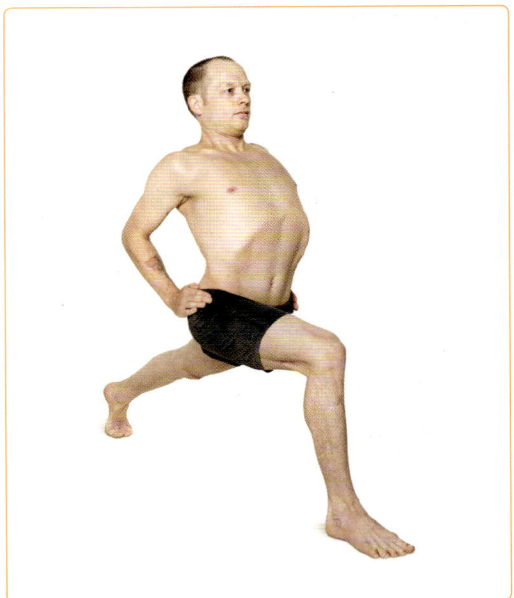

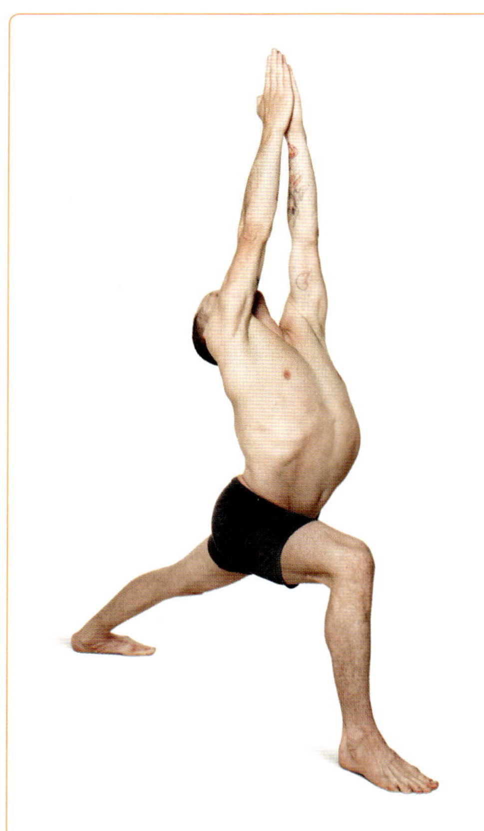

warrior 1
virabhadrasana 1

shape prep
(from mountain middle of mat, facing long edge of mat)
- Place palms together overhead; straighten arms
(more doable: separate hands shoulder-width apart).
- Take a wide stance.
- Pivot on heels—turn left foot in 60 degrees, right foot open 90 degrees.
- Point back knee in same direction as back toes.

shape pose
- Bend right knee directly above heel—shin vertical.
- Lift chin slightly, look straight ahead (more difficult: look up).

safety (strength) pose
- Press feet down—feet as evenly weighted as possible, like in mountain pose.
- Tighten glutes, press tailbone down, tone abdomen.
- Move ribs back to minimize backbend in low back.

refinement (stretch) pose
- Lift chest, stretch spine.
- Stretch arms up, back.

Repeat on the second side.

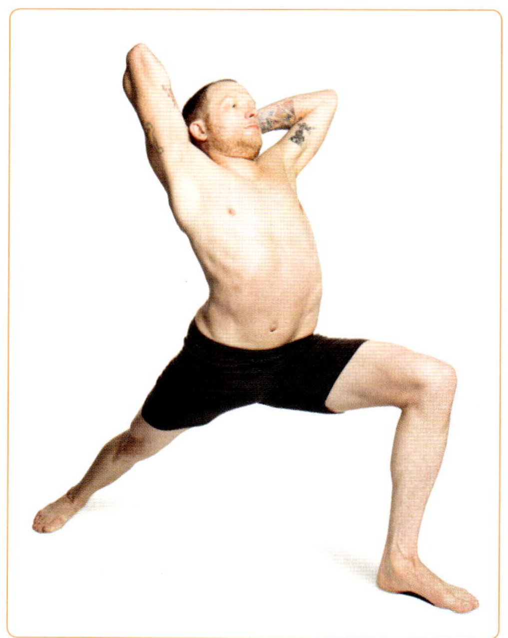

warrior 2
virabhadrasana 2

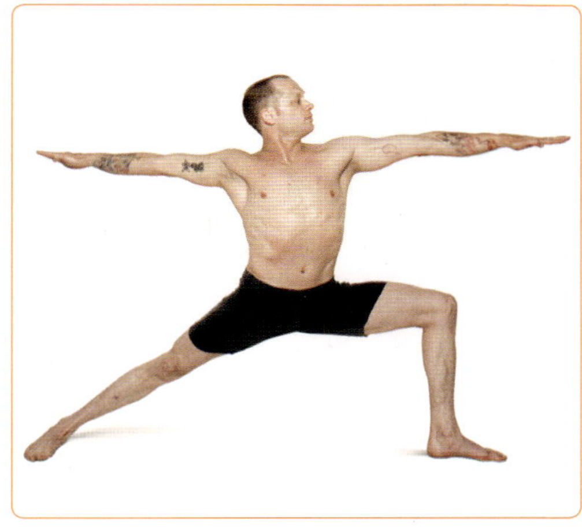

shape prep
(from mountain middle of mat, facing long edge of mat)
- Take a wide stance, arms parallel to floor.
- Point big toes straight ahead. Make outer heels widest part of pose.
- Turn right foot out 90 degrees.
- Line up front heel to center of back arch.
- Look past right hand.

shape pose
- Bend front knee above heel; move knee out slightly (knee tends to tilt in).
- Warrior 2 is a front shin vertical, thigh parallel to floor and outer edge of mat pose. If thigh parallel to floor is too intense, shorten stance so hips are higher than front knee.
- Make torso vertical (torso tends to lean toward front knee).

safety (strength) pose
- Press back foot, front heel down.
- Back leg—tone thigh, tighten kneecap, firm hamstrings.
- Lift pelvic floor; tone abdomen.
- Move ribs back.
- Minimize backbend in low back.

refinement (stretch) pose
- Lift chest, stretch spine.
- Extend arms out.

Repeat on the second side.

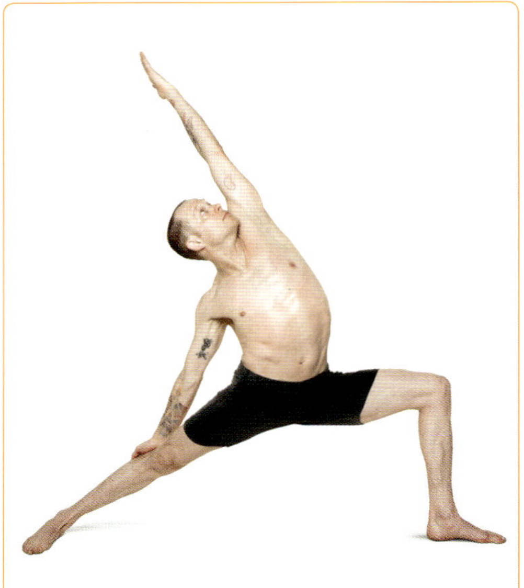

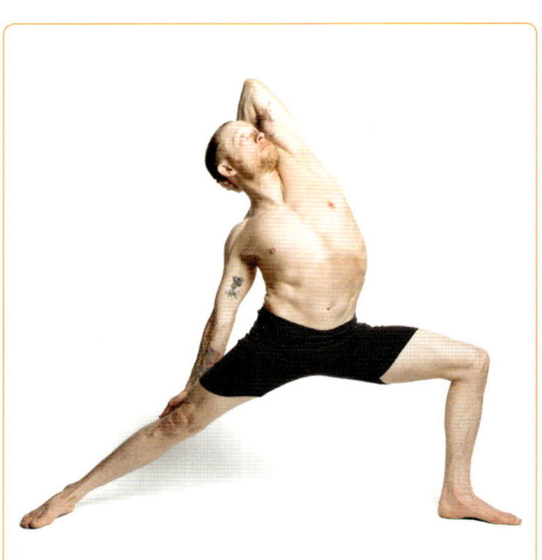

reverse warrior
viparita virabhadrasana

shape prep (from warrior 2)
- Point right palm up.
- Slide left hand down outer edge of left leg above or below knee.

shape pose
- Bring right arm across face.
- Straighten arms.
- Look straight ahead or up.

safety (strength) pose
- Press back foot down.
- Tighten glutes, press tailbone in, tone abdomen.
- Avoid overstretching or compressing either side of torso.

refinement (stretch) pose
- Lift chest, stretch spine.
- Stretch top arm.

Repeat on the second side.

elevated locust

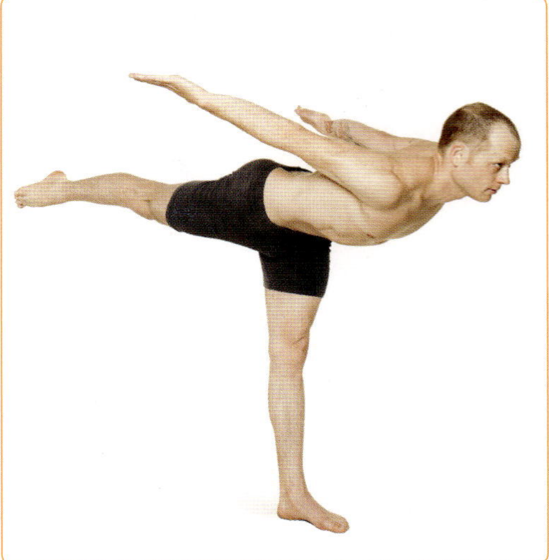

shape prep (from mountain back of mat)
- Point palms back.
- Keeping arms by side, step right foot forward to middle of mat.

shape pose
- Bring torso, back leg parallel to floor. Point lifted foot.
- Straighten legs (more doable: bend standing knee to accommodate tight hamstrings).
- Look straight ahead.

safety (strength) pose
- Lean forward slightly.
- Tone legs, tighten kneecaps, firm hamstrings.
- Press tailbone down, tone abdomen.
- Squeeze shoulders together on back.

refinement (stretch) pose
- Lift left back ankle, abdomen, chin, and wrists.
- Be soft, yet determined in eyes.

Repeat on the second side.

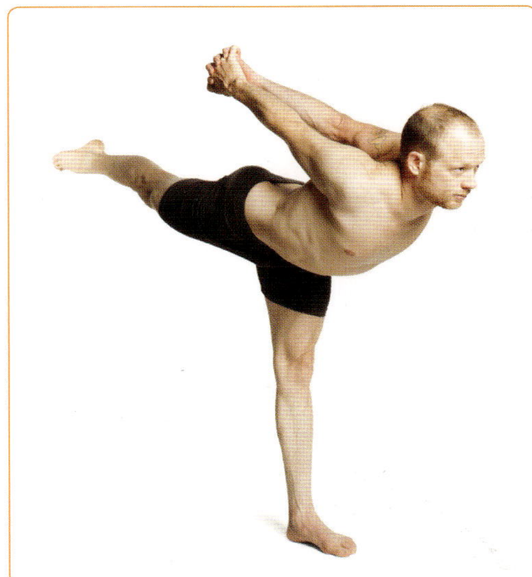

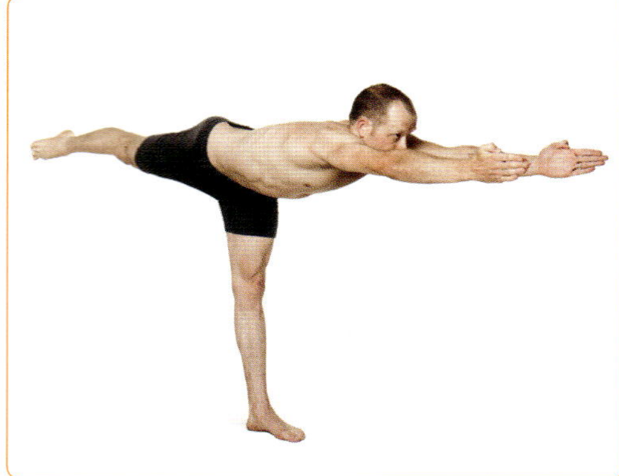

warrior 3
virabhadrasana 3

shape prep (from mountain back of mat)
◾ Lift arms overhead; straighten arms. Separate hands shoulder-width apart (more difficult: keeping arms straight, place palms together, cross thumbs).
◾ Step right foot forward to middle of mat.

shape pose
◾ Bring arms, torso, and back leg parallel to floor. Point lifted foot.
◾ Straighten legs (more doable: bend standing knee to accommodate tight hamstrings).
◾ Look straight ahead.

safety (strength) pose
◾ Lean forward slightly.
◾ Tone legs, tighten kneecaps, firm hamstrings.
◾ Press tailbone down, tone abdomen.

refinement (stretch) prep
◾ Lift chest, stretch spine

refinement (stretch) pose
◾ Lift back ankle, abdomen, chin, and wrists.
◾ Be soft, yet determined in eyes.

Repeat on the second side.

This pithy posture, like the practice of yogahour, leaves little room for kind of/sort of.

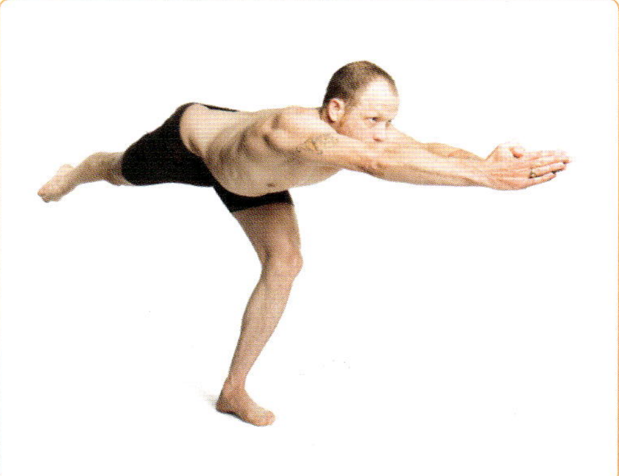

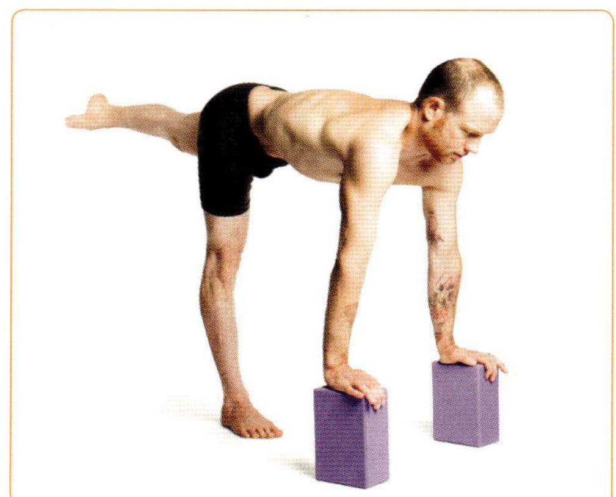

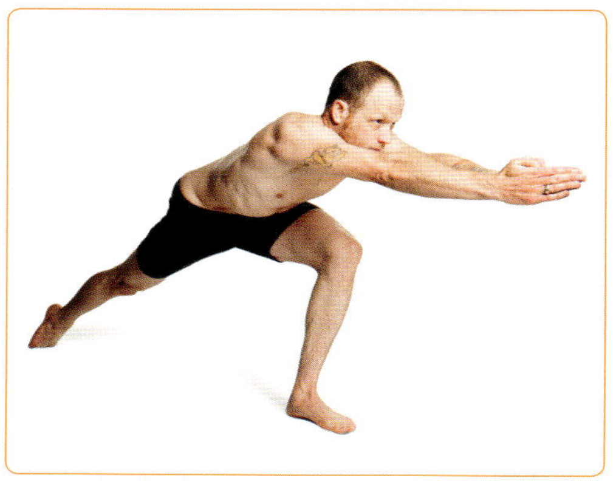

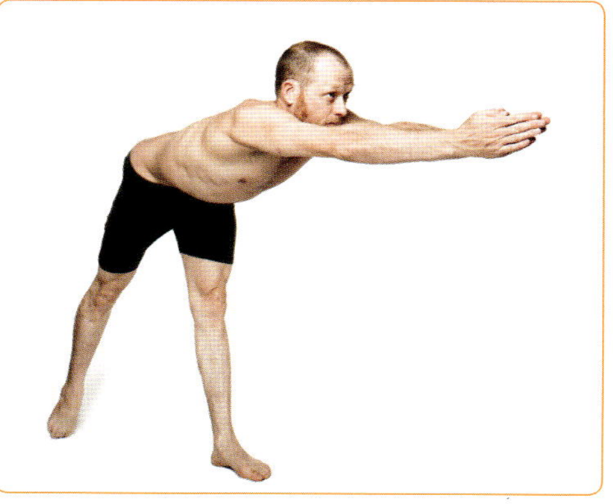

power pose
utkatasana

shape prep (from mountain)
- Look down.
- Lift arms overhead—hands shoulder-width apart (more difficult: place palms together, cross thumbs).
- Straighten arms.

shape pose
- Keeping arms vertical, head above hips, bend knees slightly.

safety (strength) pose
- Squeeze knees together, separate inner ankles.
- Tone abdomen—create a straight line from waistline to base of sternum.

refinement (stretch) prep
- Lift chest, stretch spine.

refinement (stretch) pose
- Lift arms up, back.
- Hold pose, not breath.

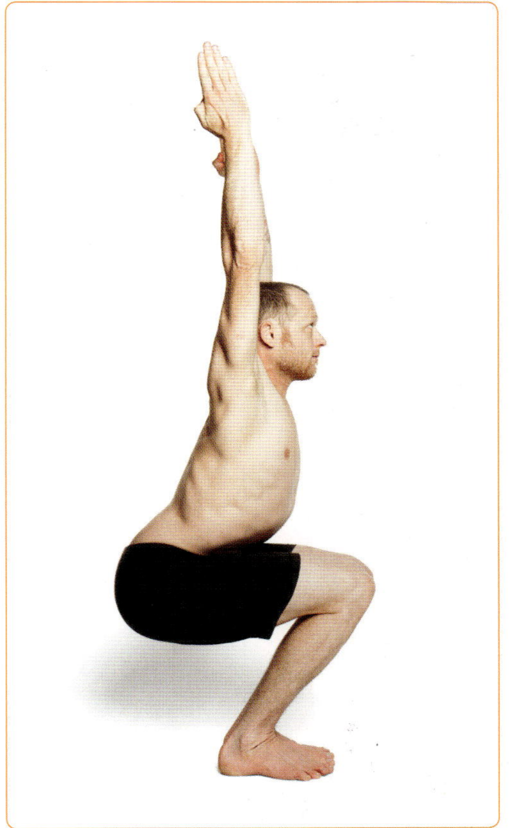

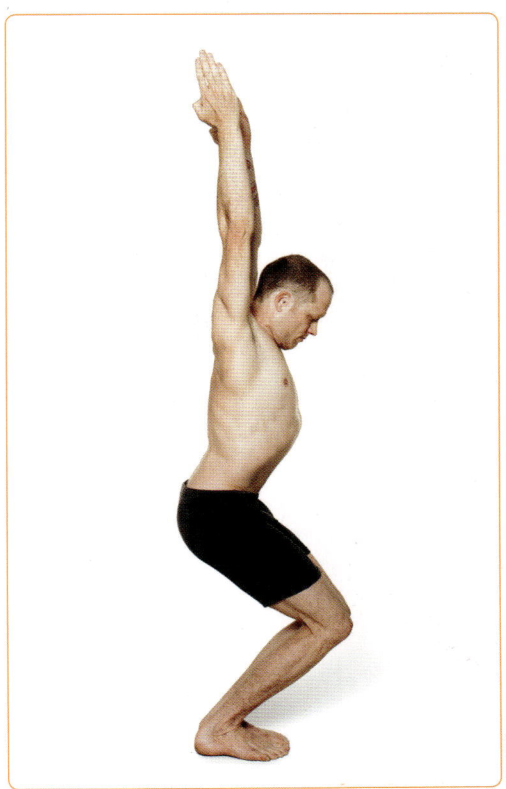

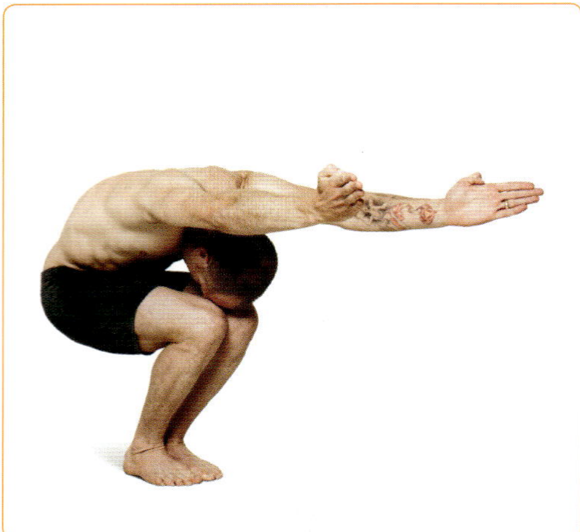

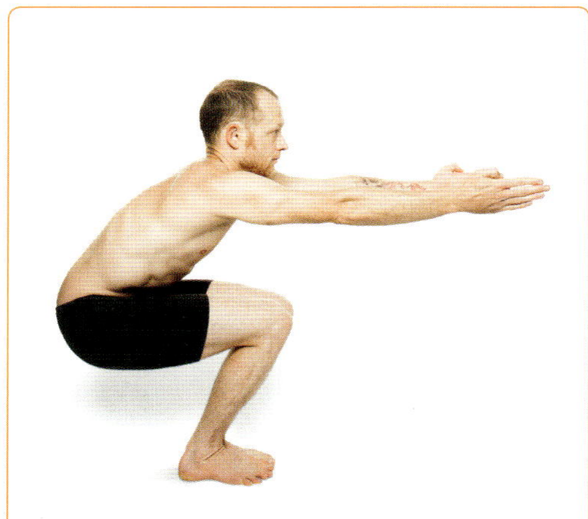

power pose *head to knee*
utkatasana

shape pose (from mountain)
- Bend knees, bring thighs and arms parallel to floor.
- Place forehead on knees (more doable: place chin on knees).
- Separate hands shoulder-width apart—close fingers, flatten palms.
- Straighten arms.

safety (strength) pose
- Squeeze knees together, separate inner ankles.
- Lift abdomen.

refinement (stretch) pose
- Round and keep rounding back.
- Lift and keep lifting wrists.

twisted power pose
parivrtta utkatasana

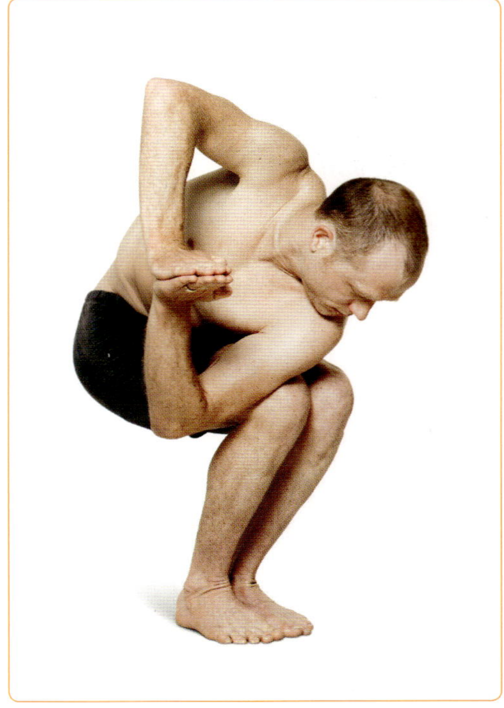

shape prep (from mountain)
- Bend knees slightly.
- Place left shoulder or arm on right knee.

shape pose
- Place palms together, point right elbow up.
- Look down.
- Line up head with feet, hips with head.
- Lower thighs parallel to floor.

safety (strength) pose
- Squeeze knees together, separate inner ankles.
- Press palms together.
- Press knee into arm, arm into knee.
- Lift abdomen.

refinement (stretch) pose
- Lift chest, stretch spine.

Repeat on the second side.

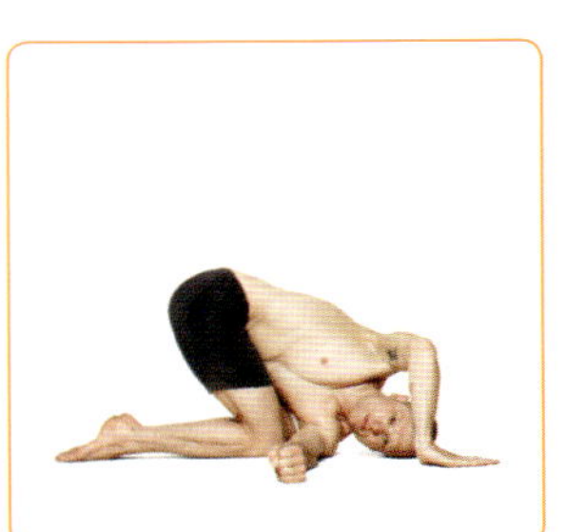 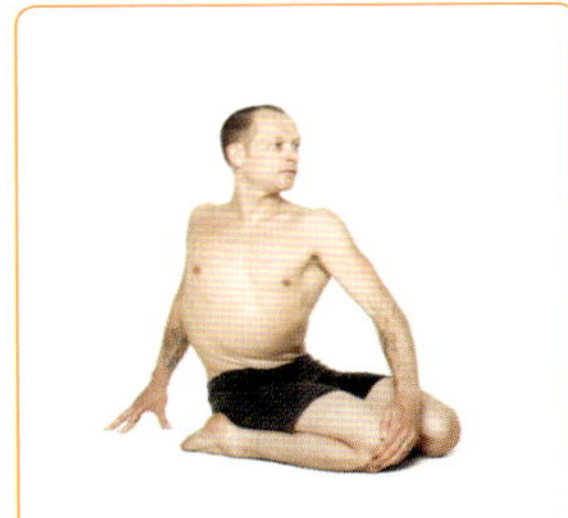 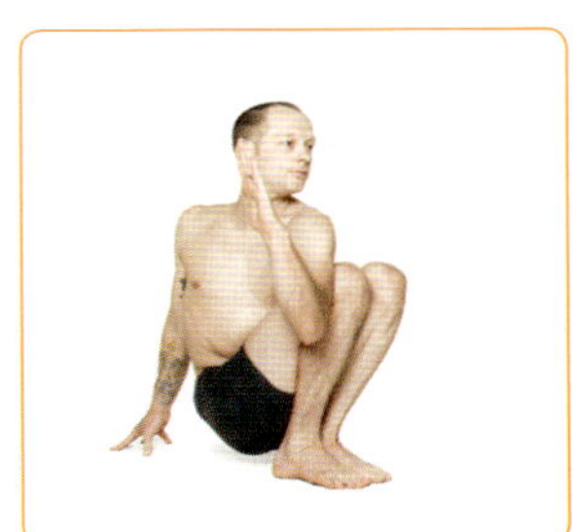 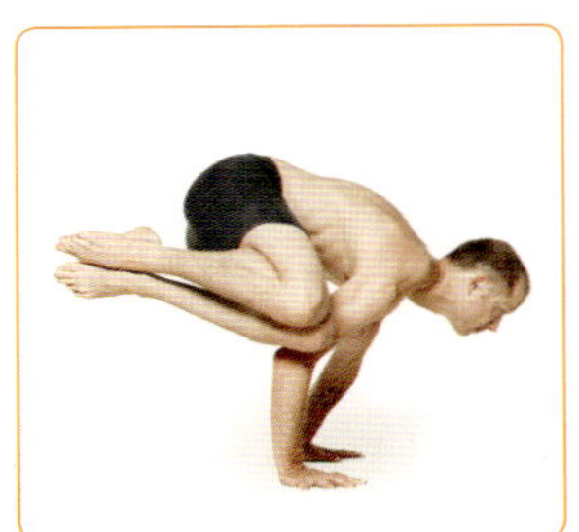

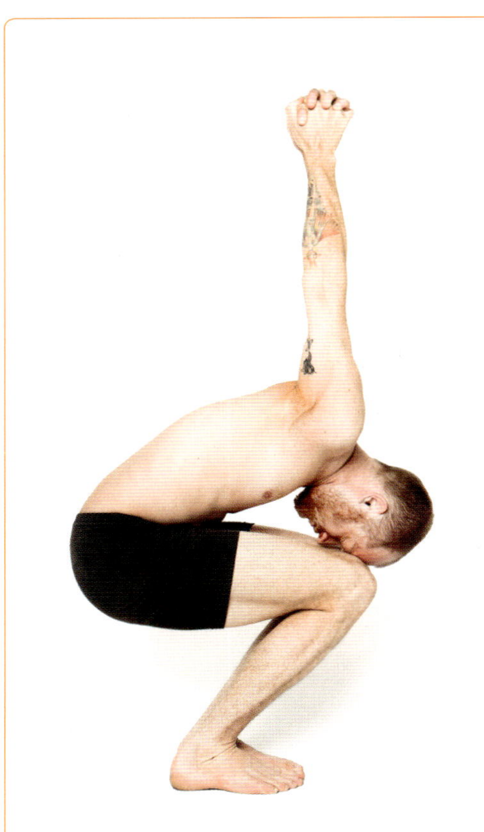

power pose *hands bound*
baddha hasta utkatasana

shape prep (from mountain)
- Interlace fingers behind back with elbows slightly bent.
- Pull palms apart; straighten arms
(more difficult: place palms together).

shape pose
- Bend knees, bring forehead to knees
(more doable: bring chin to knees).
- Lower thighs parallel to floor. Lift arms toward or beyond vertical.
- Round back evenly.

safety (strength) prep
- Squeeze shoulders together on back.

safety (strength) pose
- Squeeze knees together, separate inner ankles.
- Lift abdomen.

refinement (stretch) pose
- Move shoulders away from head.
- Stretch hands up.

standing sage
utthita hasta padangusthasana 1

shape prep (from mountain)
- Place left hand on left hip.
- Bend knees slightly.
- Clasp right big toe with first two fingers and thumb of right hand—arm inside leg.

shape pose
- Stay here or lift right shin parallel to floor.
- Stay here or straighten both legs.
- Lift chin slightly, look straight ahead.

safety (strength) pose
- Press fingers and big toe together to help strengthen lifted leg.
- Tone thighs, tighten kneecaps, firm hamstrings.
- Move right hip down, in.
- Allow right shoulder to move forward; hold it steady in that position.

refinement (stretch) pose
- Lift chest, stretch spine.

Repeat on the second side.

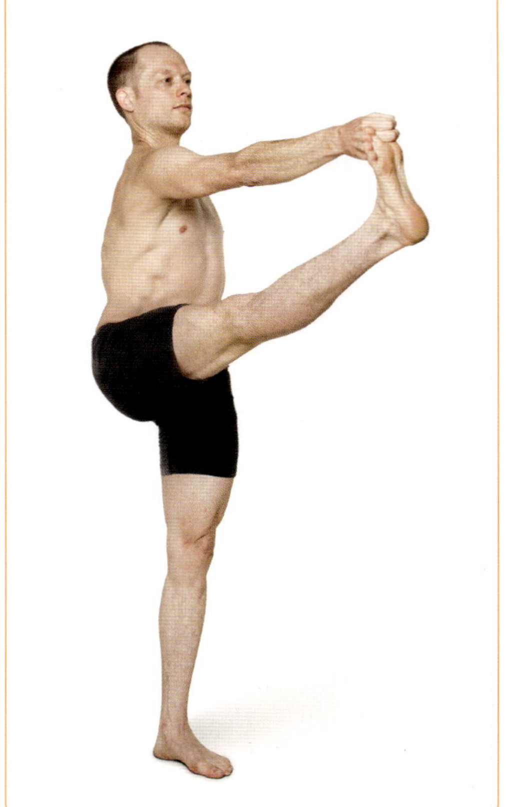

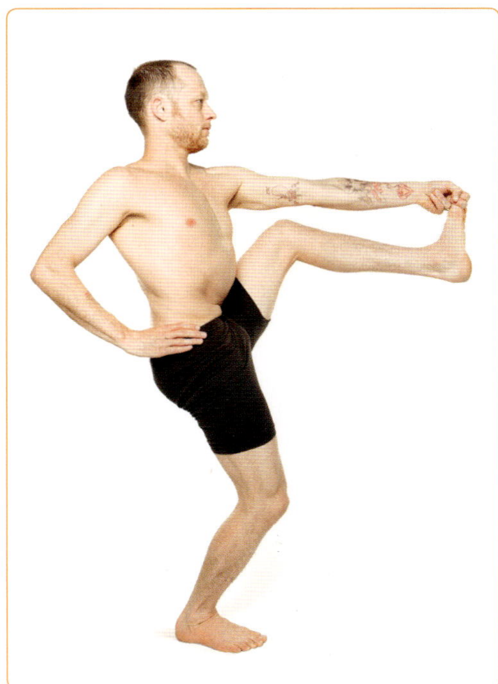

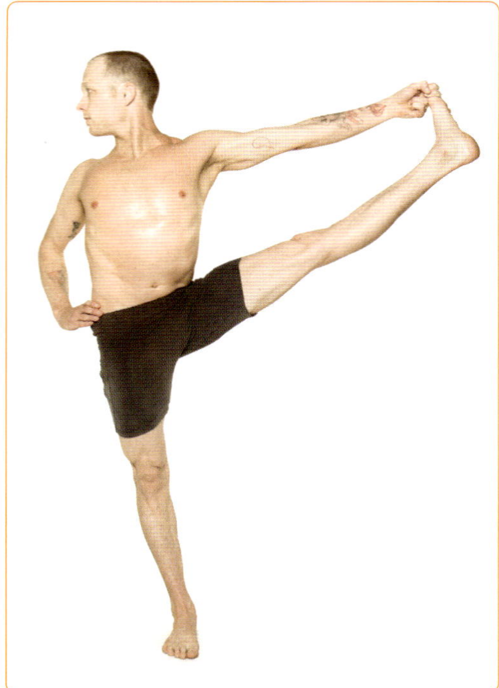

standing sage *leg to side*
utthita hasta padangusthasana 2

shape prep (from mountain)
■ Place left hand on left hip (more doable: extend arm out to side for better balance).
■ Bend knees slightly.
■ Clasp right big toe with first two fingers and thumb of right hand—arm inside leg (different variation: hold outer edge of foot).

shape pose
■ Keep right knee bent, move leg out to side.
■ Stay here or lift right shin parallel to floor.
■ Stay here or straighten standing leg.
■ Stay here or straighten lifted leg.
■ Look to left (more doable: look straight ahead or at a single point on floor).
■ Move standing thigh back—leg straight up and down.

safety (strength) prep
■ Press fingers and big toe together to help strengthen lifted leg.

safety (strength) pose
■ Extend top foot down.
■ Tone thighs, tighten kneecaps, firm hamstrings.
■ Move right hip down, in, so top foot tilts out slightly.

refinement (stretch) pose
■ Lift chest, stretch spine.

Repeat on the second side.

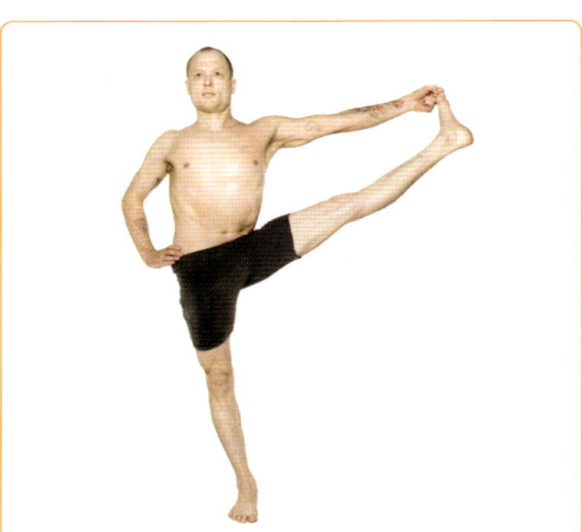

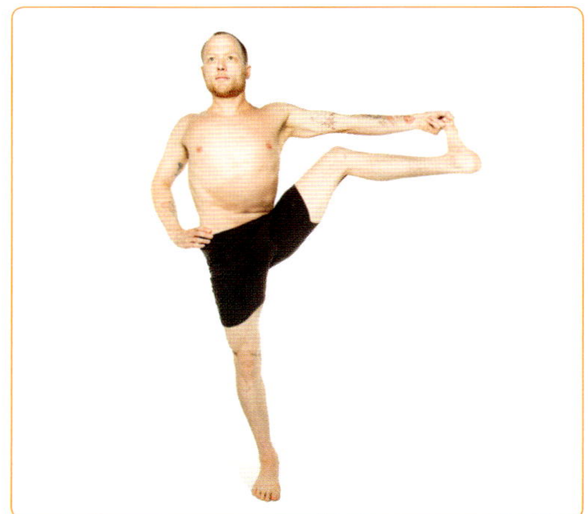

bowing sage *stage 1*
dwi hasta padasana

shape prep (from mountain)
■ Bend knees slightly.
■ Hold right foot with hands—arms inside leg.
■ For safety of low back, lift foot as high as hips, bring head above hips.

shape pose
■ Lift foot as high as hips, bring head above hips.
■ Stay here or straighten standing leg.
■ Stay here or straighten lifted leg—leg parallel to floor.
■ Straighten arms.
■ Move standing thigh back.

safety (strength) prep
■ Press hands and foot together.

safety (strength) pose
■ Tone thighs, tighten kneecaps, firm hamstrings.
■ Press top foot down.
■ Tone abdomen.

refinement (stretch) pose
■ Lift chest, stretch spine.

Repeat on the second side.

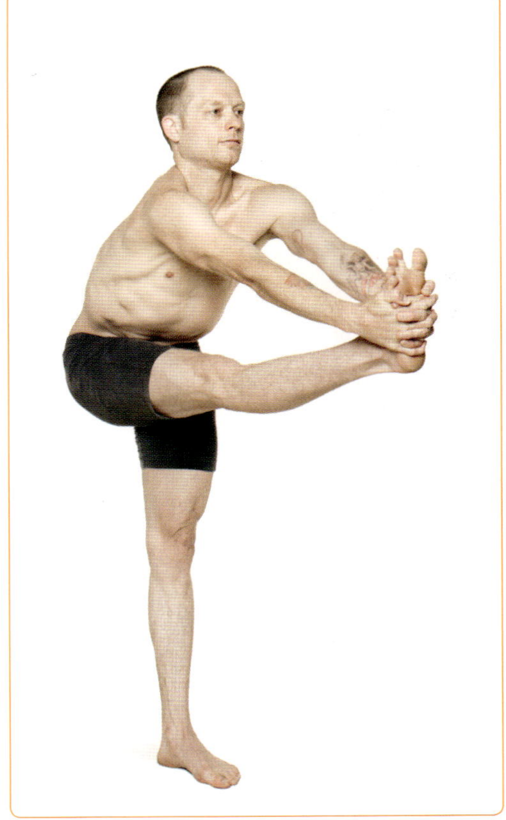

To improve balance, focus on a single point on the floor. This pose strengthens the standing leg. Done properly, it also strengthens and stretches the lifted leg. As far as I understand, one of the original purposes of Hatha Yoga was to create a strong vessel (body). That vessel is often compared to a clay pot after it's been fired (gone through tapasya—the fire of yoga). Think about the difference between a clay pot prior to and after going into the kiln. Prior: pliable. Post: strong. The point of yogahour is not to get flexible but to be strong in every pose, which paradoxically requires flexibility.

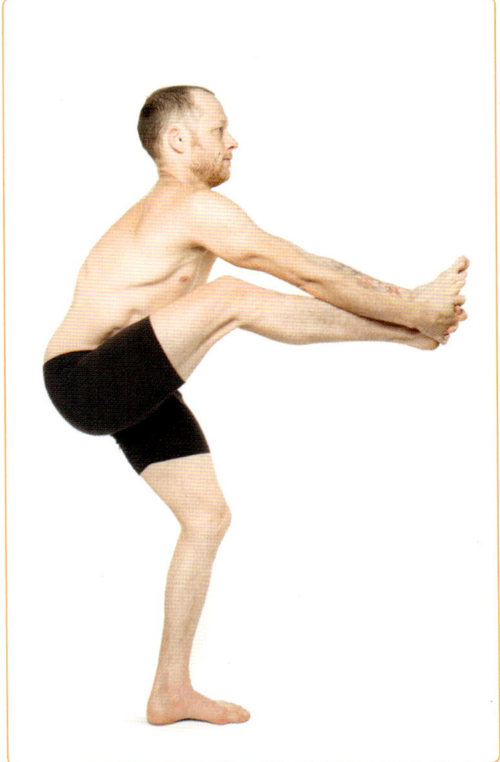

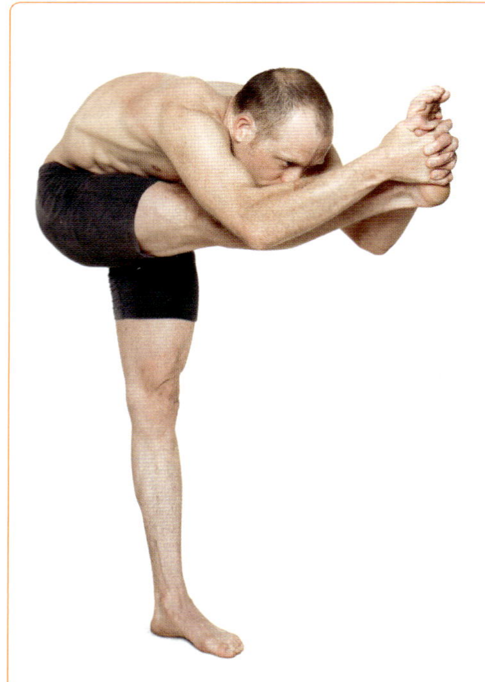

bowing sage
dwi hasta padasana

shape prep (from mountain)
- Bend knees slightly.
- Hold right foot with hands—arms inside leg.
- For safety of the low back, lift foot as high as hips, bring head above hips.
- Stay here or straighten standing leg.
- Stay here or straighten lifted leg—leg parallel to floor.
- Straighten arms.

shape pose
- Stay here or bring forehead to knee or chin to shin.
- Bend and point elbows down.
- Round back evenly.
- Take standing thigh back—leg straight up and down.

safety (strength) prep
- Press hands, top foot together.
- Tone thighs, tighten kneecaps, firm hamstrings.
- Press top foot down.
- Tone abdomen.

refinement (stretch) pose
- Pay attention to your breath. Allow your breath to breathe itself.

Repeat on the second side.

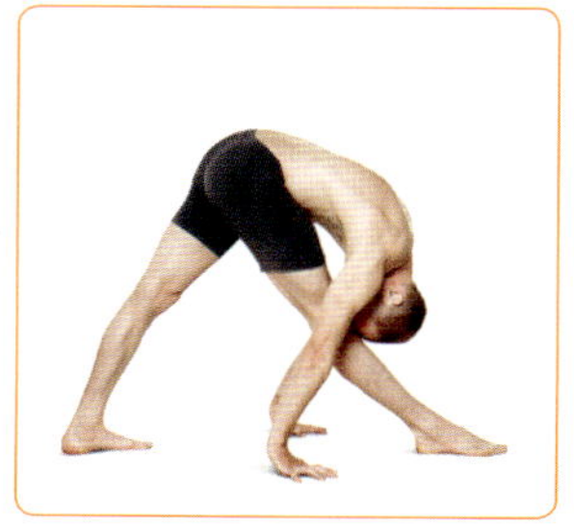
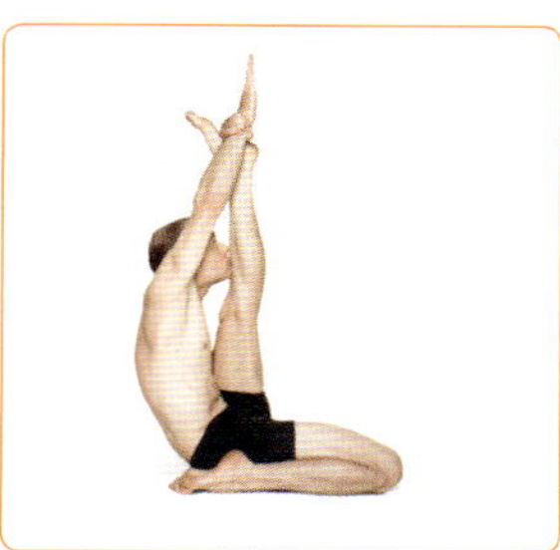
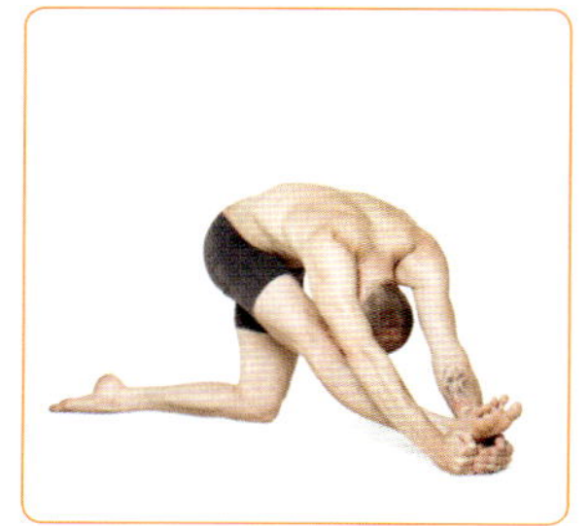
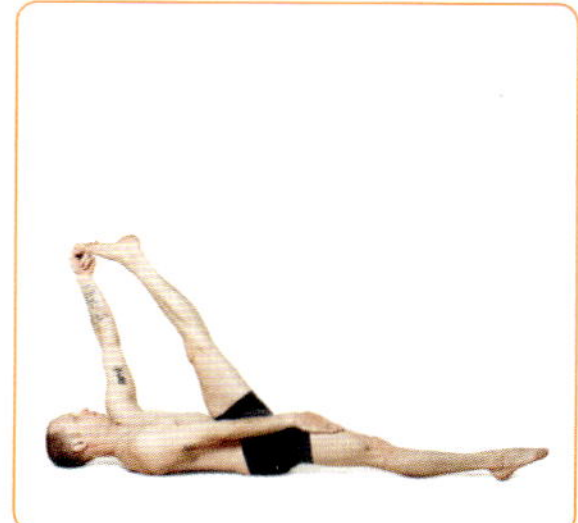

revolved sage
parivrtta hasta padangusthasana

shape prep (from mountain)
- Bend knees slightly.
- Hold outside of right foot with left hand.
- Lift foot as high as hips, head directly above hips.
- Stay here or straighten standing leg.
- Stay here or straighten lifted leg—leg parallel to floor.
- Straighten arms.

shape pose
- Twist torso to right, extend right arm straight back—arm parallel to floor.
- Look straight ahead (more difficult: look back past right hand).
- Stay here or lift right shin parallel to floor.
- Stay here or straighten right leg.
- Move standing thigh back.

safety (strength) prep
- Press foot, hand together.

safety (strength) pose
- Tone thighs, tighten kneecaps, firm hamstrings.

refinement (stretch) pose
- Lift chest, stretch spine.

Repeat on the second side.

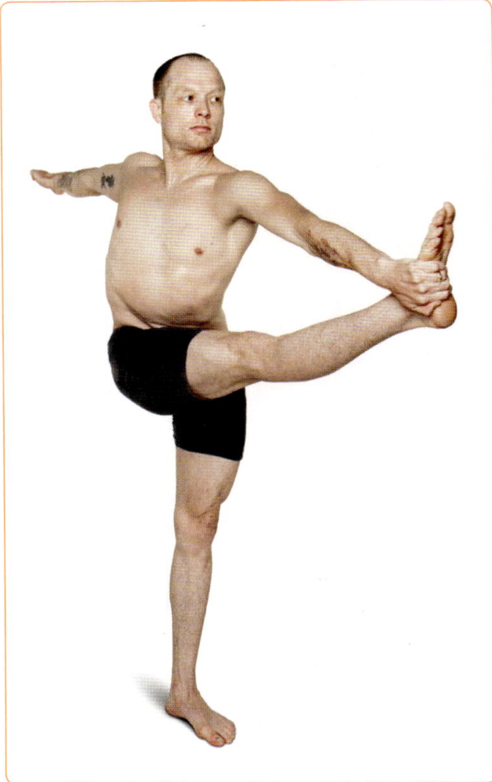

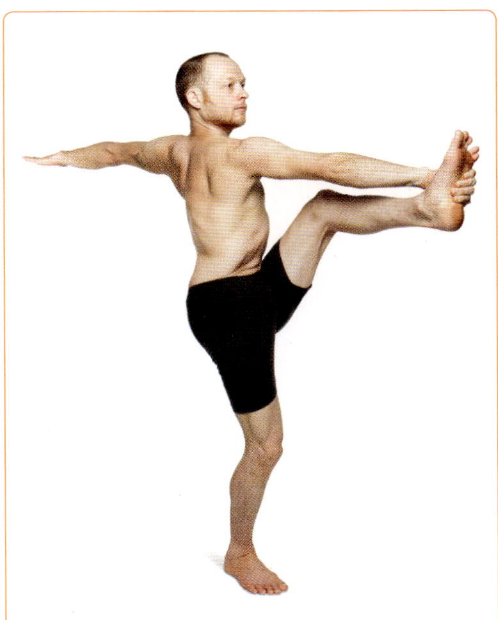

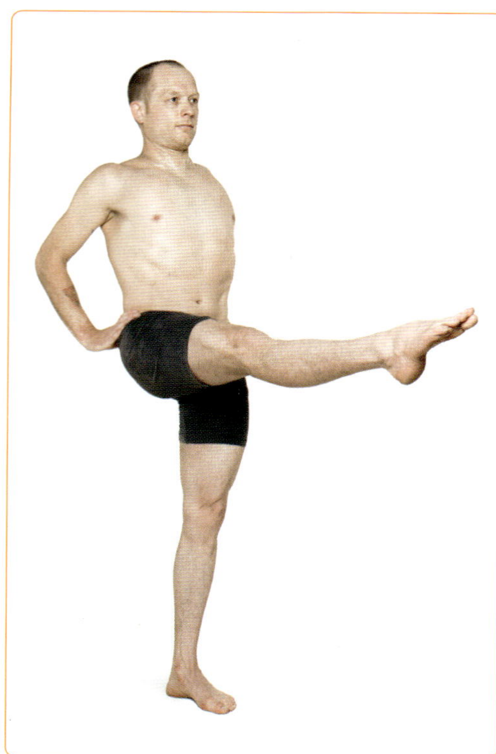

levitating sage
utthita eka padasana

shape prep (from mountain)
- Place hands on hips.

shape pose
- Lift right leg parallel to floor.
- Point right foot, straighten leg; turn leg out slightly.
- Look at lifted foot.

safety (strength) pose
- Use abdomen, hamstrings, and glutes to support lifted leg.
- Press abdomen towards spine.

refinement (stretch) pose
- Lift chest, stretch spine.

Repeat on the second side.

Yogahour inspired me to practice this pose on a regular basis. Thanks to this pose, along with boat and half boat, my weak hip flexors have become strong.

tree
vrksasana

shape prep (from mountain)
- Hold right ankle with right hand—arm inside leg.
- Place right foot against inner left thigh well above knee (more doable: bring right heel to left ankle).
- Point right foot down, knee out.

shape pose
- Place palms together above head—cross thumbs.
- Straighten arms.
- Lift chin slightly—look straight ahead (more doable: look at a single point on floor).

safety (strength) prep
- Do not touch standing knee with lifted foot.
- Make standing leg strong like the trunk of a tree.
- Press foot into thigh, thigh into foot.

safety (strength) pose
- Tighten glutes, press tailbone down, tone abdomen, move ribs back.

refinement (stretch) pose
- Press left foot down.
- Lift chest, stretch spine.
- Stretch arms up, back—touch ears with shoulders.

Repeat on the second side.

Tree pose develops balance and poise.

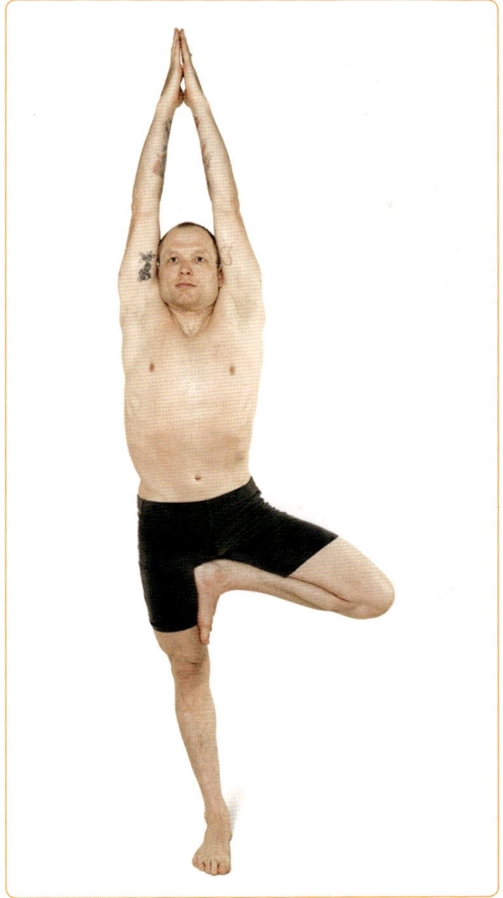

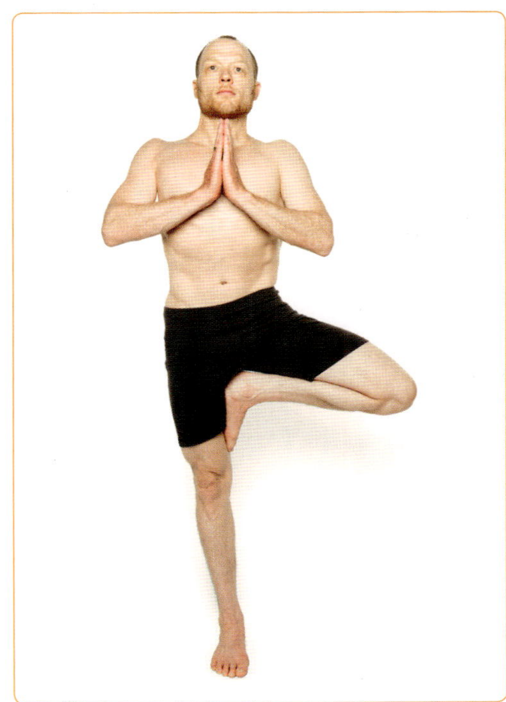

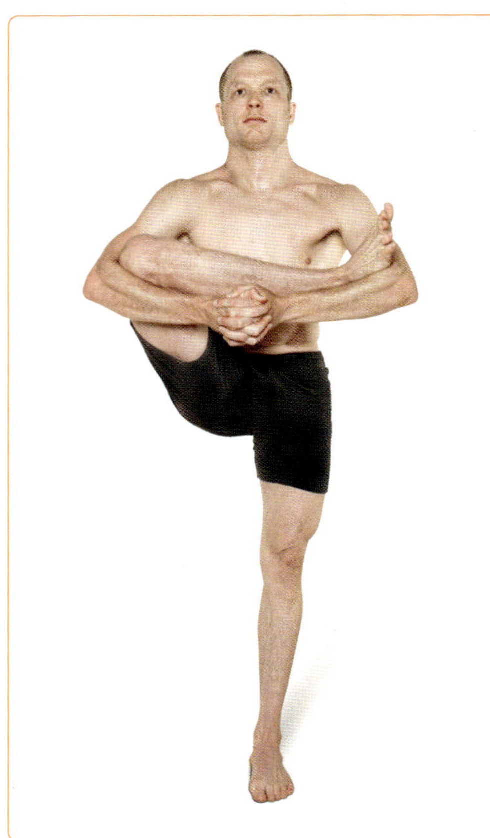

elevated pigeon
utthita hindolasana

shape prep (from mountain)
- Bend knees slightly.
- Hold right ankle with right hand.
- Lift foot as high as hips, point right knee out.

shape pose
- Wrap left elbow around right foot, right elbow around right knee, interlace fingers mid shin (more doable: hold right knee with right hand, right foot with left hand).
- Bend standing leg more, lift head above hips.
- Stay here or straighten standing leg; keep head above hips.

safety (strength) prep
- Flex right foot, flare toes.

safety (strength) pose
- Press inner edge of right foot against biceps.
- Press right foot, left arm together. Drag heel down.

refinement (stretch) pose
- Lift chest, stretch spine.

Repeat on the second side.

eagle
garudasana

shape prep (from mountain)
- Bend knees slightly—knees in line with toes.
- Wrap right leg around left leg—bring right big toe to Achilles tendon, flatten right foot against left calf (more doable: single cross legs; do not wrap foot around calf).

shape pose
- Wrap right elbow under left elbow, place palms together (more doable: place backs of hands together or hold shoulders).
- Move head directly above hips.

safety (strength) pose
- If shoulders are feeling good, press palms, elbows together.
- Press elbows into abdomen, abdomen into spine (more doable: lift elbows—upper arms parallel to floor).
- Move shoulders down.
- Squeeze legs together.

refinement (stretch) pose
- Lift chest, stretch spine.

Repeat on the second side.

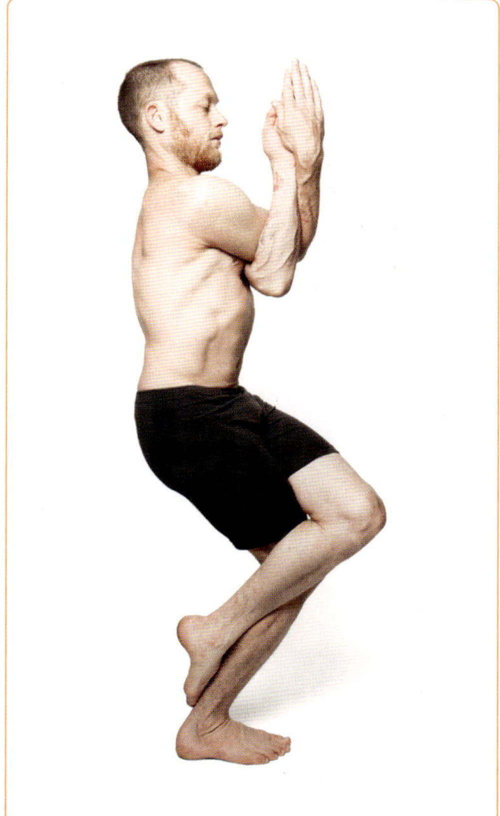

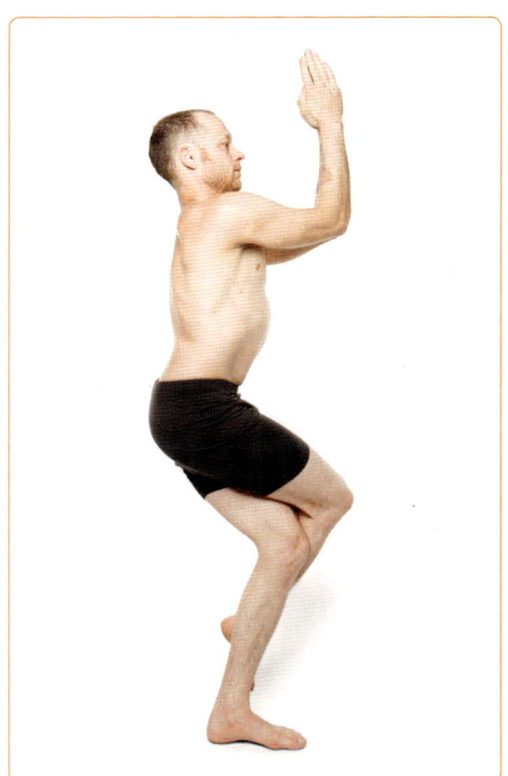

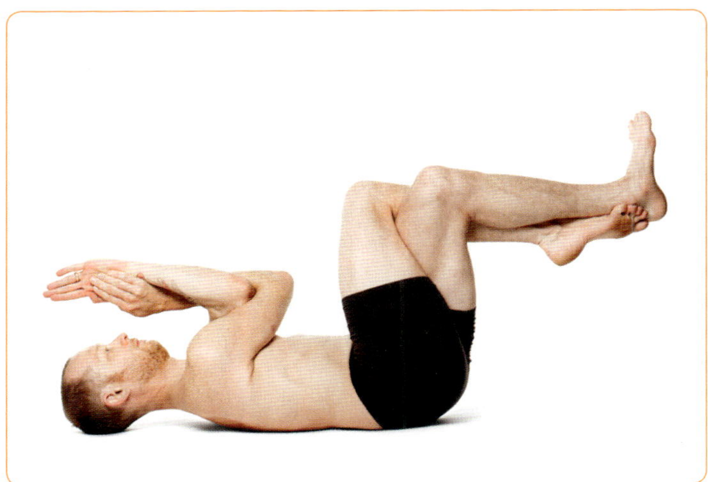

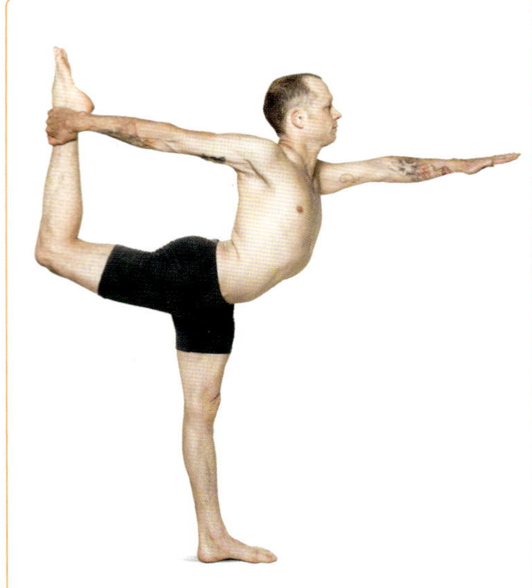

dancing yogi

natarajasana

shape prep (from mountain)
- Hold outside of right foot with right hand behind hips.
- Point right knee straight down, straighten right arm. Square hips and shoulders.
- Lift left arm parallel to floor in front of torso.

shape pose
- Stay here or kick right foot up, back—thigh parallel to floor (keep hips/shoulders square).
- Lift chin slightly, look straight ahead.

safety (strength) pose
- Tighten glutes, press tailbone down, tone abdomen.
- Lift back leg with leg—not just by kicking foot into hand (equally employ quads, inner thigh, hamstrings, and glutes).
- Lift shoulders up, back.

refinement (stretch) pose
- Lift chest, stretch spine.
- Extend out through back knee.

Repeat on the second side.

There are several variations of dancing yogi. In this variation, the torso is similar to cobra or bow pose. It's not the warrior 3 backbend variation, which is more like a standing splits.

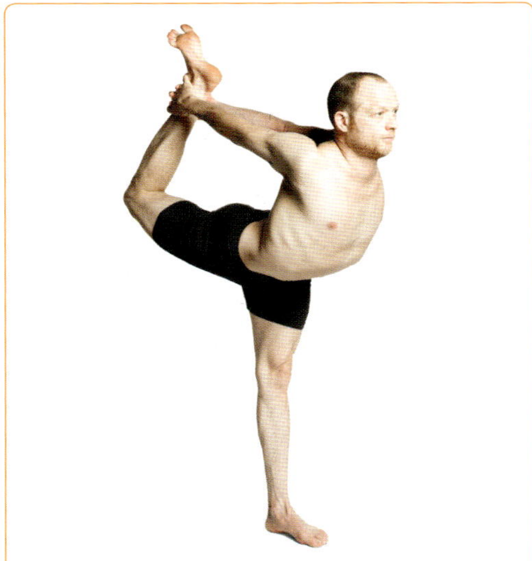

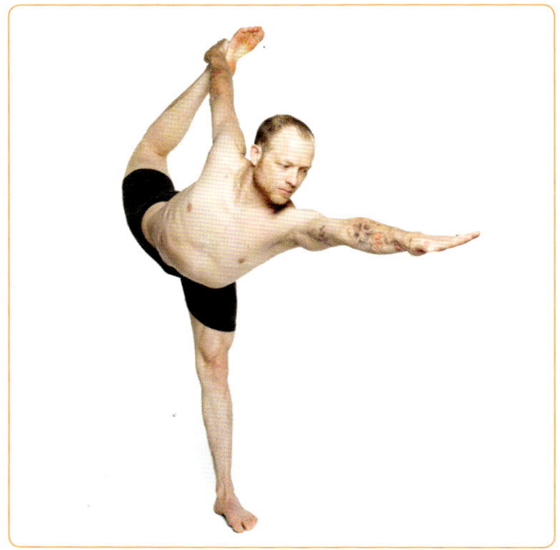

half moon
ardha chandrasana

shape prep (from mountain back of mat facing left)
- Step right foot to middle of mat with big toe facing top of mat.
- Bend right knee, place right fingertips a foot in front of right foot, tip of thumb in line with pinky toe. Move right knee out slightly.

shape pose
- Straighten right leg, lift left foot slightly higher than hips.
- Point left foot. Lift top arm vertical to floor. Close fingers.
- Look down, out, or up.
- Stack hips. Stack shoulders.
- Be as sideways as possible.
- Line up head, back foot with hips.

safety (strength) pose
- Tone thighs, tighten kneecaps, firm hamstrings.
- Press tailbone in, tone abdomen, move ribs back.

refinement (stretch) pose
- Stretch legs. Stretch spine. Stretch arms.

Repeat on the second side.

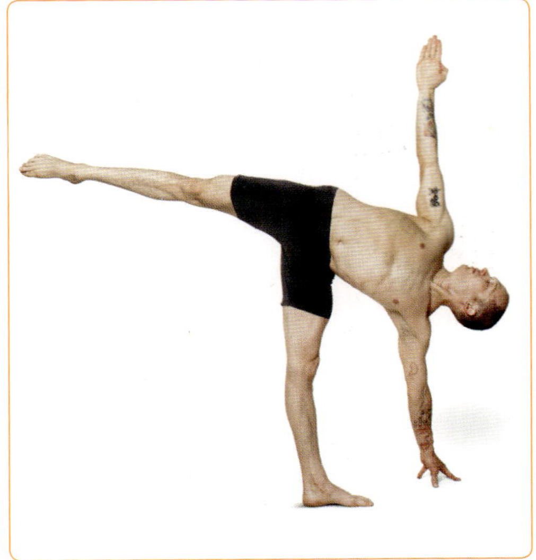

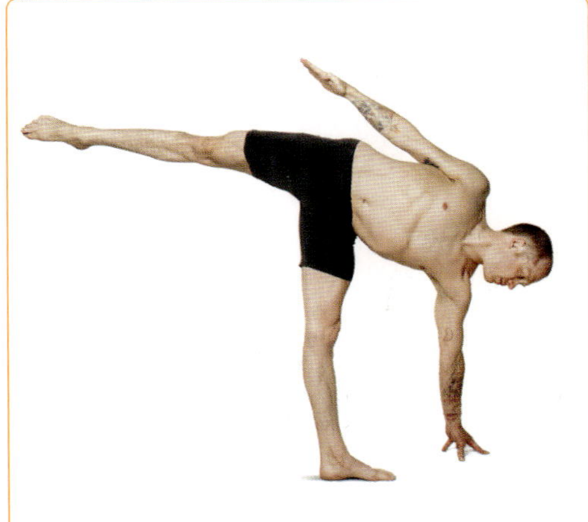

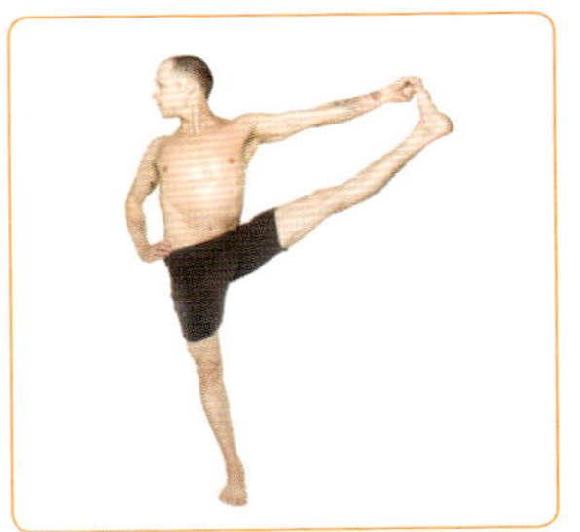

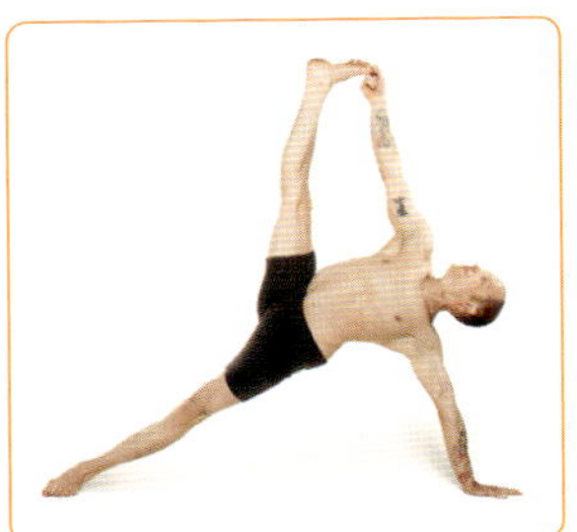

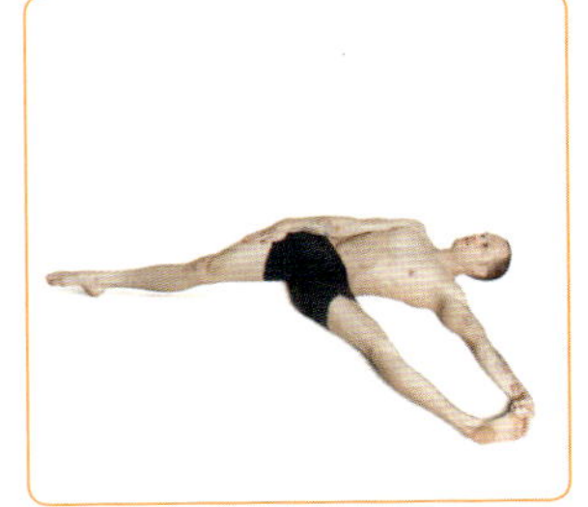

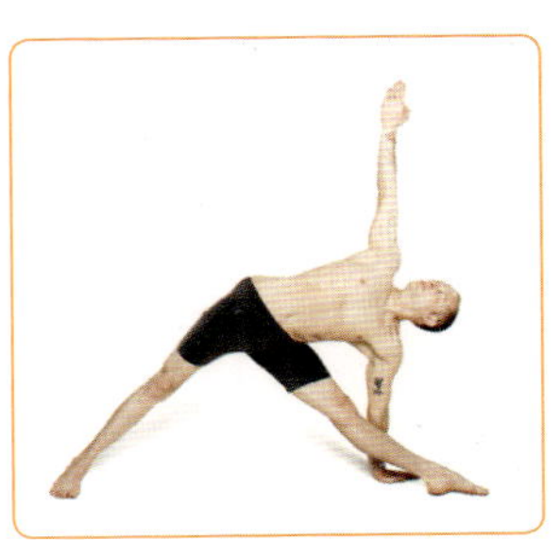

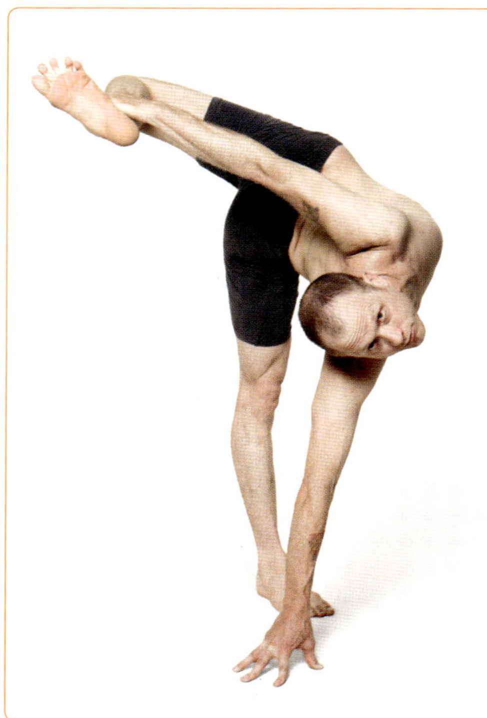

sugar cane
ardha chandrachapasana

shape prep (from half moon)
- Look down.
- Bend standing knee slightly.
- Bend top knee, hold outer edge of foot with hand.
- Bring top heel to hip.
- Point top knee straight back.
- Stay here or straighten standing leg.

shape pose
- Stay here or kick top foot straight back, extend chest forward.

safety (strength) prep
- Standing leg: tone thigh, tighten kneecap, firm hamstrings.
- Point kneecap of standing leg straight ahead (leg tends to turn in).

safety (strength) pose
- Tighten glutes, press tailbone in, tone abdomen.
- Kick back foot back with entire leg.

refinement (stretch) pose
- Lift chest, stretch spine.
- Flare toes of top foot.

Repeat on the second side.

If backbend is deep, move bottom hand out so it remains under shoulder.

revolved half moon

parivrtta ardha chandrasana

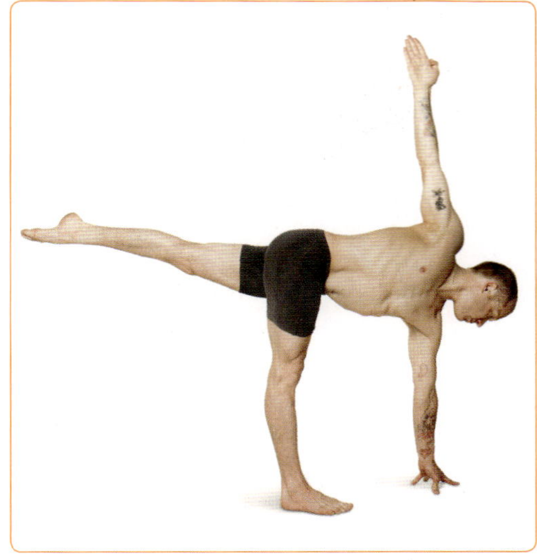

shape prep (from mountain)
- Bend knees slightly.
- Place fingertips on floor directly below shoulders.
- Lift left leg back, parallel to floor; point top foot.
- Square hips.
- Straighten standing leg (more doable: keep knee bent).
- Twist to right, stack shoulders.

shape pose
- Lift right hand up—arm vertical.
- Look up (more doable: look out or down).
- Line up head with hips.

safety (strength) pose
- Tone thighs, tighten kneecaps, firm hamstrings.
- Tighten glutes, press tailbone down, tone abdomen.

refinement (stretch) pose
- Stretch legs. Stretch spine. Stretch arms.

Repeat on the second side.

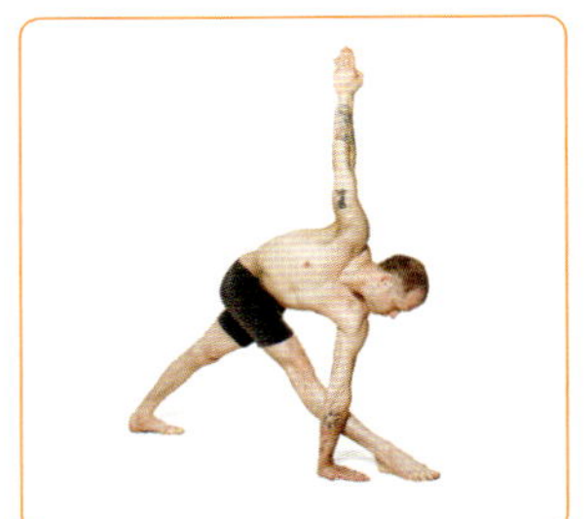
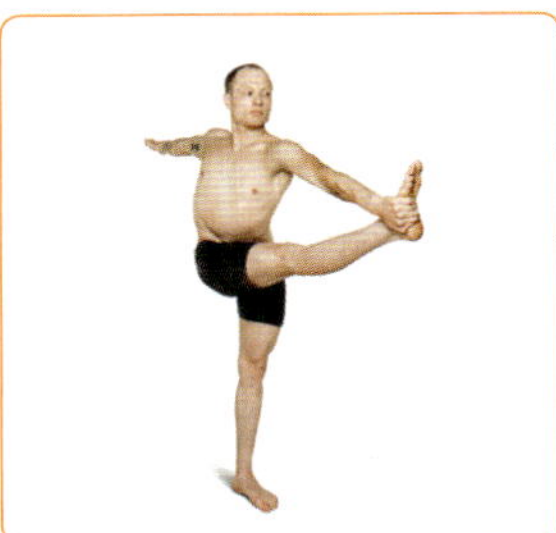
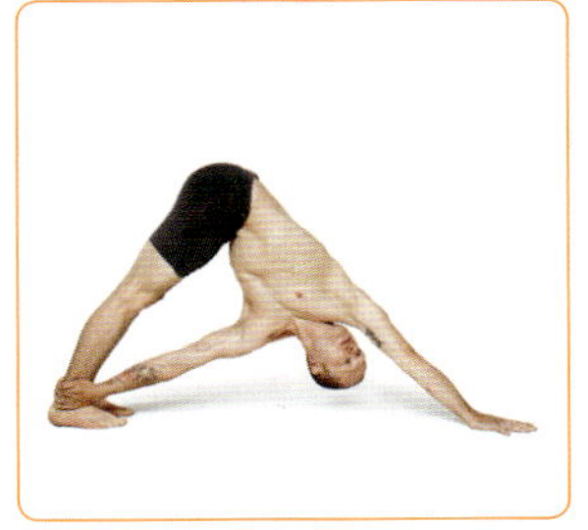
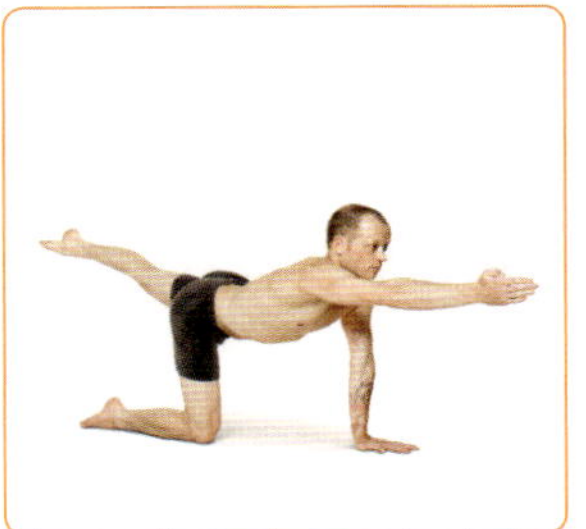

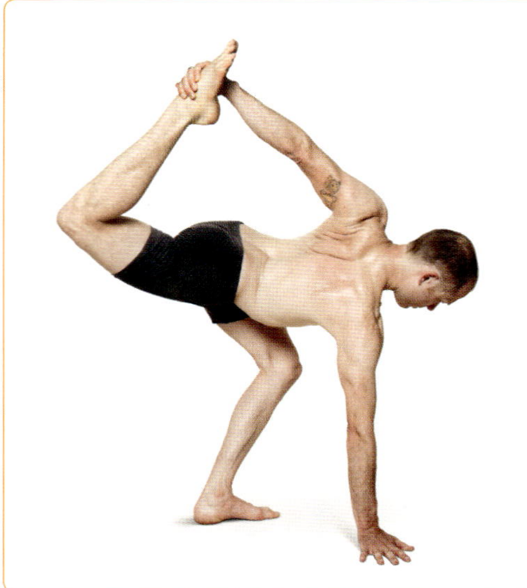

revolved sugar cane *prep*

parivrtta ardha chandrachapasana prep

shape prep (from revolved half moon)
- Bend standing knee, turn knee out slightly.
- Bend top knee, hold inner edge of foot with opposite hand. Press heel into hip.
- Bring top thigh parallel to floor (more doable: lower thigh toward floor).
- Bend standing knee more, twist torso to right—stack shoulders.

shape pose
- Stay here or kick top foot up. Bend in upper back.
- Look up (more doable: look out or down).
- Line up head with hips.

safety (strength) prep
- Keep standing knee bent.

safety (strength) pose
- Tighten glutes, press tailbone down.
- Tone, turn abdomen up.
- Use leg to lift leg.

refinement (stretch) pose
- Lift chest, stretch spine.

Repeat on the second side.

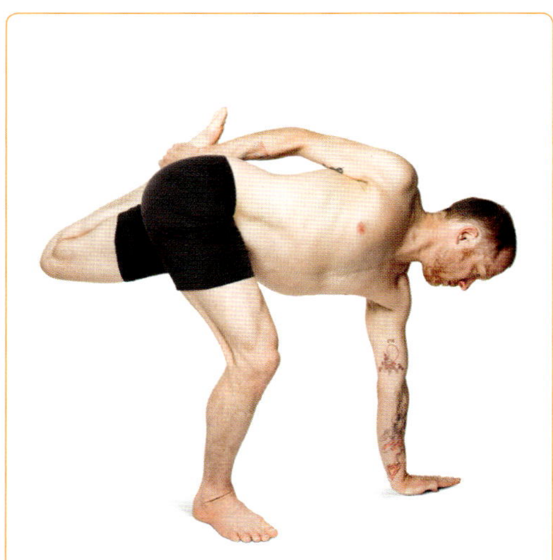

cat
marjarasana

shape prep
- Come onto hands and knees—arms, upper legs straight up and down.
- Bring knees, ankles together, or separate knees hip-distance apart—shins parallel.
- Flatten tops of feet on floor.
- Separate hands slightly wider than shoulder-width apart.
- Separate fingers evenly, point index fingers straight ahead.

shape pose
- Round back evenly, bring chin toward chest.
- Look past tip of nose.

safety (strength) prep
- Grip floor with fingertips, press inner edges of hands down.

safety (strength) pose
- Squeeze ankles, knees together.
- Squeeze elbows in.
- Press tailbone down, tone abdomen.

refinement (stretch) pose
- Press hands down.
- Stretch spine evenly.

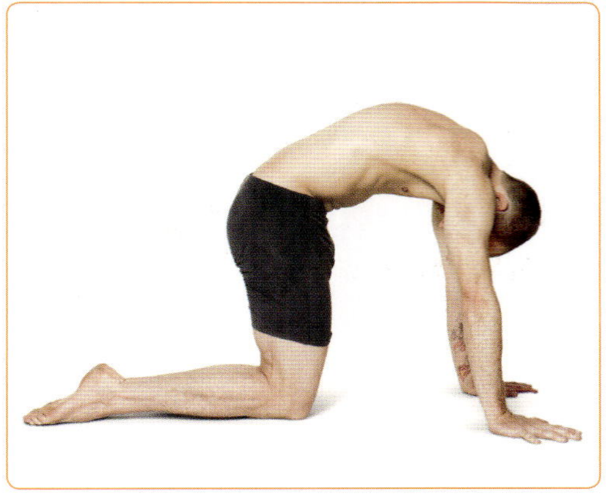

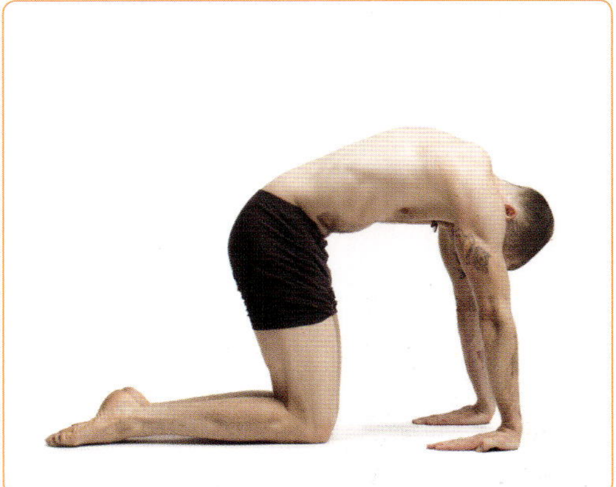

southpaw cat

In many yoga classes cat is practiced and taught in tandem with cow pose—not in yogahour. Cat and cow are often taught solo. Cat pose makes for a great shoulder, back, and spine warm-up.

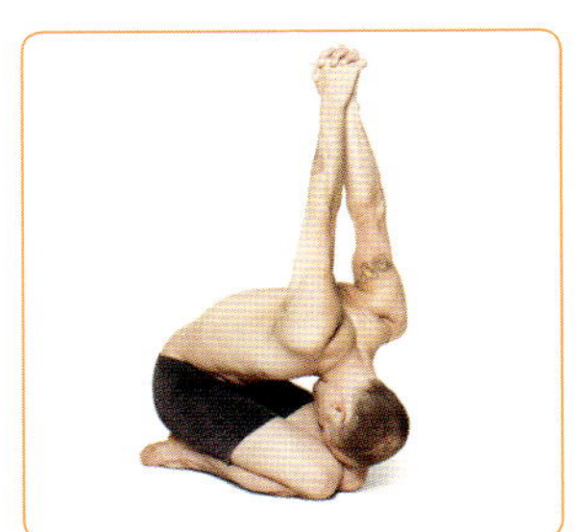
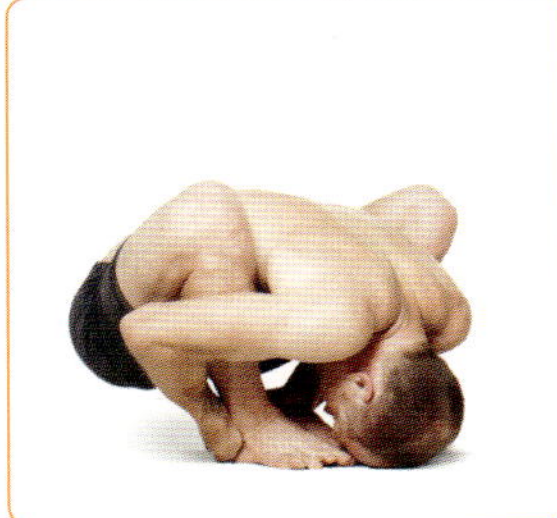
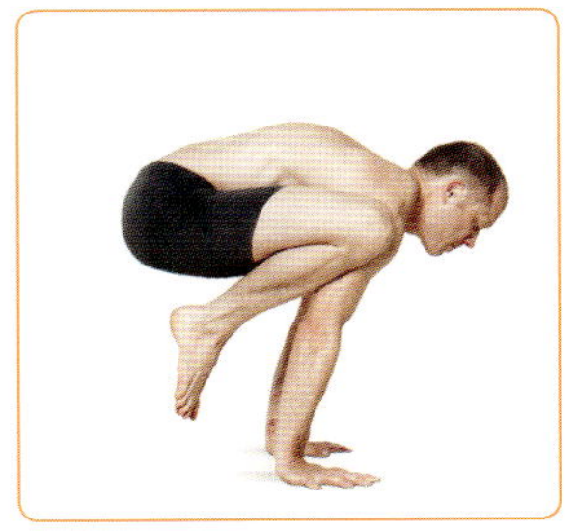
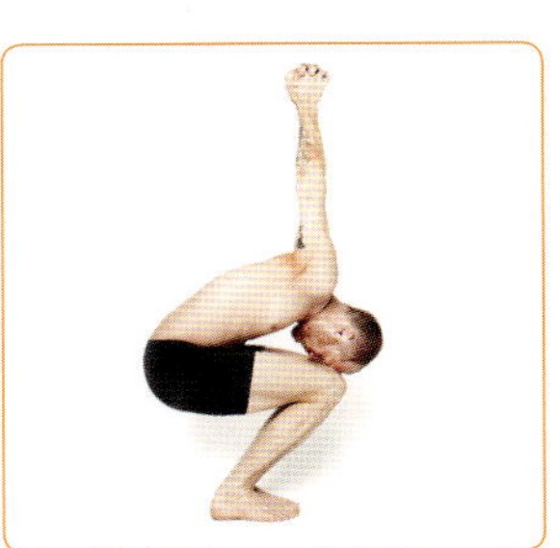

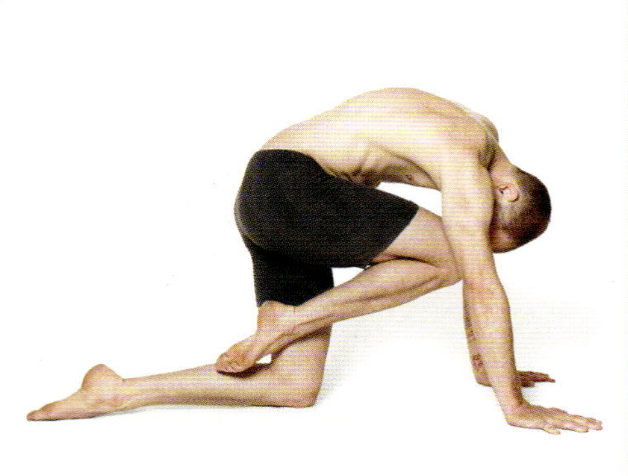

cat *forehead to knee*
vyaghrasana

shape prep
▦ Come onto hands and knees—arms, upper legs straight up and down.
▦ Bring knees, ankles together.
▦ Flatten tops of feet on floor.
▦ Separate hands slightly wider than shoulder-width apart.
▦ Separate fingers evenly, point index fingers straight ahead.
▦ Round back evenly, bring chin toward chest.
▦ Look past tip of nose.

shape pose
▦ Bring right knee to forehead; lift foot off floor—point foot.
▦ Place right foot against left inner thigh (more doable: rest right foot on floor).

safety (strength) prep
▦ Grip floor with fingertips, press inner edges of hands down.

safety (strength) pose
▦ Squeeze elbows in.
▦ Tone abdomen.
▦ Press foot, inner thigh together.

refinement (stretch) pose
▦ Press hands down.
▦ Stretch spine evenly (do not overly stretch neck).

Repeat on the second side.

downward facing dog
adho mukha svanasana

shape prep

- Come onto hands and knees—arms, upper legs straight up and down, knees and feet outer hip-width apart.
- Separate hands slightly wider than shoulder-width apart.
- Separate fingers evenly, point index fingers straight ahead.
- Move knees back four to six inches, curl toes under.

shape pose

- Lift knees, straighten legs. Create a natural curve in low back (if hamstrings are tight: bend knees slightly).
- Create a straight line from wrists, shoulders, to hips.
- Downward facing dog is a forward fold on hands and feet: hands and feet 4 to 4.5 feet apart; hands slightly wider than shoulders; feet outer hip-width apart.

safety (strength) pose

- Press hands down, lift shoulders up (especially inner edge of shoulders).
- Tone calves.
- Tone thighs, tighten kneecaps, firm hamstrings.

refinement (stretch) pose

- Press hands down, forward.
- Stretch shoulders.
- Stretch spine.
- Extend heels down to stretch backs of legs.

I've been to plenty of classes where the down dogs were many and seemingly aimless; not in yogahour! In yogahour, downward facing dog is usually ONLY practiced once or twice (aside from the times it's used as a transition). When down dog does ha-tha-happen it's not of the wait-in-line for the next pose variety. But wait, what about surya namaskar (sun salutations), isn't down dog incorporated into that? Yes, you've got me there. But, keep in mind, only 1 out of the first 10 yogahour set sequences utilizes surya namaskar as the warm-up. Why? That's easy: forward fold, cobra/up dog, and going from down dog to warrior 1 require warm-up in and of themselves for many if not most. The warm-ups in yogahour, and the entire practice for that matter, are aimed at the fit beginner (students without major limitations or injuries). Most fit beginners are not flexible begin-ners. The poses that make up surya namaskar are often just too extreme for them, unless modifications are given. And if there is one thing yogahour is not, it's extreme. Actually, that's not true at all. Yogahour is extremely doable and difficult; extremely consistent and creative; extremely punctual (starting class 15 seconds late is late; holding students 3 seconds too long in a pose is too long).

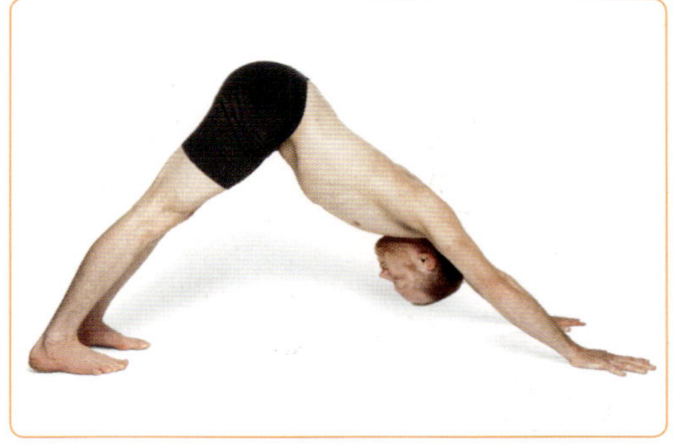

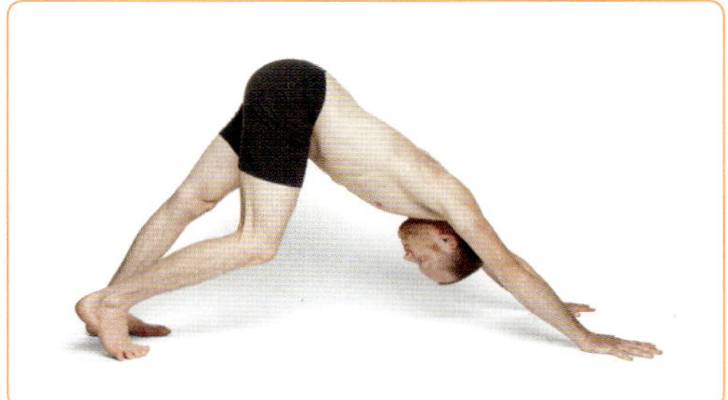

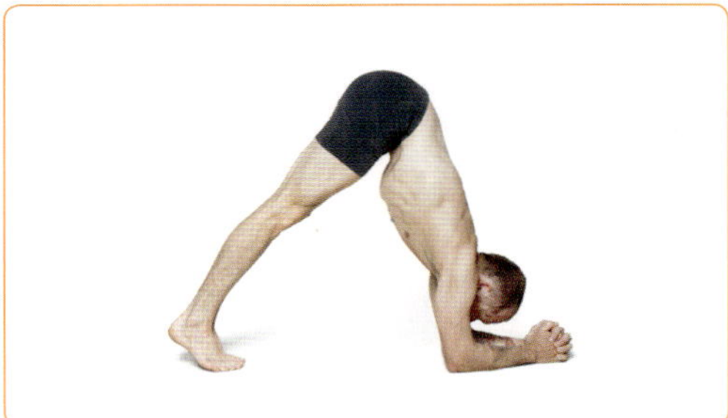

dolphin

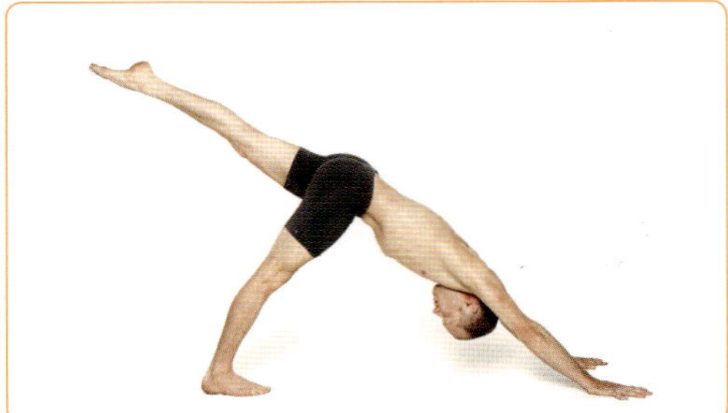

three leg dog

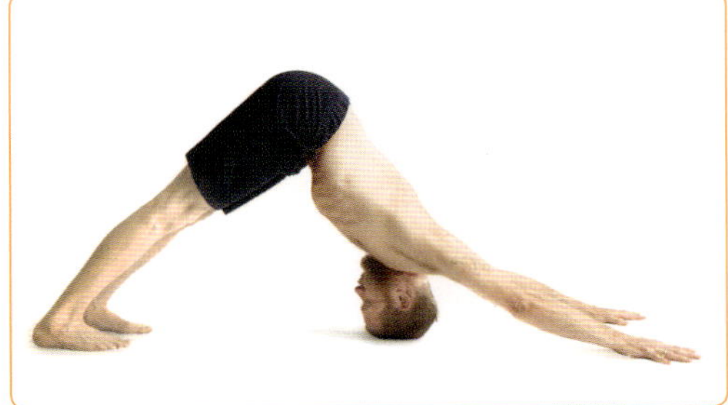

downward facing dog *head on floor*

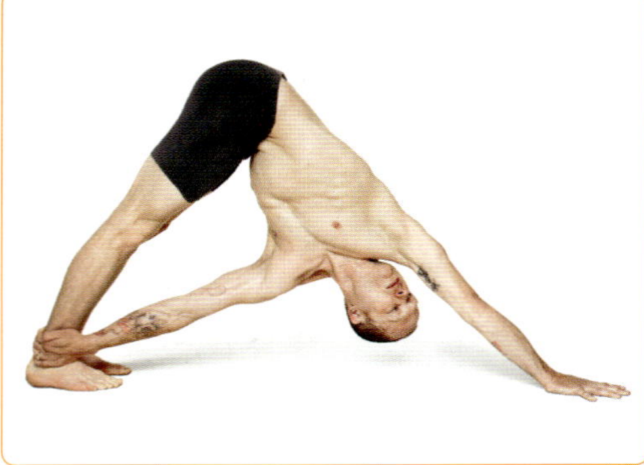

twisted downward facing dog
parivrtta adho mukha svanasana

shape pose (from downward facing dog)
▢ Bend left knee slightly; hold outer left ankle or shin with right hand.
▢ Stay here or straighten leg.
▢ Square hips.
▢ Turn chin toward left armpit.

safety (strength) pose
▢ Press front hand down, lift shoulder.
▢ Tone abdomen.
▢ Tone calves.
▢ Tone thighs, tighten kneecaps, firm hamstrings.

refinement (stretch) pose
▢ Press front hand down, forward.
▢ Extend hips back, heels towards floor.

Repeat on the second side.

This pose is a good prep for arm balances such as v sage and k sage 1.

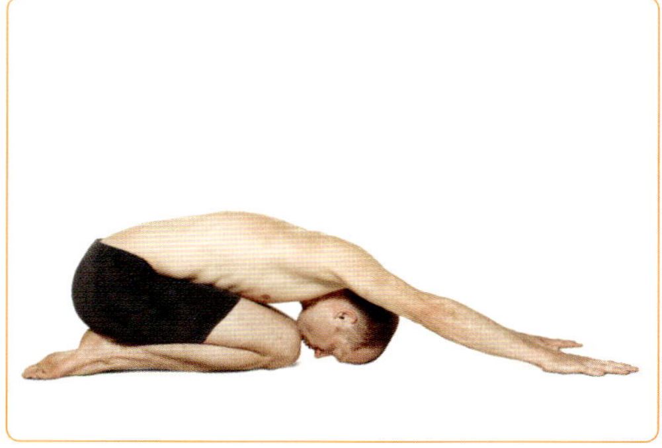

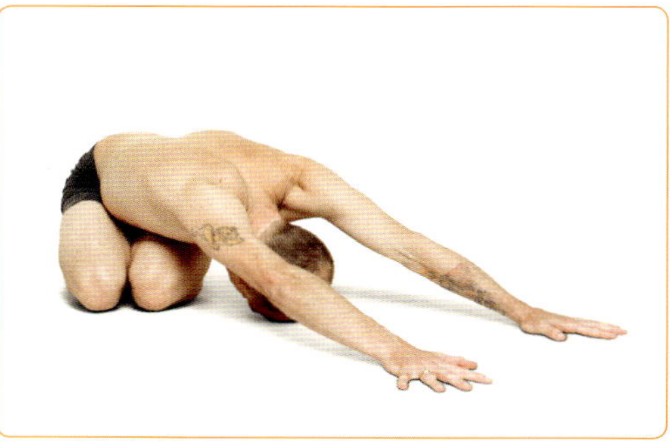

child's pose
balasana

shape prep
▢ Have a seat on feet—tops of feet on floor.
▢ Bring thighs parallel to each other.
▢ Lower forehead to floor; rest torso on thighs.

shape pose
▢ Bring hands, arms into down dog position (more doable: rest forehead on block).

safety (strength) pose
▢ If hip flexors are uncomfortable, lift torso upright; press tops of thighs down, out with hands; stay there or fold forward again.

refinement (stretch) pose
▢ Soften face.
▢ Notice breath.
▢ Relax.

twisted child's pose
parivrtta balasana

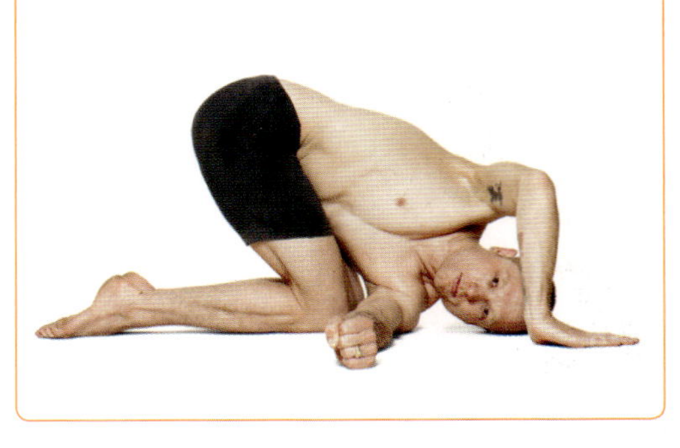

shape prep
- Come onto hands and knees—arms, upper legs straight up and down.
- Bring knees, ankles together (more doable: separate knees and feet outer hip-width apart).
- Point feet. Flatten tops of feet on floor.
- Lift right arm out to side.

shape pose
- Swing right arm under torso, lower shoulder to floor in line with knees, place right side of face on floor.
- Straighten right arm—right arm parallel to top of mat.
- Bend left elbow—forearm vertical to floor.

safety (strength) prep
- Squeeze knees, ankles together.

safety (strength) pose
- Place equal weight under knees.
- Lift without lifting feet to engage hamstrings.
- Do not allow hips to move right or left.
- Press tailbone down, tone abdomen.
- Press right arm down, back. Press left hand down, out.
- Move shoulders back.

refinement (stretch) pose
- With each inhalation, expand torso.

Repeat on the second side.

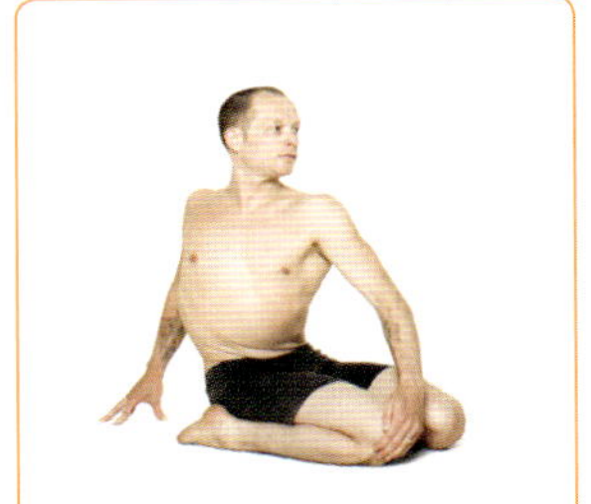
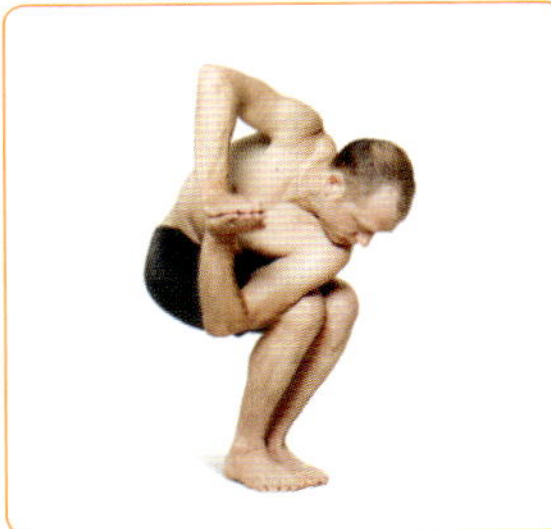
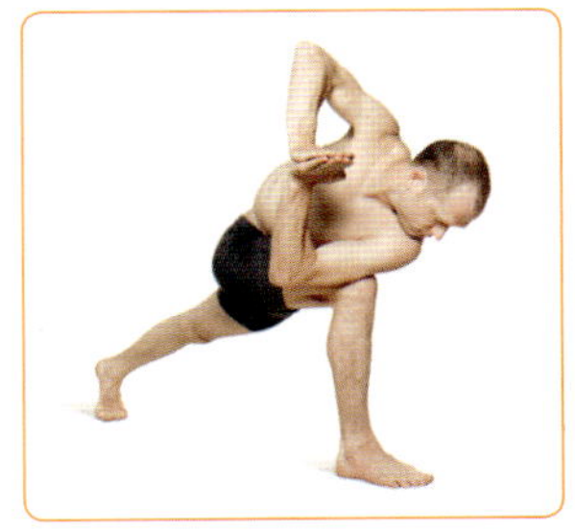
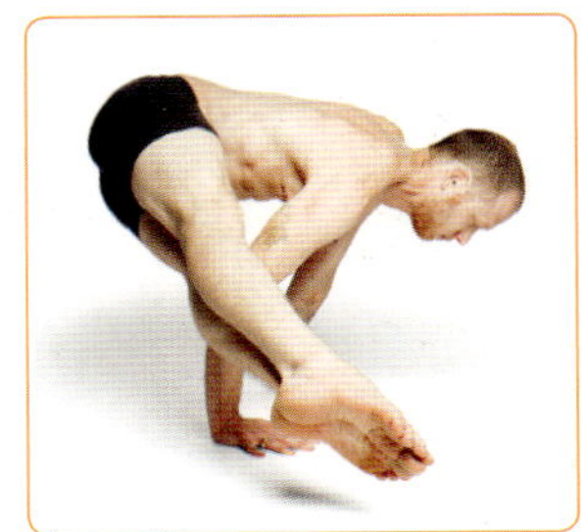

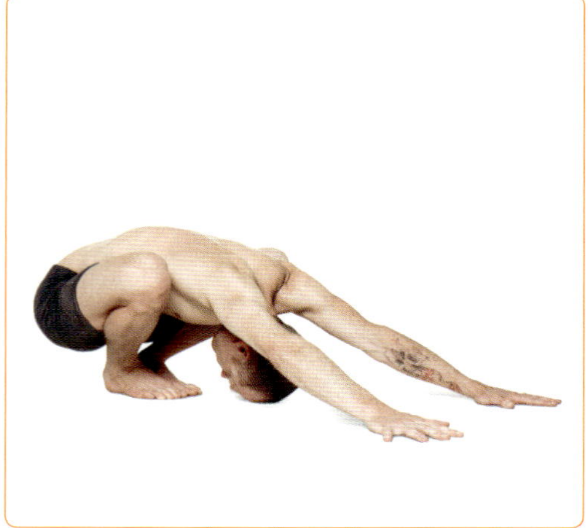

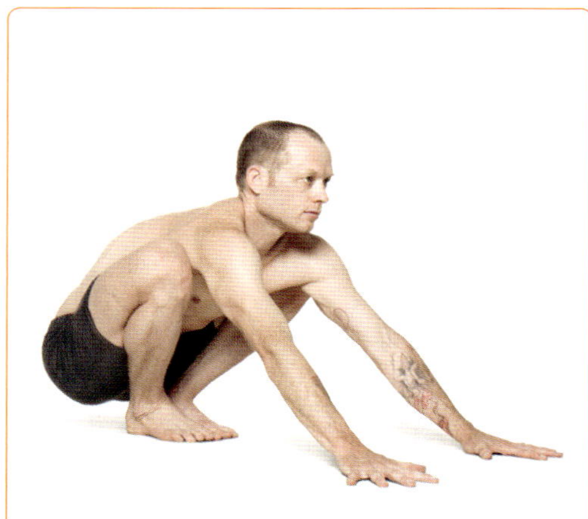

garland 1 prep
malasana prep

shape prep (from mountain)
■ Lower into a squat position (more doable: separate feet outer hip-width apart, point feet in line with knees.) If heels hover above floor put rolled up mat underneath them or lift heels vertical, shins parallel to floor, then walk hands out more.

shape pose
■ Fold torso inside thighs, slide hands forward, straighten arms.
■ Place palms flat on floor shoulder-width apart.
■ Look down (more difficult: rest forehead on floor).
■ Round back evenly.

safety (strength) pose
■ Press inner edges of feet down, grip floor with toes, press ankles together.
■ Squeeze torso with thighs.
■ Press hands down, lift shoulders.
■ Tone abdomen.

refinement (stretch) pose
■ Press hands down, forward; move hips down, back.

garland 2
malasana 2

shape prep (from mountain)
- Bend knees slightly.
- Widen knees slightly wider than hips.
- Fold forward, hold backs of heels with hands, bring armpits to shins just below knees.
- Stay here or lower hips to heels.

shape pose
- Stay here or lean forward, place forehead on floor (more difficult: forehead to big toes).
- Round back evenly.

safety (strength) pose
- Press inner edges of feet down, ankles in, grip floor with toes.
- Squeeze torso with thighs.
- Tone abdomen.

refinement (stretch) pose
- Pull forward and up on heels with hands.
- Stretch spine; stretch shoulders toward ears.

Garland 2 sets the tone and tenor for bound angle, crane pose and formidable forearm pose.

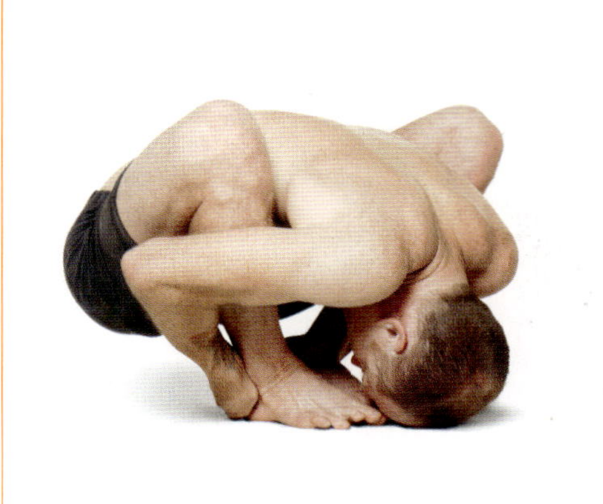

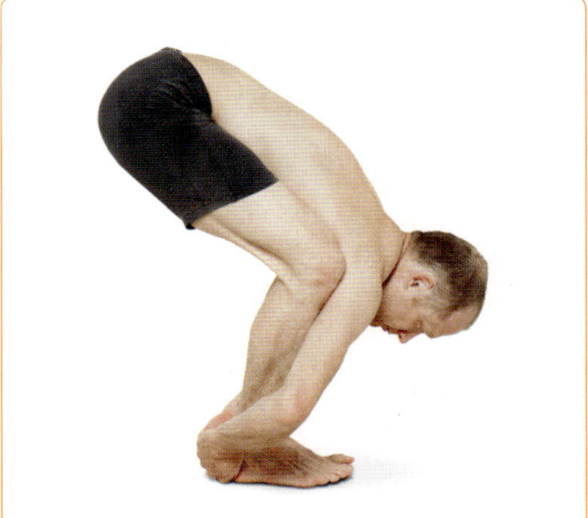

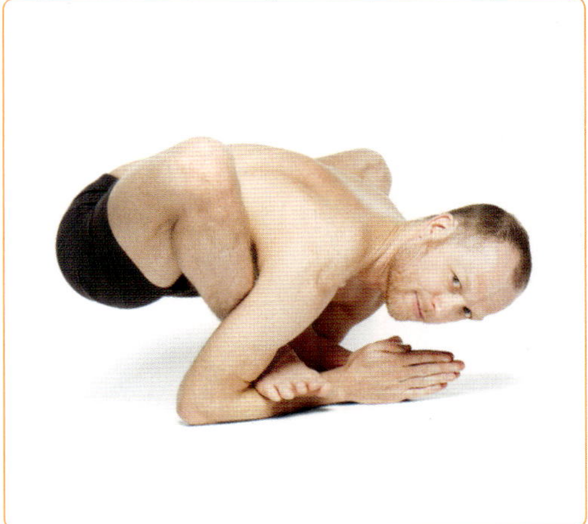

formidable forearm pose

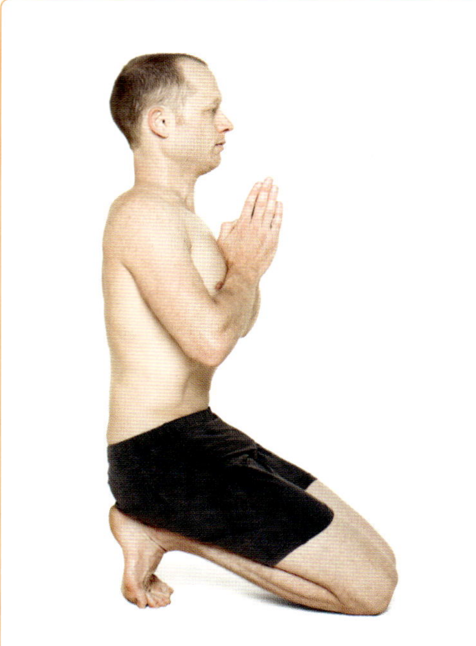

elevated thunderbolt
vajrasana

shape pose
■ Have a seat on heels with toes curled under—torso upright.
■ Bring knees together, ankles as close together as possible (more doable: separate knees as much as needed and/or lean forward, lift hips, and place hands on floor in front of knees).
■ Place palms together in front of chest.
■ Lift chin slightly, look straight ahead.

safety (strength) pose
■ Squeeze knees in.
■ Press tailbone down, tone abdomen, move ribs back.

refinement (stretch) pose
■ Lift chest, stretch spine.
■ Relax jaw, soften eyes, notice breath.

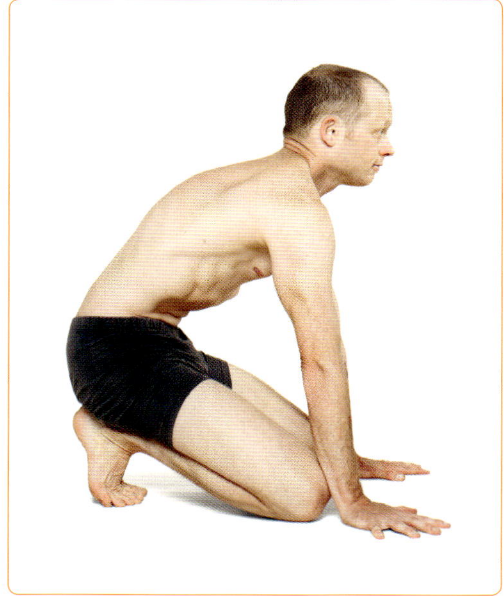

thunderbolt *arms extended*
vajrasana

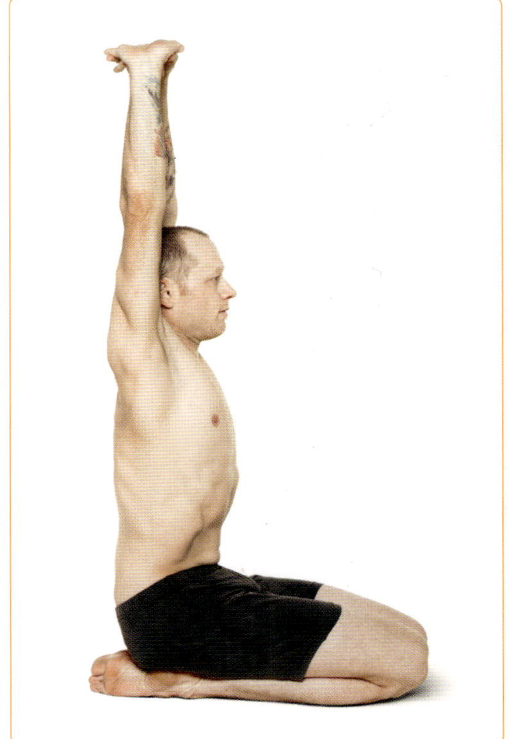

shape pose
- Have a seat on heels with toes curled under—torso upright.
- Bring knees together, ankles as close together as possible (more doable: separate knees as much as needed and/or lean forward, lift hips, and place hands on floor in front of knees).
- Interlace fingers, extend arms overhead, point palms up.
- Lift chin slightly, look straight ahead.

safety (strength) pose
- Squeeze knees in.
- Press tailbone down, tone abdomen, move ribs back.

refinement (stretch) pose
- Lift chest, stretch spine.
- Extend shoulders up, back.
- Relax jaw, soften eyes, notice breath.

thunderbolt *hands bound*
baddha hasta vajrasana

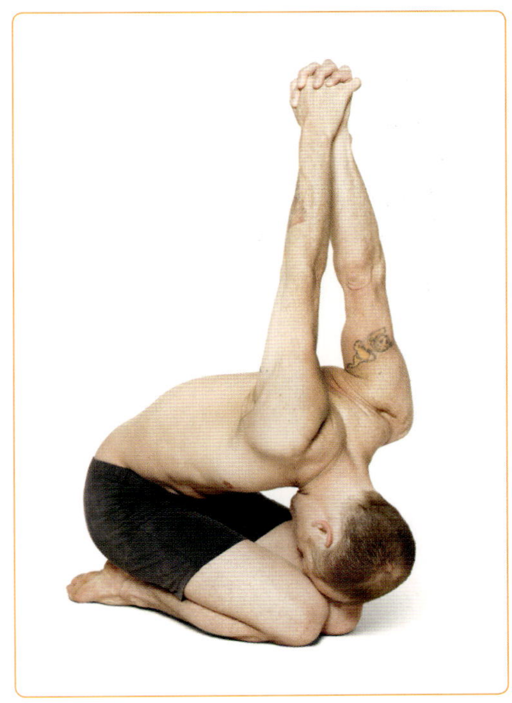

shape prep
- Have a seat on feet—tops of feet on floor.
- Interlace fingers behind back with elbows slightly bent.
- Pull palms apart. Straighten arms to capacity (more difficult: place palms together).

shape pose
- Bring forehead to knees (more doable: bring chin to knees).
- Round back evenly.

safety (strength) pose
- Squeeze knees, shoulders in.
- Lift abdomen.

refinement (stretch) pose
- Move shoulders away from head.
- Stretch hands up.

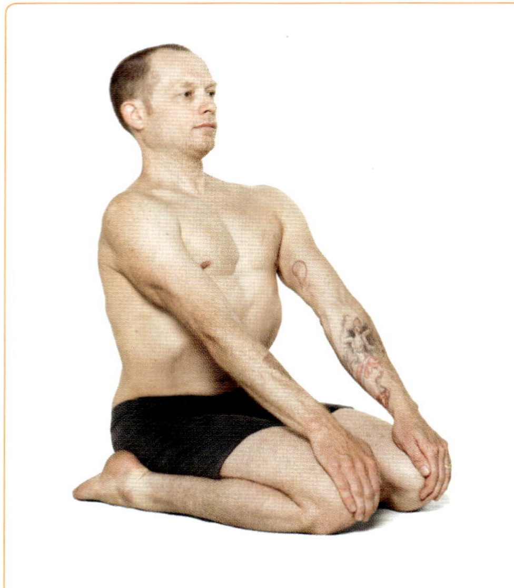

hero
virasana

shape pose
- Have a seat between feet—tops of feet on floor (more doable: sit on a block).
- Bring inner heels against outer hips; point feet.
- Bring thighs parallel or widen knees as much as necessary.
- Hold knees with hands, straighten arms.
- Look forward or down.

safety (strength) pose
- Move abdomen in.

refinement (stretch) prep
- To reduce ankle stretch, place knees and shins on one to three yoga blankets--tops of feet on floor.

refinement (stretch) pose
- Lift low back, lift chest, stretch spine.

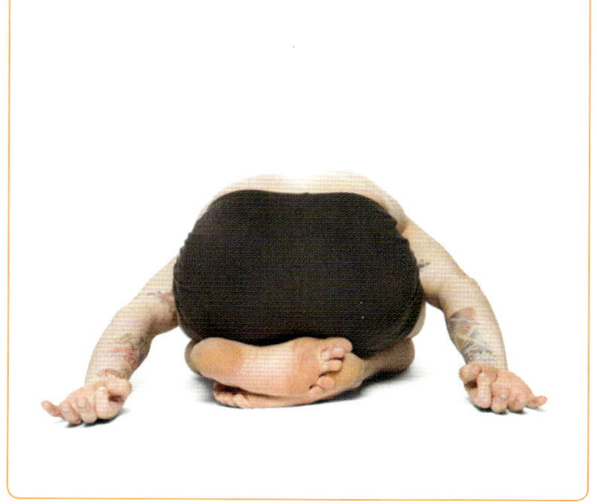

twisted hero
parivrtta virasana

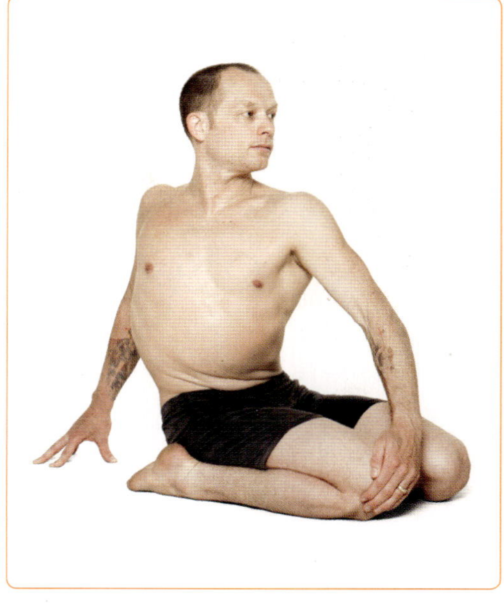

shape prep (from hero—hips on floor or block)
- Place right hand on left knee, left fingertips on floor behind hips.

shape pose
- Twist to left; look over back or front shoulder.

safety (strength) prep
- Keep knees flush—do not let either knee move forward or back.

safety (strength) pose
- Tone, turn abdomen to left.
- Move ribs back.
- Lift left shoulder up, back.

refinement (stretch) prep
- To reduce ankle stretch, place knees and shins on one to three yoga blankets—tops of feet on floor.

refinement (stretch) pose
- Lift low back, lift chest, stretch spine.

Repeat on the second side.

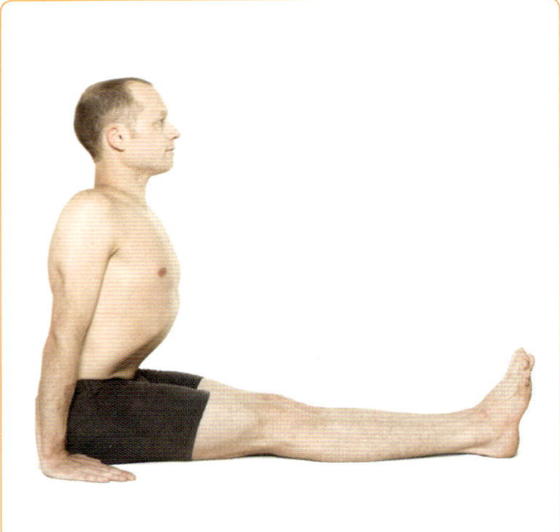

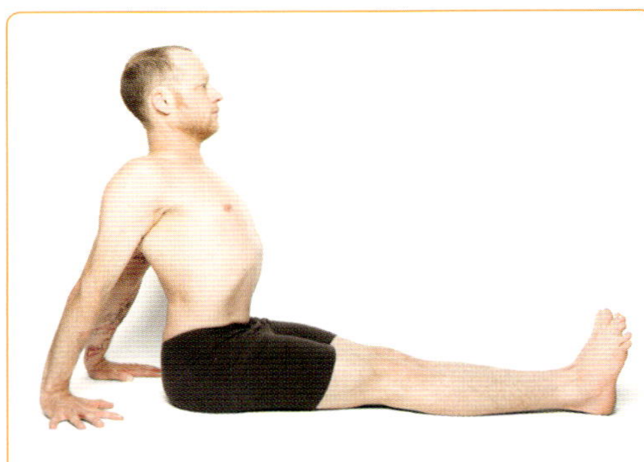

staff
dandasana

shape prep
- Come into a seated position toward back of mat.
- Straighten legs, bring ankles together.
- Place palms or fingertips on floor outside hips.

shape pose
- Flex feet, straighten arms, lift torso upright.
- Extend inner edges of feet forward, pull outer edges of feet back.
- Curve low back in so that spine is in a neutral position (more doable: bend knees 4-6 inches, separate feet outer hip-width apart or sit on a yoga block and straighten legs).
- Lift chin slightly, look straight ahead.

safety (strength) pose
- Tone thighs, tighten kneecaps, firm hamstrings.
- Press legs into floor.
- Squeeze legs together.

refinement (stretch) pose
- Lift chest, stretch spine.

Staff is a stage 1 forward fold. It's not a pre-forward fold; it's a forward fold in its own right. In dandasana, straight legs + tight hamstrings = rounded low back. If the low back starts off rounded in stage 1, it will end up compressed in stage 2. Instead of bending knees, sitting on a block or blankets is also an option.

The shape of the body in staff is similar to that of downward facing dog. The primary difference between them: the body's relationship to gravity; the position of the arms; the shape of the feet. Seeing similar shapes in different poses is key to understanding the art of sequencing. You might also notice a similar relationship between downward facing dog/ forward fold and staff/west stretch. In an expertly taught asana class, one pose leads and paves the way to another. Shape alone is not enough; safety and strength are equally essential.

intense west stretch *knees bent*
paschimottanasana

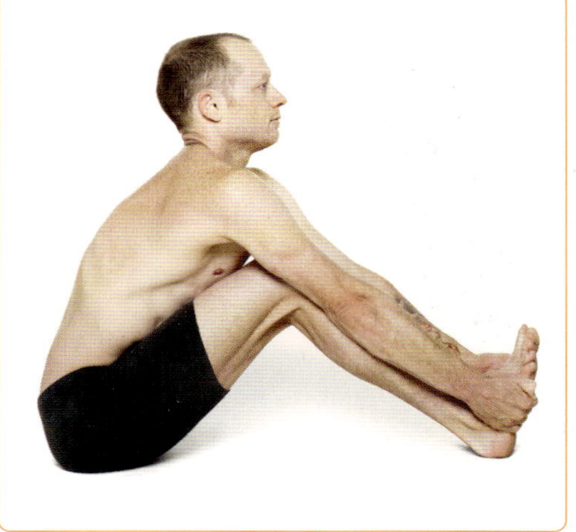

shape prep (from staff)
■ Keep legs straight or knees bent (if hamstrings are tight, separate feet outer hip width apart).

shape pose
■ Hold big toes with first two fingers/thumbs, or hold outer edges of feet.
■ Straighten arms.
■ Lift chin slightly, look straight ahead.

safety (strength) prep
■ If legs are straight: tone thighs, tighten kneecaps, firm hamstrings, press thighs and heels down.
■ If knees are bent: dig heels into floor.

safety (strength) pose
■ Press hands, feet together to strengthen legs.
■ Squeeze legs together.
■ Tone abdomen.
■ Lift shoulders up.

refinement (stretch) prep
■ Lift chest, stretch spine.

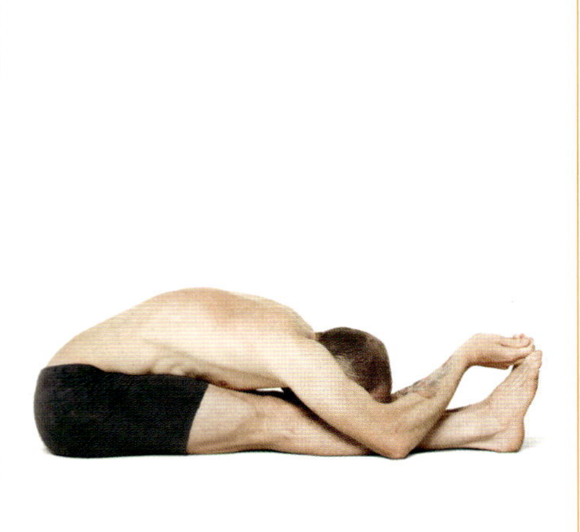

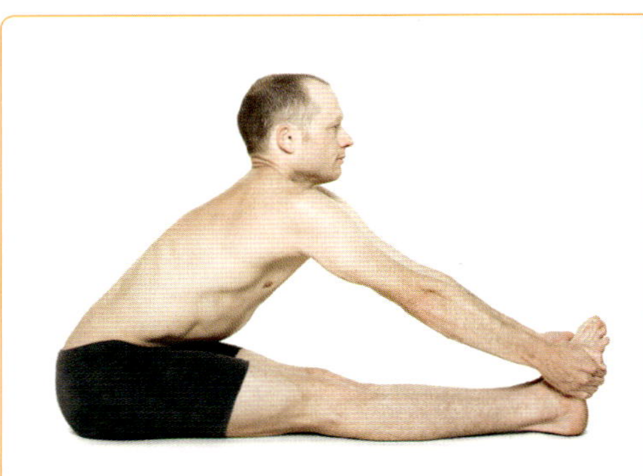

intense west stretch
paschimottanasana

shape prep (from staff)
■ Keep knees bent or legs straight (if hamstrings are tight separate feet outer hip width apart).
■ Hold big toes with first two fingers, thumbs.
■ Straighten arms.
■ Lift chin slightly, look straight ahead.

shape pose
■ Place torso against thighs, face against shins.
■ Round back evenly.
■ Point elbows down, palms up.

safety (strength) prep
■ If legs are straight: tone thighs, tighten kneecaps, firm hamstrings, press thighs and heels down.
■ If knees are bent: dig heels into floor.
■ Lift pelvic floor.

safety (strength) pose
■ Press fingers, big toes together to help strengthen legs.
■ Squeeze legs together.
■ Tone abdomen.

refinement (stretch) prep
■ Lift chest, stretch spine.

refinement (stretch) pose
■ Use arms to help lengthen spine.
■ Extend shoulders forward, elbows down.

In Light On Yoga on page 166 B.K. S. Iyengar states Paschima literally means west. Implying that this pose stretches the entire back of the body from the head to the heels. Ugrasana is another name for Paschimottansana. Mr. Iyengar defines Ugra as formidable, powerful and noble.

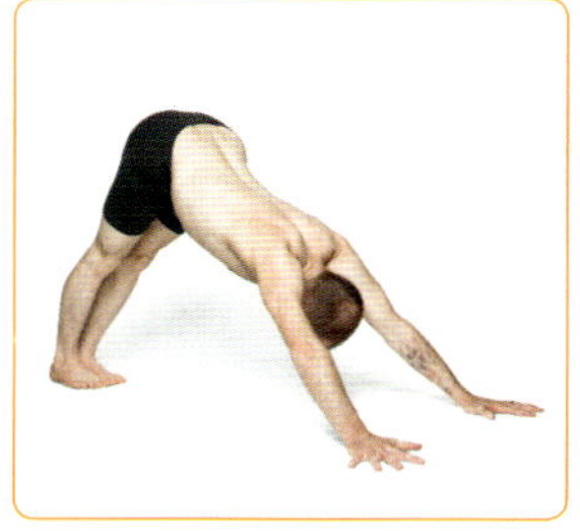

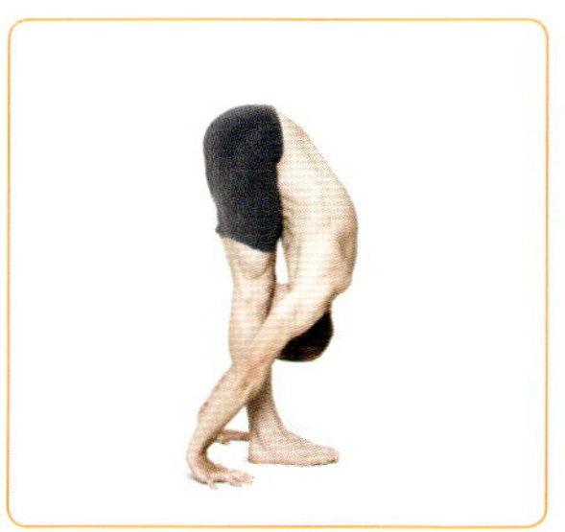

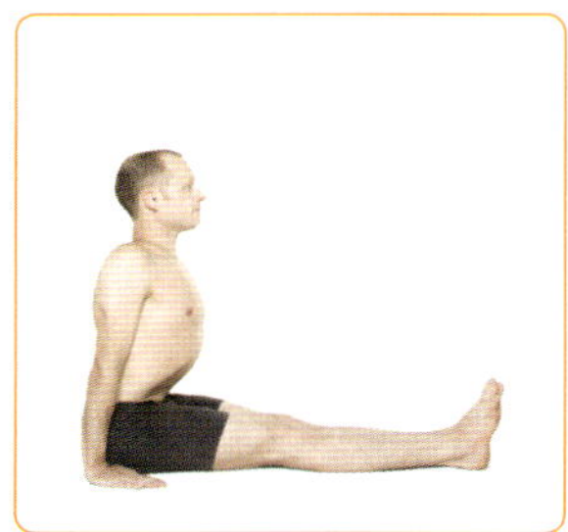

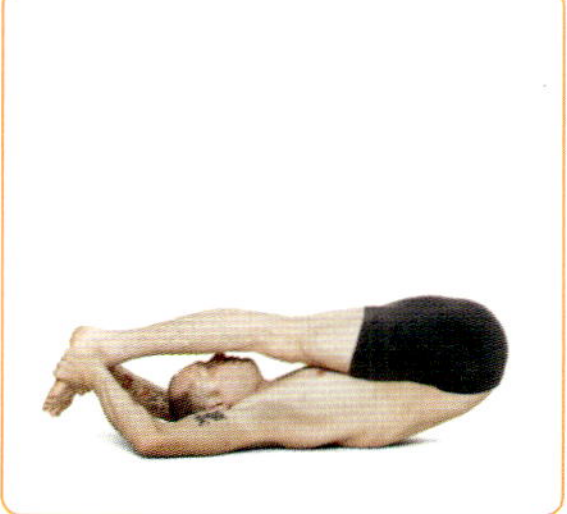

both-big-toes pose
ubhaya padangusthasana

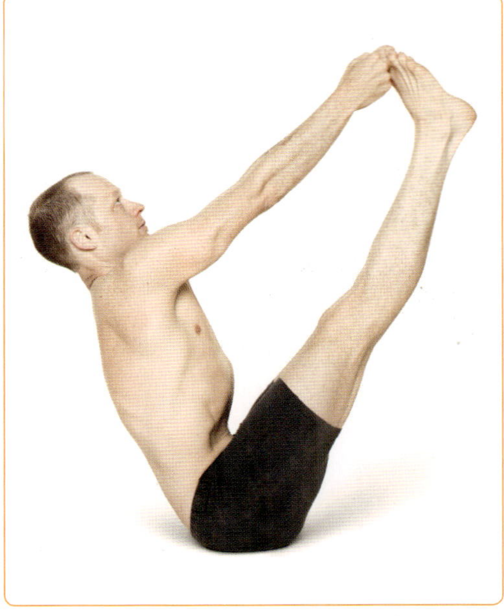

shape prep (from staff)
- Stage 1: bend knees, bring heels in front of hips; hold big toes with first two fingers and thumbs—arms inside legs. Separate feet outer hip-width apart.
- Curve low back in.

shape pose
- Stage 2: lift shins parallel to floor—feet outer hip-width apart.
- Stage 3: straighten legs.
- Stage 4: bring inner edges of feet together.
- Lift chin, look up.

safety (strength) prep
- Before lifting feet off floor, low back must curve in.

safety (strength) pose
- If legs are straight, tone thighs, tighten kneecaps, firm hamstrings.
- Tone abdomen.

refinement (stretch) pose
- Lift chest, stretch spine.

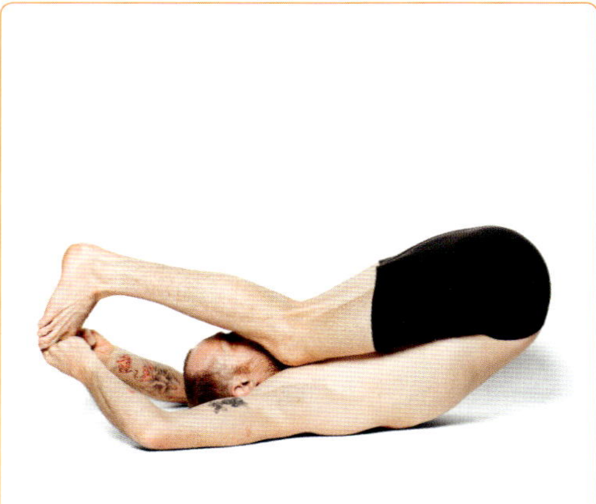

reclined west stretch knees bent

reclined west stretch
urdhva mukha paschimottanasana 2

shape prep
- Lie down on back.
- Bring thighs to ribs, shins vertical.
- Hold outer edges of feet with hands.

shape pose
- Stay here or roll onto upper back with legs slightly bent. Bring hips and feet equidistant to floor.
- Stay here or straighten legs, legs parallel to floor.
- Point elbows out.

safety (strength) pose
- If legs are straight, tone thighs, tighten kneecaps, firm hamstrings.
- Press hands, feet together.
- Squeeze legs together (more doable: separate feet outer hip-width apart).

refinement (stretch) pose
- Extend elbows out, shoulders towards head.

boat
navasana

shape prep (from staff)
- Point feet.

shape pose
- To gain momentum, swing torso forward then back; lift legs up off floor at a 60-65% angle (more doable: bend knees—shins parallel or feet on floor).
- Lift arms up, parallel to floor.
- Close fingers, point palms in.

safety (strength)
- Tighten glutes, squeeze legs together, tone abdomen.
- Minimize rounding in low back.

refinement (stretch) pose
- Extend arms out.
- Soften face, eyes. Breathe as evenly as possible.

In boat, low back must float. You must lift your chest, stretch your spine start to finish. For the sake of your low back, do not allow any part of your spine to collapse.

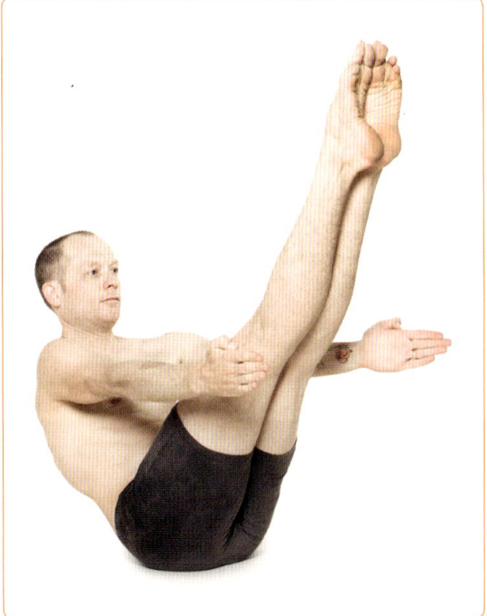

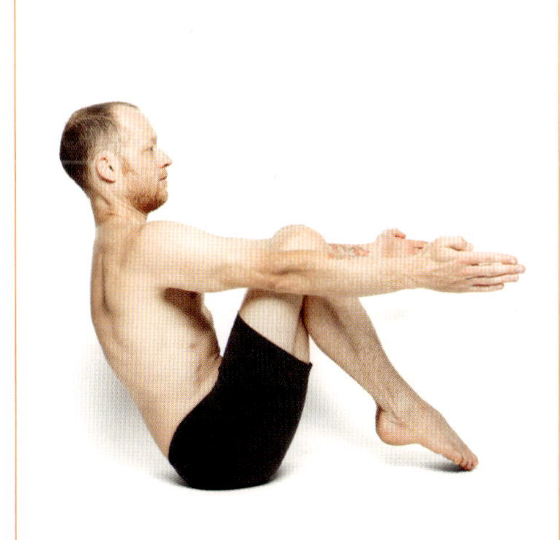

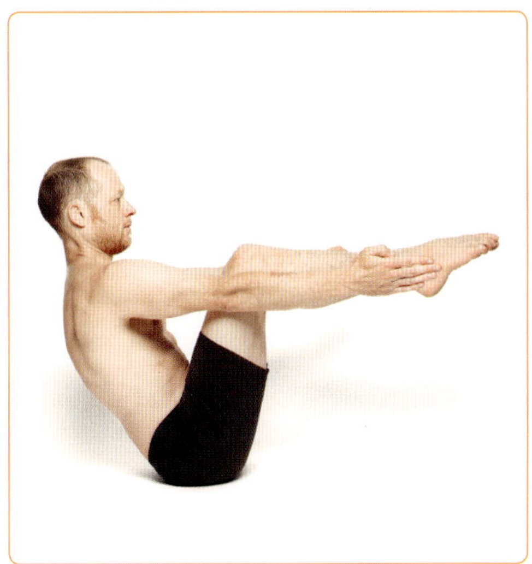

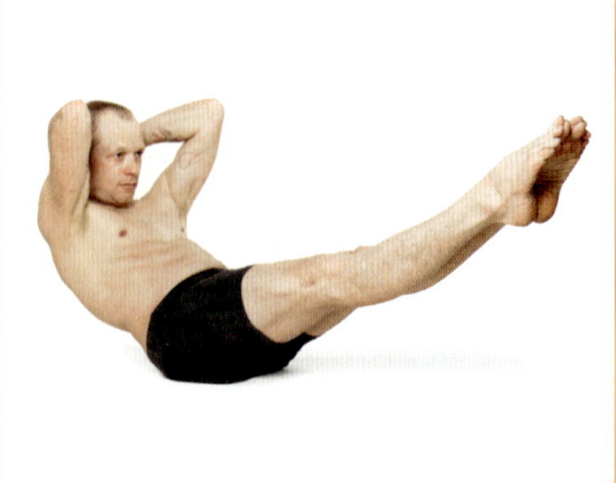

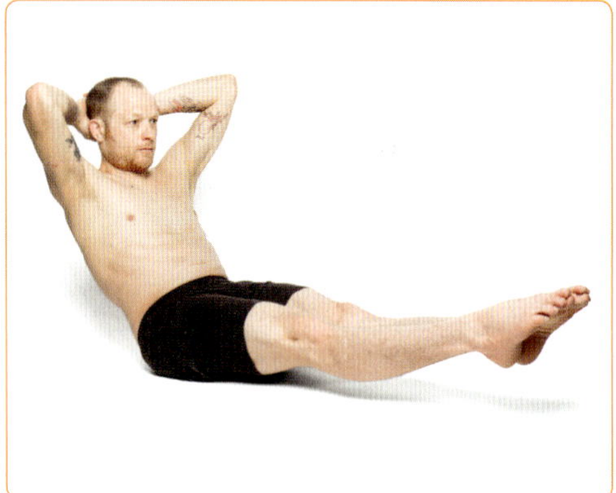

half boat

ardha navasana

shape prep (from dandasana)
- Point feet.
- Interlace hands behind head.
- Lean back.

shape pose
- Stay here or lift feet up in line with face (more doable: bend knees until big toes touch floor).

safety (strength) prep
- Squeeze legs together, tighten glutes, firm hamstrings, tone abdomen.

safety (strength) pose
- Minimize rounding in low back.

refinement (stretch) prep
- Lift chest, stretch spine.

refinement (stretch) pose
- Extend legs out.
- Soften face, eyes. Breathe as evenly as possible.

Like boat, in half boat, low back must float. You must lift your chest, stretch your spine, start to finish. For the sake of your low back, do not allow any part of your spine to collapse. I almost always say in class, "Half boat, twice as hard as boat."

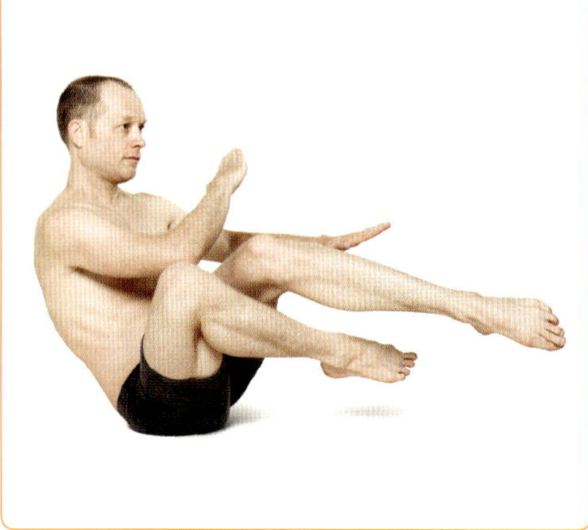

cosmic abs

shape prep
- Have a seat on right hip only; bend knees, elbows.
- Turn knees to right, torso to left.

shape pose
- Move arms and legs slowly.
- Move intermittently from right hip to left hip every few seconds.

safety (strength) prep
- Tone abdomen.
- Minimize rounding in low back.

This pose is best done to music with a good beat. Move to the rhythm.

leg lifts
urdhva prasarita padasana

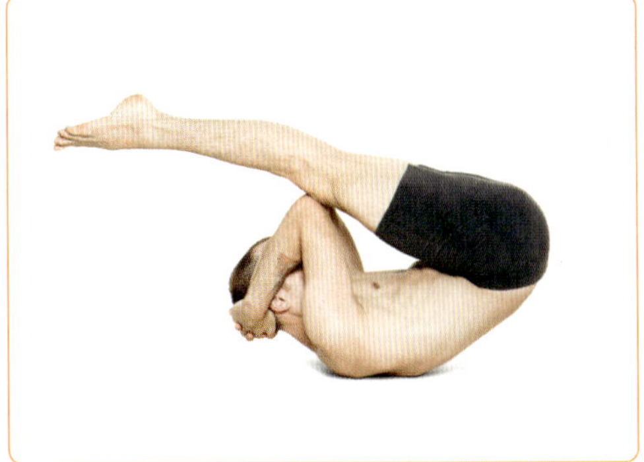

shape prep (from dandasana)
- Lie down on back.
- Interlace fingers behind head, not neck.
- Lift head off floor, squeeze face with forearms.
- Lift feet above head, point feet, straighten legs (more doable: bend knees).
- For extra back support wedge arms along outer edge of body—point palms down.

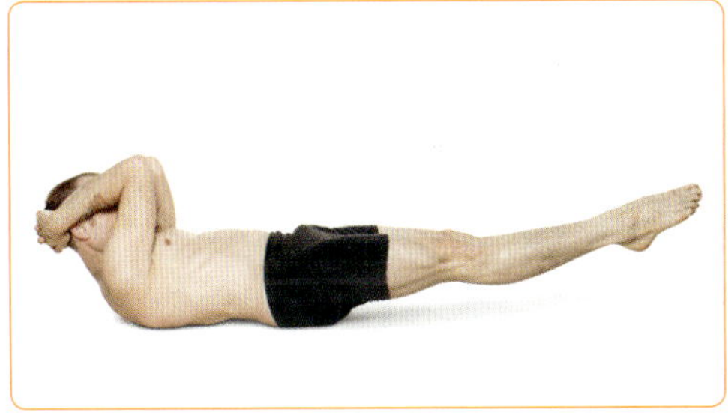

shape pose
- Inhale, lower heels just above floor; exhale, bring knees to elbows so that hips momentarily lift off floor (lifting hips off floor promotes length in low back as heels move back down toward floor).

safety (strength) pose
- Press heels together.
- Tone legs, tighten kneecaps, firm hamstrings.
- Tone abdomen, lift pelvic floor, tighten glutes.

refinement (stretch) pose
- Soften face, relax jaw.

To effectively develop strength in this pose move slowly and smoothly. Be sure to at least partially inhale and exhale with each movement of the legs.

leg lifts / twist variation

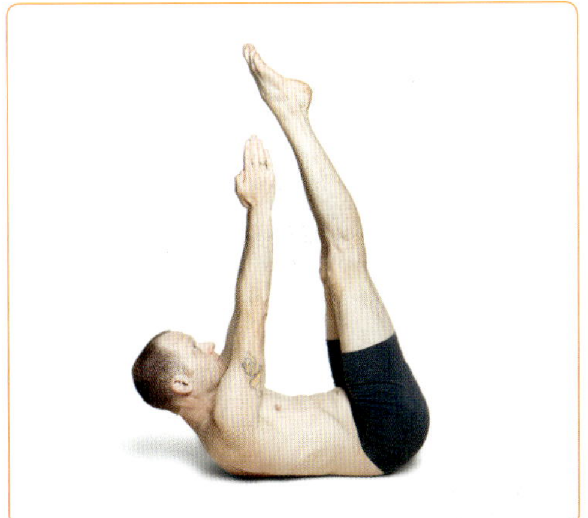

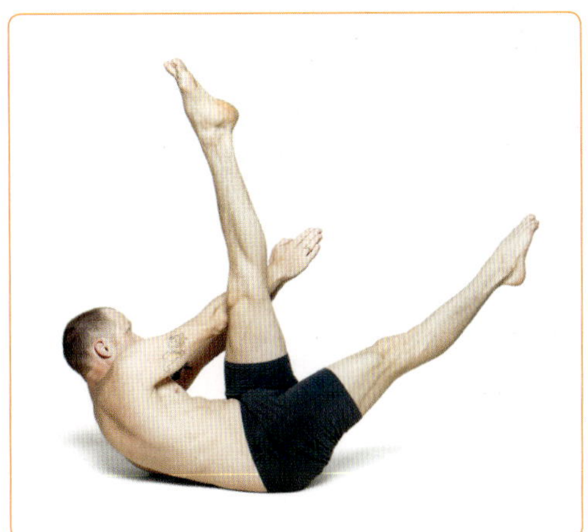

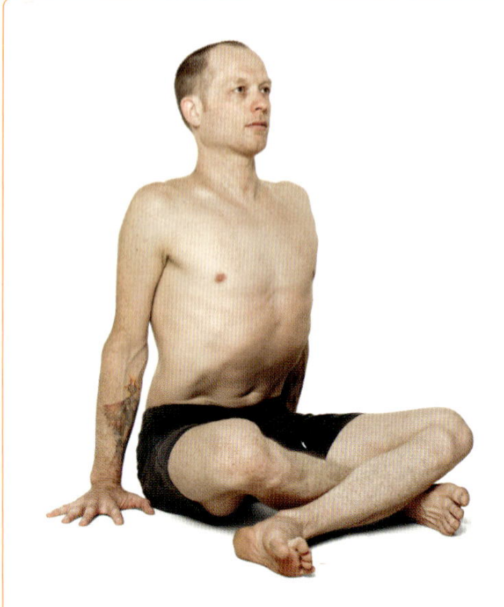

easy pose
sukhasana

shape prep (from staff)
- Cross shins, bring feet under knees.
- Move feet forward and apart until shins are parallel to front of mat.
- Place hands next to hips; curve low back in.

shape pose
- Stay here or fold forward, place hands on floor like in down dog.
- Rest forehead on floor.
- Round back evenly.

safety (strength) prep
- Press outer edges of feet down, lift ankles up.
- Isometrically, moving without movement, squeeze heels toward hips to tone hamstrings.

safety (strength) pose
- Press hands down, lift shoulders up.
- Tone abdomen.

refinement (stretch) pose
- Press hands down, forward.
- Extend knees out.

Repeat on the second side—change cross of legs.

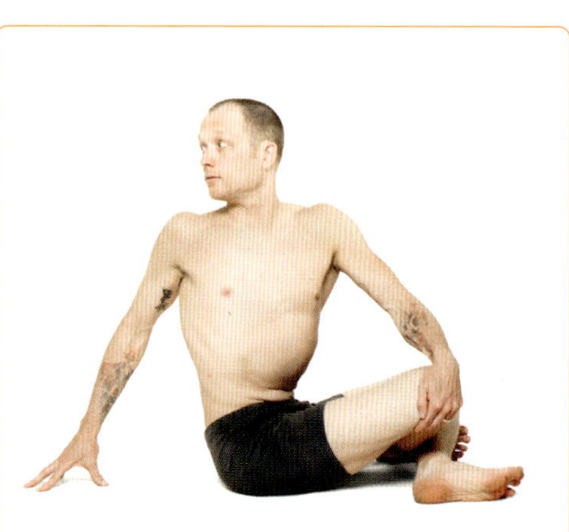

Easy pose (maybe more aptly named: easier-said-than-done pose) is an excellent asana alternate to fire logs pose.

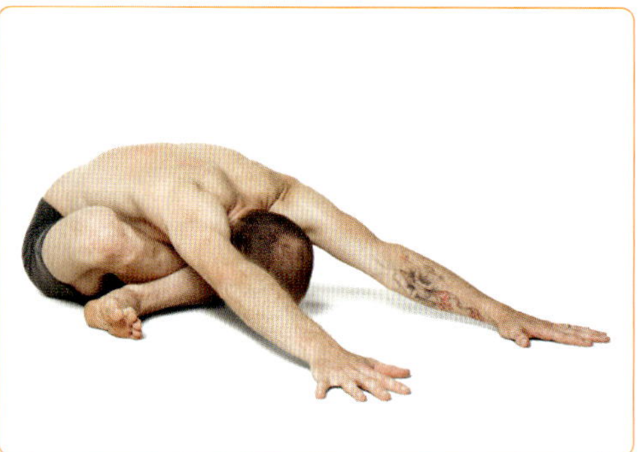

meditation pose

shape pose (from staff)
■ Bring right heel against pubic bone. Place left foot against right foot with heels in line with each other (and/or vice versa).
■ Place hands on knees, straighten arms.
■ Curve low back in (more doable: sit up on a yoga block or several folded blankets).

safety (strength) pose
■ Press outer edges of feet down.
■ Squeeze heels in.
■ Tone abdomen.

refinement (stretch) pose
■ Lift chest, stretch spine.
■ Close eyes, turn attention inward.

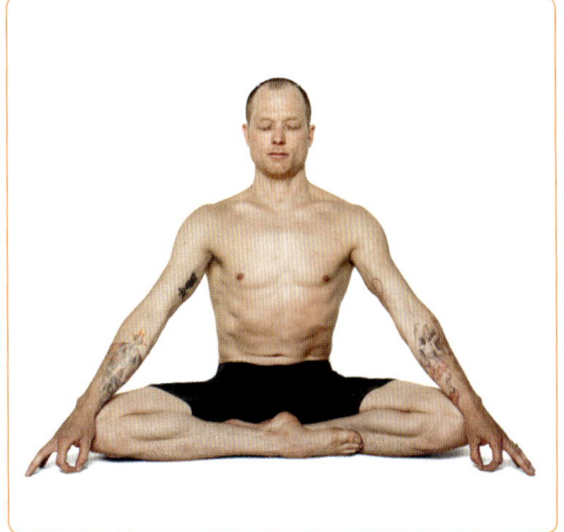

It's often said that hatha yoga is a preparation for meditation. Another perspective: hatha yoga creates an interest in meditation. Ready, sit, go!

If this pose is too intense on knees or hips, do easy pose instead.

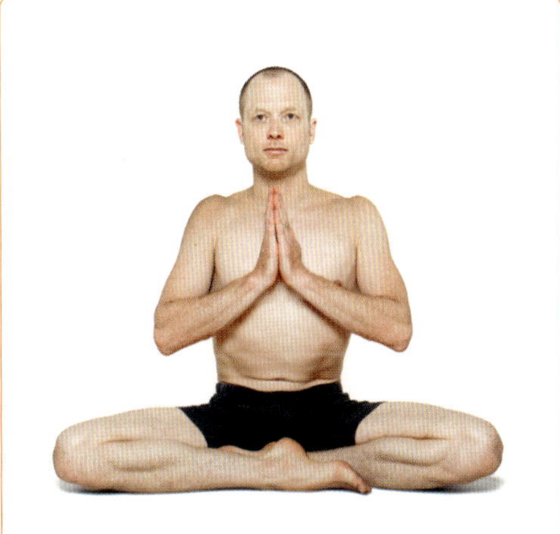

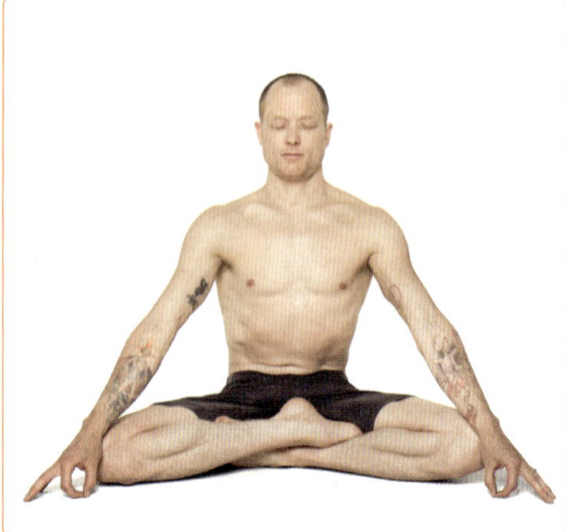

accomplished pose
siddhasana

shape prep (from meditation pose)
- Place left ankle on top of right ankle.
- Lift knees.
- One at a time, use hands to help slide feet between calves and thighs—point left foot down, right foot up.
- Return knees to floor.

shape pose
- Place hands on knees, straighten arms.
- Curve low back in.
- Close eyes.

safety (strength) pose
- Clamp knees closed, squeeze knees in, press feet into thighs.
- Press low belly in.

refinement (stretch) pose
- Lift chest, stretch spine.

bound angle
baddha konasana

shape prep (from staff)
- Place soles of feet together just in front of hips; point knees out.
- Place hands behind hips, slide hips forward slightly.
- Hold feet with hands.
- Curve low back in (if low back is rounded or knees are higher than waistline sit up on a block or blankets).

shape pose
- Stay here or open feet, round back evenly, and lower forehead to floor (more difficult: lower chin and tip of nose to floor).

safety (strength) prep
- Turn skin of inner ankles forward, skin of outer ankles backward.
- Press feet together.
- Squeeze heels toward hips.
- Move inner thighs down.

safety (strength) pose
- Tighten glutes.
- Tone abdomen.

refinement (stretch) prep
- Lift chest, stretch spine.

refinement (stretch) pose
- Extend knees out.
- Stretch spine evenly.

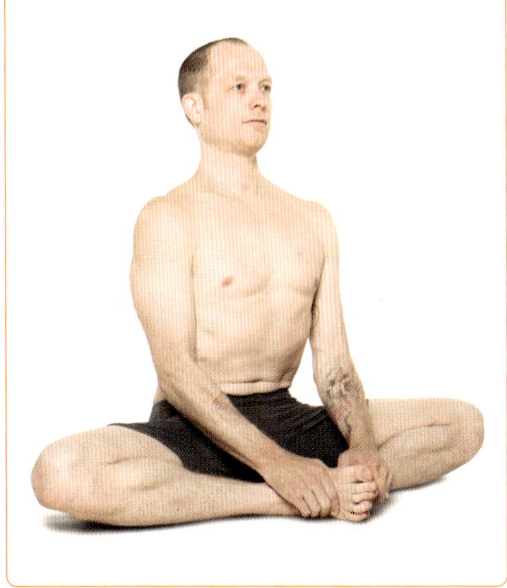

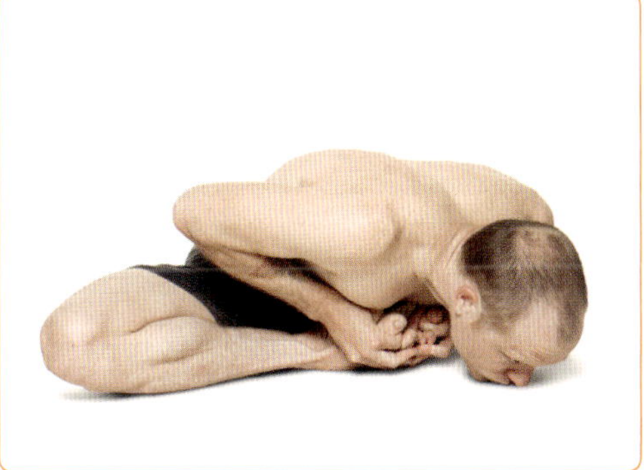

A forward fold misnomer = don't round your back in forward folds. That's like saying, don't backbend in backbends or twist in twists. Do round your back in forward folds; don't overly round it. That asana applies to all poses across the syllabus— too much is in fact too much. Once your back is evenly rounded, hinge from hips to proceed further into a given forward fold, without rounding back further.

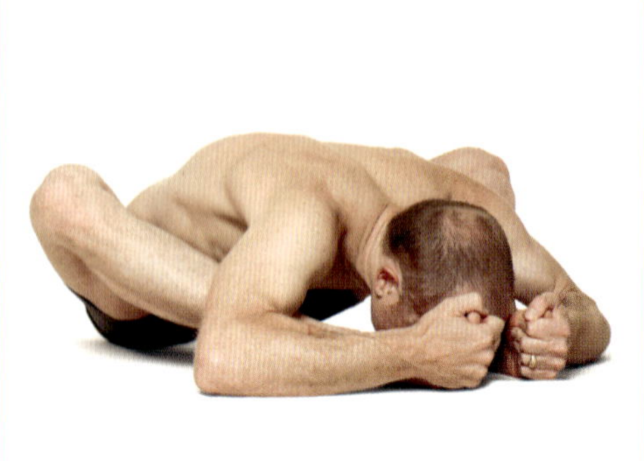

star
tarasana

shape prep (from bound angle)
- Slide feet 1.5 feet forward; separate feet 6 inches.

shape pose
- Hold tops of feet with hands, place forehead on floor between feet. Point elbows out.
- Round back evenly.

safety (strength) prep
- Press outer edges of feet down, lift ankles up.
- Squeeze feet toward hips.
- Tone low belly.

refinement (stretch) prep
- Lift chest, stretch spine.

refinement (stretch) pose
- Stretch shoulders towards head.

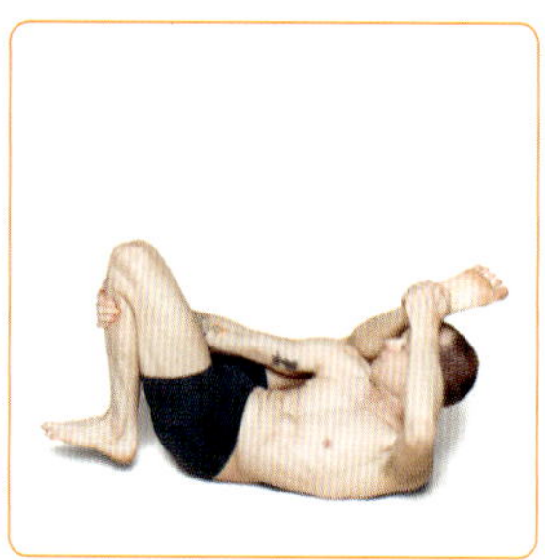
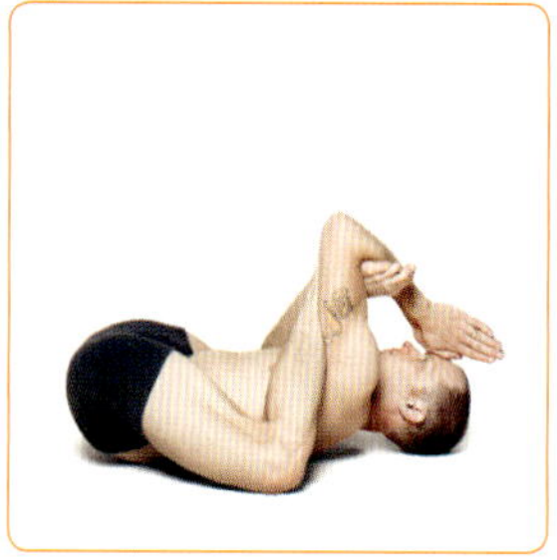
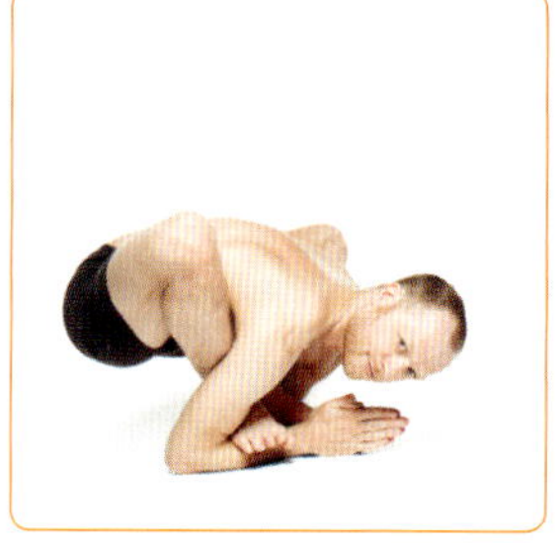
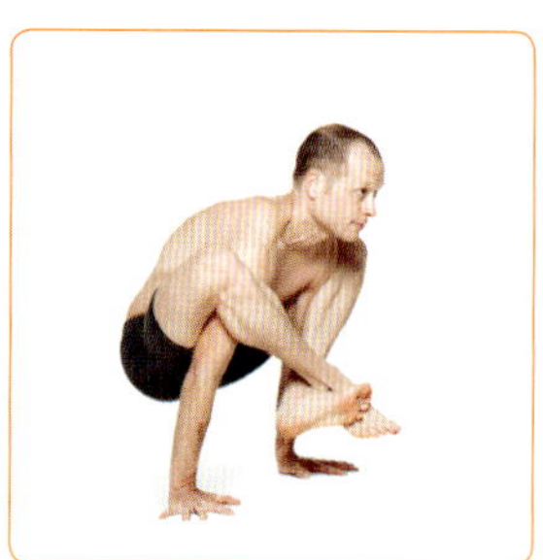

head knee pose

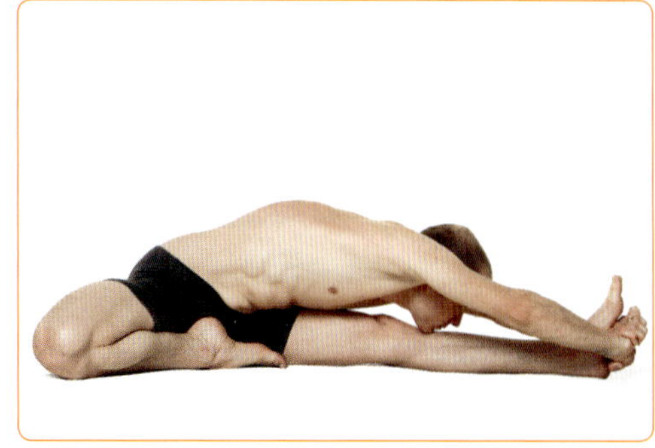

shape prep (from staff)
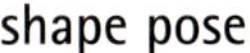 Bring left foot into tree pose—sole of foot against right inner thigh well above knee (more difficult: move left knee back so that thighs are in an obtuse angle; bring top of left foot on floor so that heel is vertical, like in hero).

Straighten right leg. Point right kneecap, foot straight up (more doable: bend right knee enough to curve low back in).

Place hands by hips, straighten arms, and curve low back in.

shape pose
Stay here or hold right foot with hands, place forehead on knee or chin on shin (more doable: place forearms or hands on floor between knees; place elbows under shoulders; interlace fingers; look down).

Round back evenly.

safety (strength) prep
Press outer edge of left foot down, squeeze heel in.

Make front thigh the heaviest part of pose—tone thigh, tighten kneecap, firm hamstrings.

Before folding forward, low back must curve in. If low back starts off rounded, it could end up compressed.

safety (strength) pose
Press hands and foot together.

Tone, turn abdomen to right.

refinement (stretch) prep
Lift chest, stretch spine.

refinement (stretch) pose
Extend elbows out.

Repeat on the second side.

This pose is often translated as head to the knee or head of the knee pose. An Iyengar teacher once sadhana scolded me: "It's head knee pose!" There you have it.

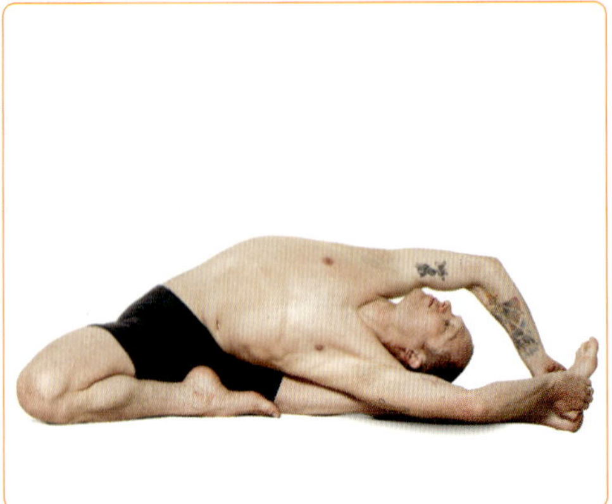

revolved head knee pose
parivrtta janu sirsasana

shape prep (from head knee right)
- Place right forearm on floor inside right shin, hold inner edge of foot with right hand; outer edge with left hand (more doable: place right hand or elbow inside right knee; bring left arm across face or hold top of foot with hand).

shape pose
- Twist torso, lift left elbow vertical.
- Look up (more difficult: place back of head on shin).

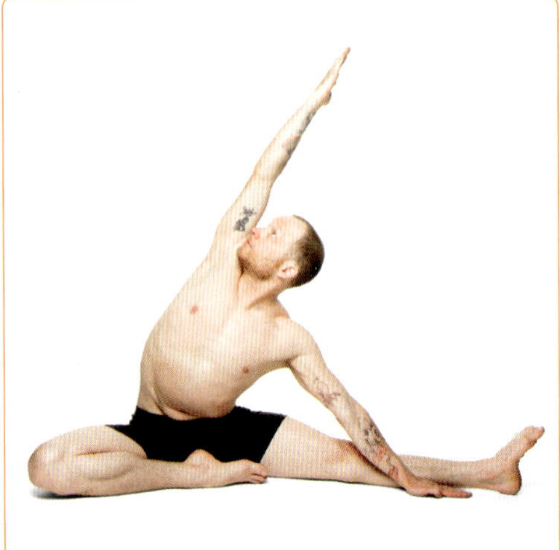

safety (strength) prep
- Press outer edge of left foot down, squeeze heel into hips.
- Tone thigh, tighten kneecap, firm hamstrings. Make front thigh heaviest part of pose.
- Press hands and foot together (or bottom hand/elbow and front knee together).

safety (strength) pose
- Tighten glutes.
- Press tailbone in.
- Tone, turn abdomen up.
- Move ribs back.

refinement (stretch) pose
- Twist and stretch spine evenly.
- Extend elbows out.

Repeat on the second side.

Many twists require the opposite shoulder and knee to touch (left to right) such as half lord of the fishes and m sage 3. Such twists are considered "closed twists" because the abdomen compresses in order to perform the twist. In this pose, however, the same shoulder and knee touch (right to right), which is considered an "open twist" because the abdomen expands, obliques stretch.

endless pose
anantasana

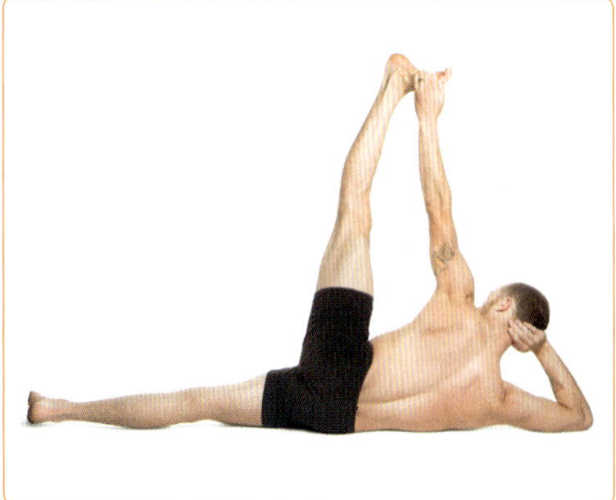

shape prep
- Lie down on right side of body.
- Place back of head on right hand—point right elbow at top of mat.
- Make a straight line from right elbow to hips, from hips to feet.
- Grasp left big toe with first two fingers and thumb of left hand or hold outside edge of left foot—arm inside leg.

shape pose
- Stay here or straighten left leg (more difficult: stack hips, be as sideways as possible).

safety (strength) prep
- Press outer edge of right foot into floor, lift ankle.
- Press fingers and big toe together.

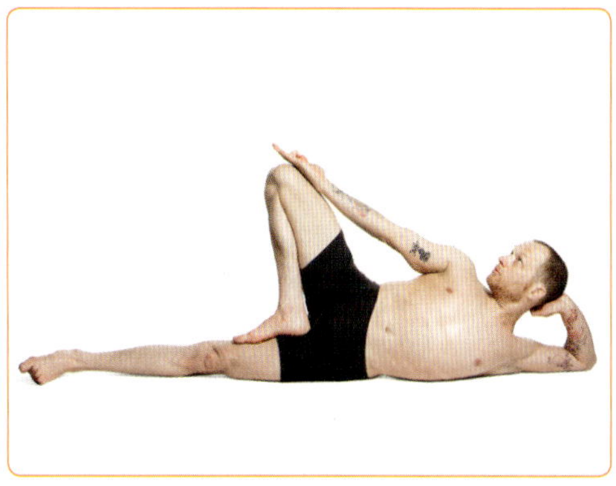

safety (strength) pose
- Tone thighs, tighten kneecaps, firm hamstrings.
- Press bottom elbow down, lift shoulder up.
- Engage glutes, press tailbone in, tone abdomen.

Repeat on the second side.

If you stack hips, endless pose can be among the more difficult balancing poses. This pose can be a good alternate to v sage.

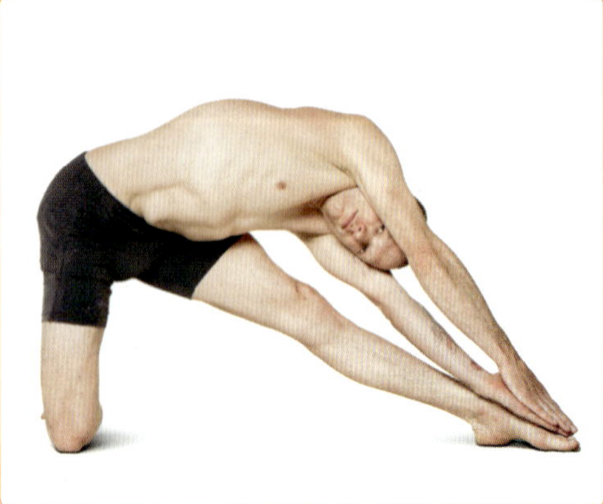

gate keeper
parighasana

shape prep

- Come into an upright kneeling position, middle of mat facing long edge of mat. Bring knees, ankles, outer hip-width apart.
- Extend right leg out to side, foot in line with left knee.
- Straighten right leg.
- Turn right foot in until big toe contacts floor.
- Point left foot, squeeze ankle in, flatten foot to floor.

shape pose

- Place palms together, cross thumbs. Bring back of right hand onto right foot.
- Straighten arms, bring heels of hands together.
- Look down.
- Stay here or move head between arms, turn torso up.

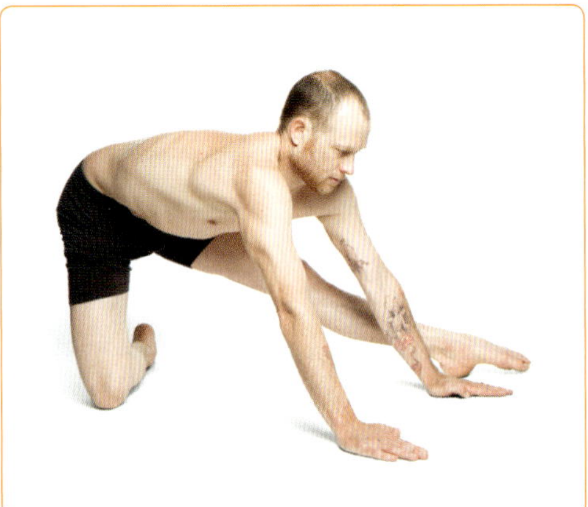

safety (strength) prep

- Tone right thigh, tighten kneecap, firm hamstrings (more doable: bend right knee slightly).

safety (strength) pose

- Tone, turn abdomen up.
- Move shoulders back.

refinement (stretch) pose

- Press front foot, back shin down and apart.

Repeat on the second side.

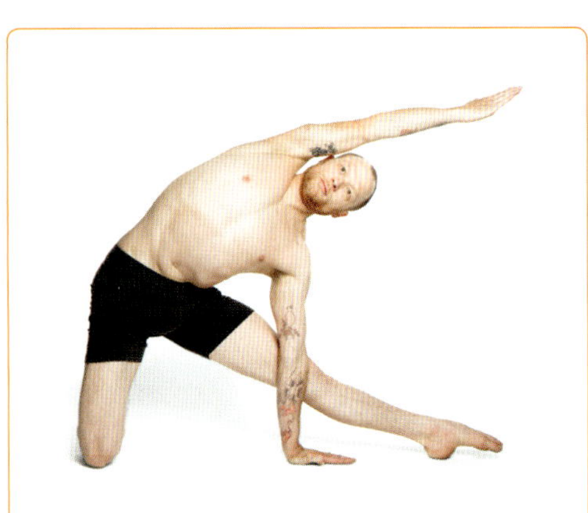

Pull this dusty pose off the shelf and practice it (if you practice yogahour on a regular basis, no need, as it shows up in many of the set sequences). Parighasana, more than almost any other pose, invites me into alignment with my asana aim.

kneeling sage
ardha hanumanasana

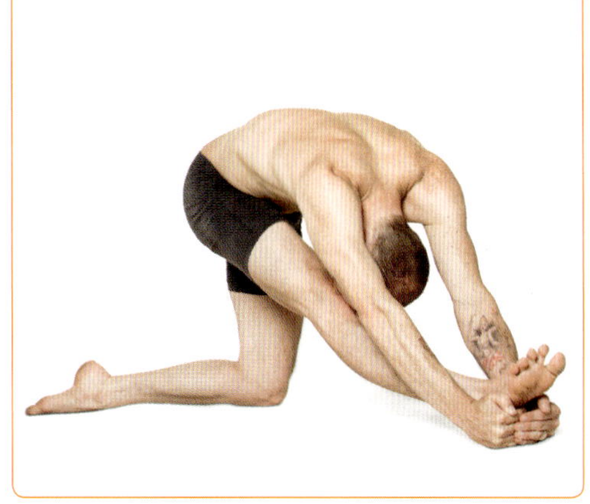

shape prep
▓ Come into an upright kneeling position middle of mat, facing front of mat.
▓ Step right foot forward, place right heel on floor, and flex foot.
▓ Straighten right leg.

shape pose
▓ Fold forward, bring hands to floor under shoulders; straighten arms (more doable: bend front knee slightly or place hands on blocks).
▓ Line up back foot with front heel.
▓ Stay here or hold front foot with hands, place forehead on knee or chin to shin.
▓ Round back evenly.

safety (strength) prep
▓ Press front heel down, back—back knee down, forward.
▓ Tone front thigh, tighten kneecap, firm hamstrings.

safety (strength) pose
▓ Tone abdomen.

refinement (stretch) pose
▓ Stretch spine.

Repeat on the second side.

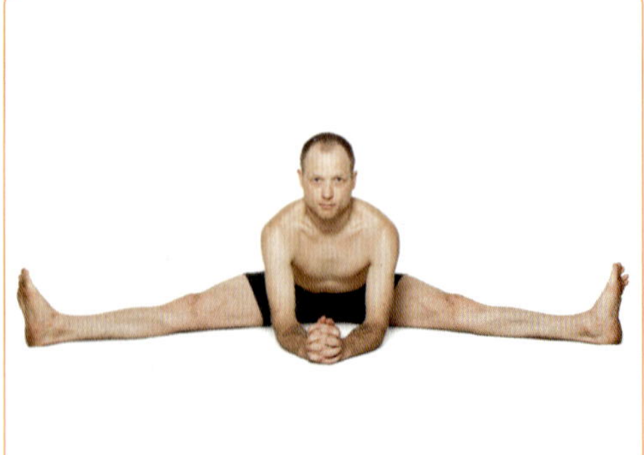

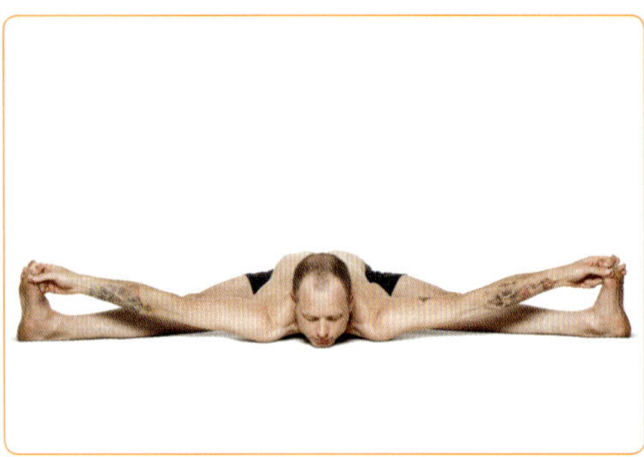

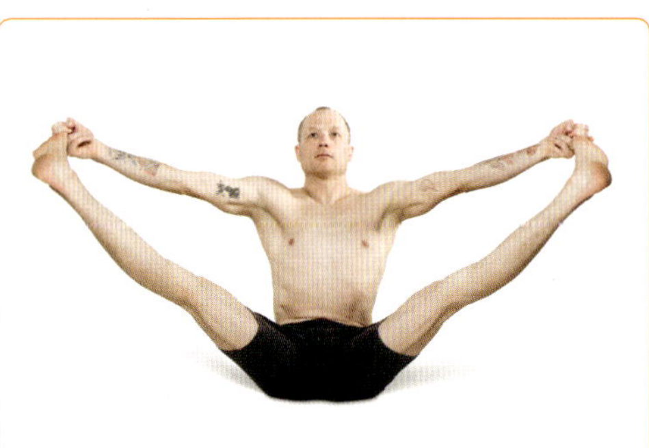

seated angle
upavistha konasana

shape prep
- Have a seat middle of mat, facing long edge of mat.
- Bring heels in line with far corners of mat so that legs are at a 90-degree angle or beyond.
- Place hands on floor beside hips.
- Flex feet, point knees up.
- Curve low back in (more doable: bend knees or sit up on a block/blankets).

shape pose
- Stay here, or hold big toes with first two fingers and thumbs; lower chin to floor (more doable: place forearms—or hands—on floor, elbows under shoulders. Interlace fingers, press palms together).
- Round back evenly.

safety (strength) prep
- Tone thighs, tighten kneecaps, firm hamstrings.
- Press thighs down.

safety (strength) pose
- Press fingers, big toes together (if forearms on floor, press them down, back).
- Tighten glutes, press tailbone down, tone abdomen.
- Do not allow legs to tilt in or out.

refinement (stretch) pose
- Stretch legs.
- Stretch spine.

lateral seated angle

parsva upavistha konasana

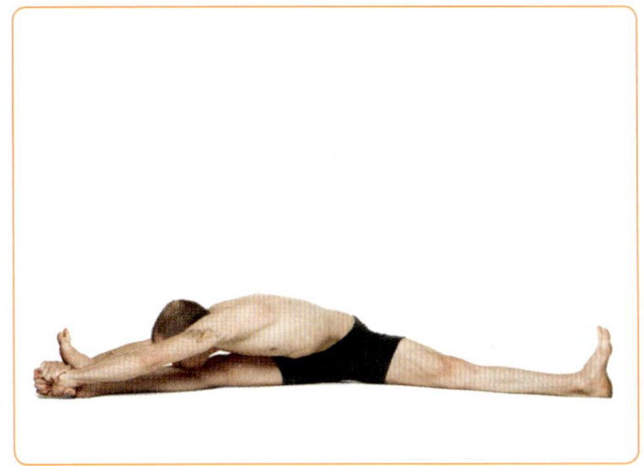

shape pose (from seated angle)
- Hold right foot with hands, fold over right leg, place chin on shin (more doable: place hands on either side of right leg, straighten arms, look straight ahead).

safety (strength) prep
- Tone thighs, tighten kneecaps, firm hamstrings.
- Make thighs heaviest part of pose.

safety (strength) pose
- Press hands, foot together.
- Tone, turn abdomen to right.
- Do not let right leg tilt in or out.

refinement (stretch) pose
- Stretch spine.
- Extend elbows out.

Repeat on the second side.

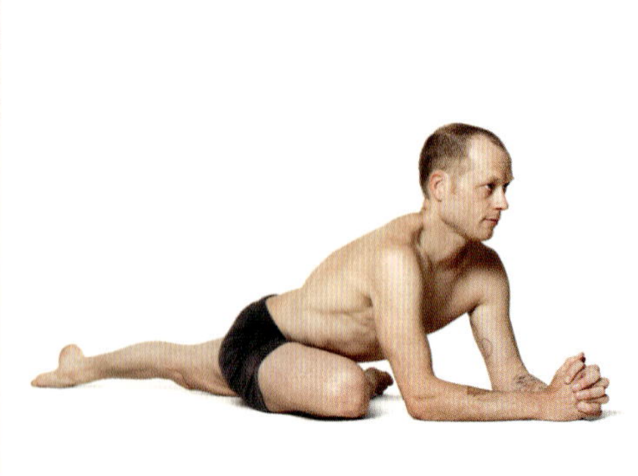

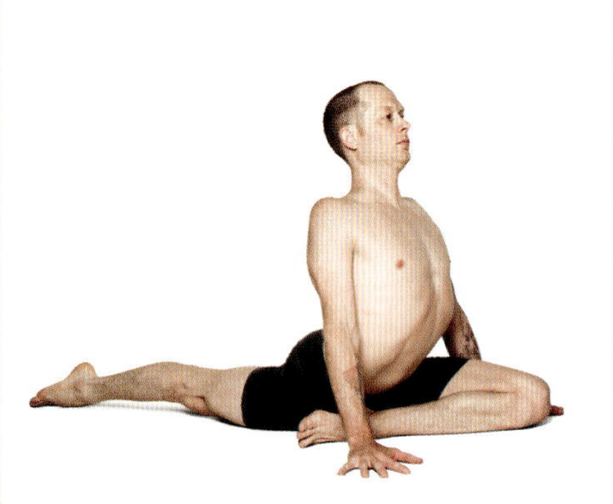

pigeon *prep*
eka pada rajakapotasana prep

shape prep (from downward facing dog)
▐ Bring right knee to right wrist; lower hips, back leg to floor.
▐ Bring right heel against left hip.
▐ Straighten and bring back leg parallel to long edge of mat; point kneecap down.
▐ Point back foot, squeeze ankle in.

shape pose
▐ Lower elbows to floor under shoulders, interlace fingers, place palms together (more difficult: extend arms into down dog position, rest forehead on floor).
▐ More doable: lean onto right hip, fold over front knee instead of shin.

safety (strength) prep
▐ Front foot: press outer edge down, lift ankle up; squeeze heel into hip.

safety (strength) pose
▐ Press back foot down, lift knee up.
▐ Move right hip toward left inner thigh.
▐ Tighten glutes, press tailbone down, tone abdomen.

refinement (stretch) pose
▐ Press forearms down/forward. Press hips down/back.

Repeat on the second side.

In Light On Yoga, B.K.S. Iyengar instructs this pose from dandasana. Check it out.

twisted pigeon 1 *shoulder to knee*
eka pada rajakapotasana prep

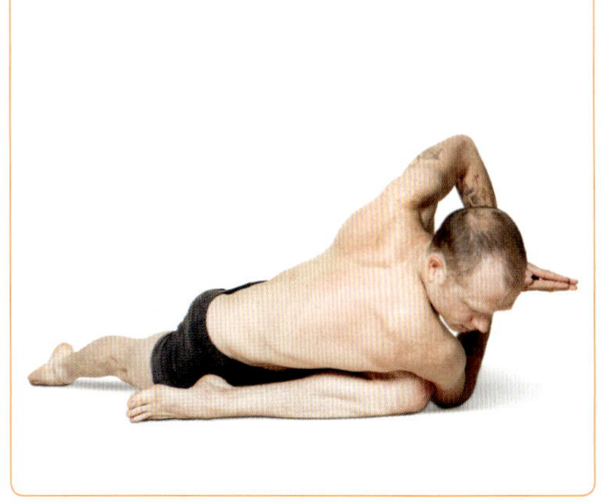

shape prep (from pigeon prep, forward fold)
- Bring left shoulder to right knee (more doable: bring elbow or chest to knee).

shape pose
- Place palms together.
- Look down.
- Line up head with hips.
- Keep back leg parallel to long edge of mat.
- Point back foot, squeeze heel in.
- Straighten back leg.

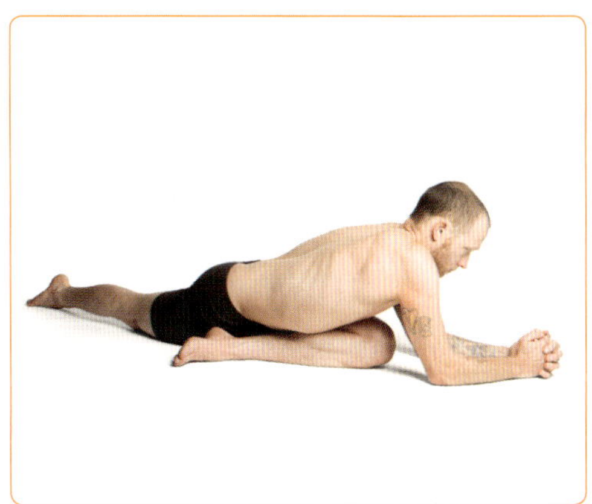

safety (strength) prep
- Press front foot down, lift ankle, squeeze heel in.
- Squeeze right hip, inner left thigh toward each other.

safety (strength) pose
- Tighten glutes, press tailbone down.
- Tone, turn abdomen up.
- Press left elbow into floor, press palms together.

refinement (stretch) pose
- Lift chest.

Repeat on the second side.

This is a good preparatory pose for revolved side angle, which recently got taken off the yogahour syllabus because it just tips the scales to more difficult than doable.

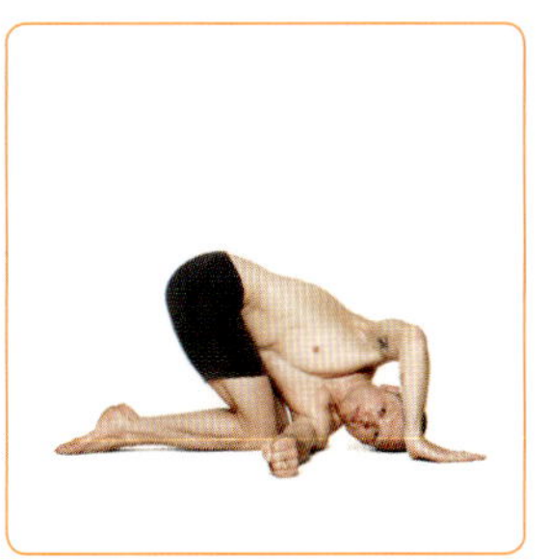
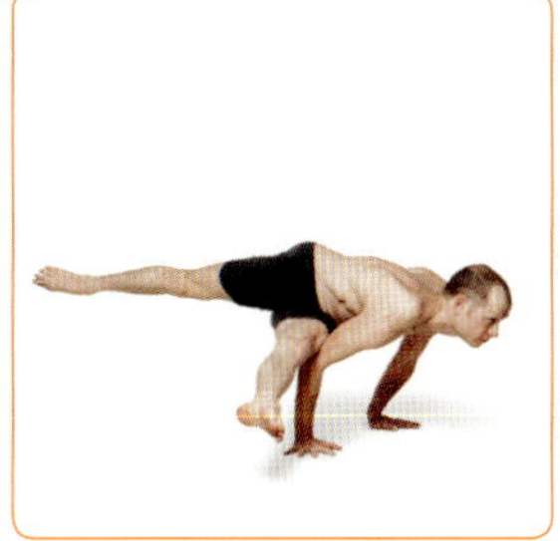
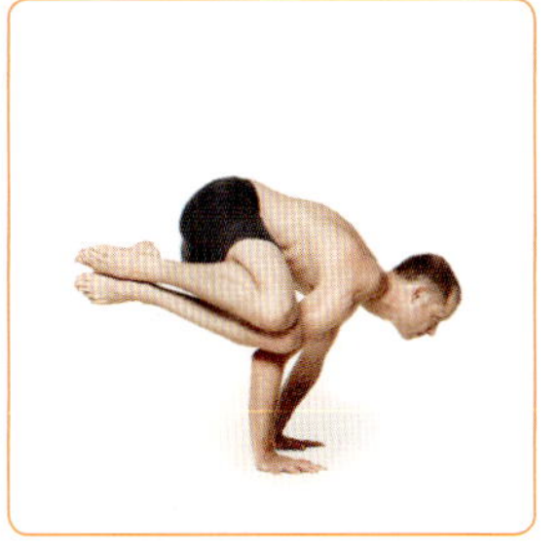
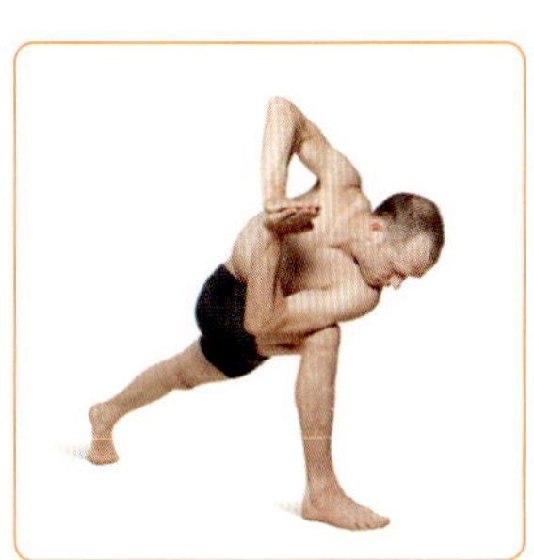

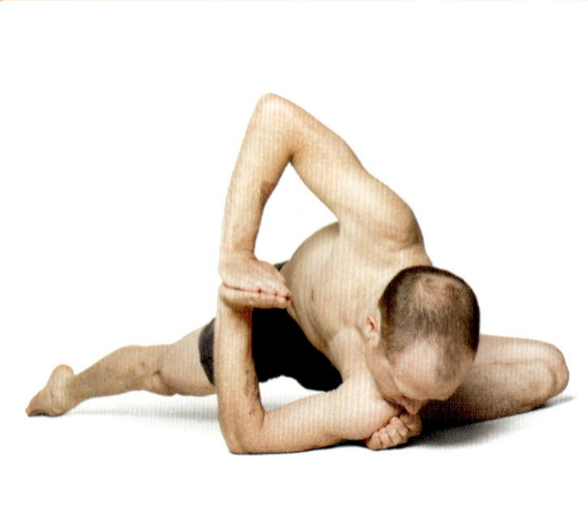

twisted pigeon 2 *shoulder to arch of foot*
eka pada rajakapotasana prep

shape prep (from twisted pigeon 1)
- Lift torso, straighten arms, lean onto right hip.
- Move right hand forward, out.
- Bring front shin parallel to top of mat; flex foot.

shape pose
- Bring right shoulder to sole of right foot. Place palms together—keep back leg in pigeon (more doable: bring right elbow/sternum to front foot).
- Point back foot, squeeze heel in (more doable: bend back knee slightly).
- Straighten back leg.
- Look down.

safety (strength) pose
- Press palms together, press bottom elbow into floor.
- Press front foot, bottom shoulder together.
- Tighten glutes, press tailbone down.
- Tone abdomen.

refinement (stretch) pose
- The stretch comes with the territory. 

Repeat on the second side.

This pose is a good preparatory pose for yogadandasana if you want to go there. Although yogahour features a limited syllabus, it can serve to create a solid foundation for poses with a higher degree of difficulty.

fallen sage

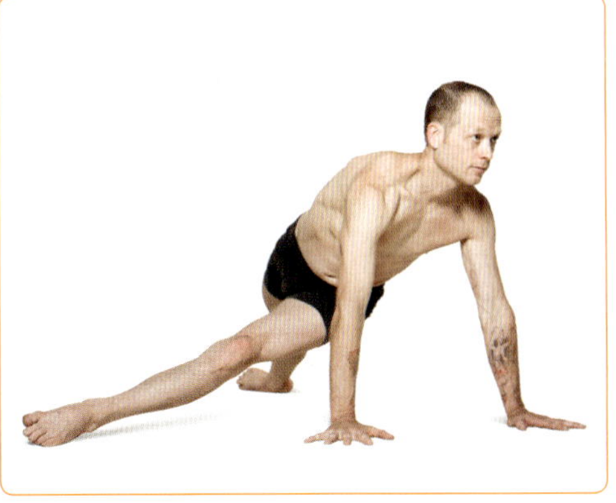

shape prep (from downward facing dog)
- Separate feet as wide as hands. Point right foot out at long edge of mat.
- Swing left leg under and across torso. Place outer edge of left foot on floor to the right, leg parallel to top of mat.
- Straighten legs, arms, spine.
- Keeping arms straight, lower outer left hip to floor (more doable: slide left foot toward back of mat so leg is no longer parallel to top of mat).

shape pose
- Bend elbows, lower right side of face to floor.
- At this point the inner edge of the right foot, outer edge of the left foot, outer edge of left hip, will be in contact with floor.
- Straighten legs.
- Lift shoulders to capacity.

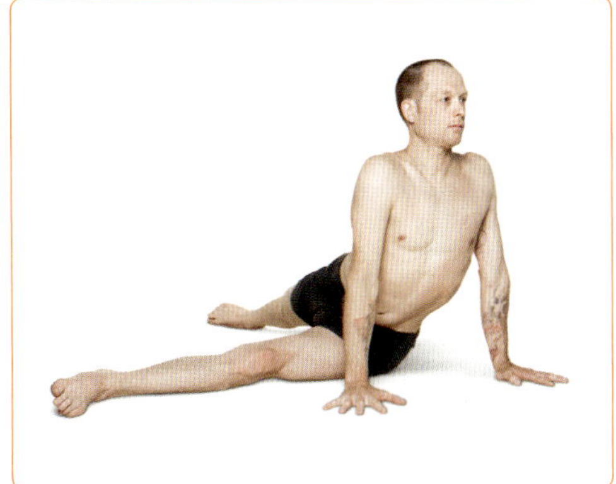

safety (strength) pose
- Squeeze feet toward each other.
- Tone thighs, tighten kneecaps, firm hamstrings.
- Tighten glutes, press tailbone in. Tone, turn abdomen to left.

Repeat on the second side.

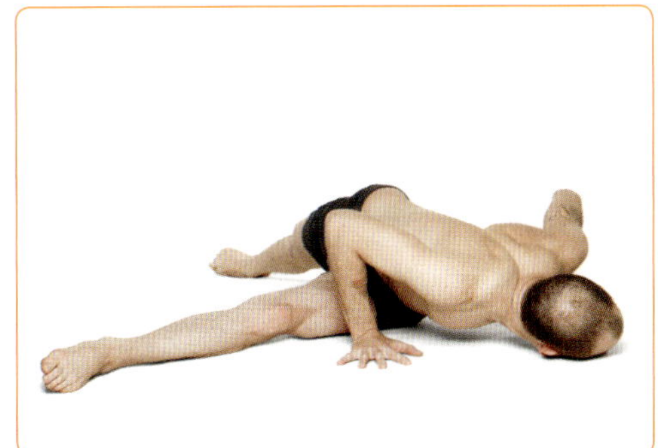

A unique feature of this pose is that the twist is initiated from the hips rather than the torso/shoulders. This is a good preparatory/alternate pose for k sage 1.

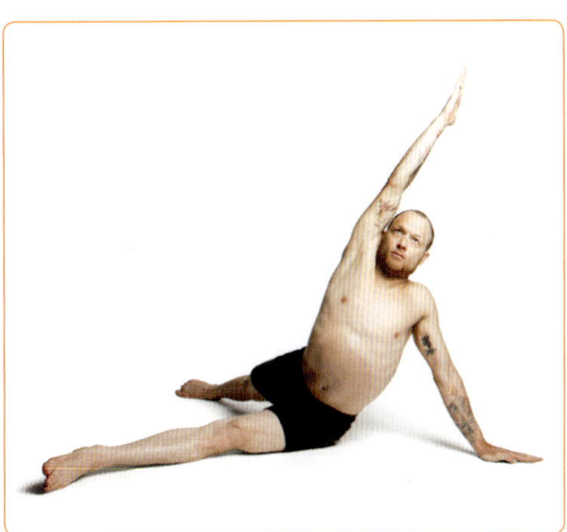

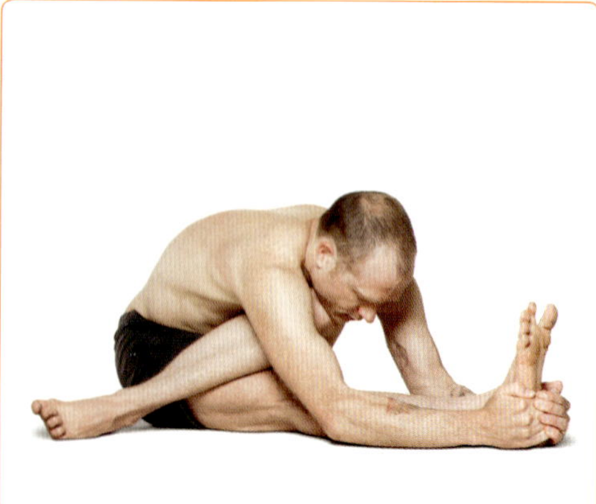

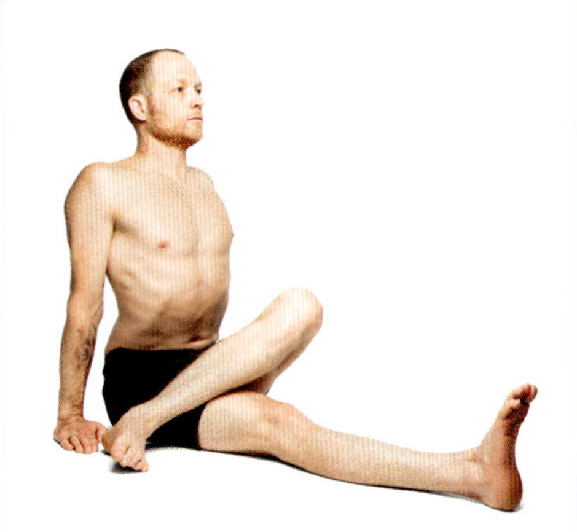

holy cow pose
eka pada gomukha paschimottanasana

shape prep (from staff)
- Cross right thigh over left thigh, place right heel against outer left hip; stack knees.

shape pose
- Hold front foot with both hands (more doable: place hands by hips with torso upright).
- Straighten arms—stay here, or:
- Place chin on right knee—forearms to floor.
- Round back evenly.

safety (strength) prep
- Press outer edge of right foot down, squeeze heel in.
- Tone left thigh, tighten kneecap.
- Press left thigh and heel down.

safety (strength) pose
- Press hands and foot together.
- Tone abdomen.

refinement (stretch) pose
- Stretch spine.

Repeat on the second side.

cowface 1
gomukhasana 1

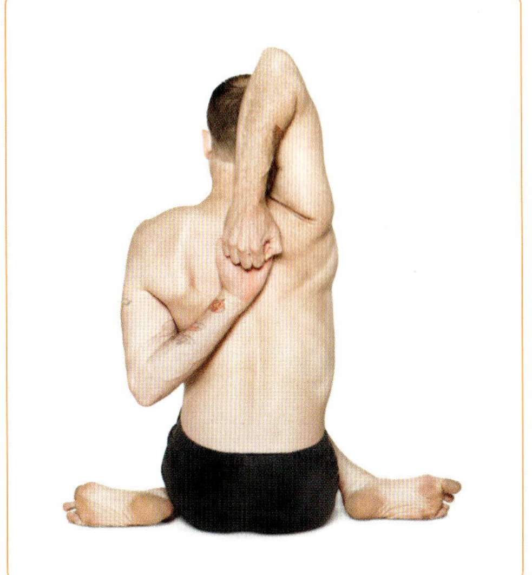

shape prep
- Come onto hands and knees.
- Lift left leg up and back, parallel to floor.
- Take left knee to outer edge of right knee with both knees bent.
- Have a seat between feet—feet against outer hips.

shape pose
- Take right arm out to side, parallel to floor. Point right thumb down. Place back of right hand behind left shoulder blade. Lift left arm up overhead. Bend left elbow. Clasp hands (more doable: use strap to bind).
- Curve low back in.
- Lift chin slightly.

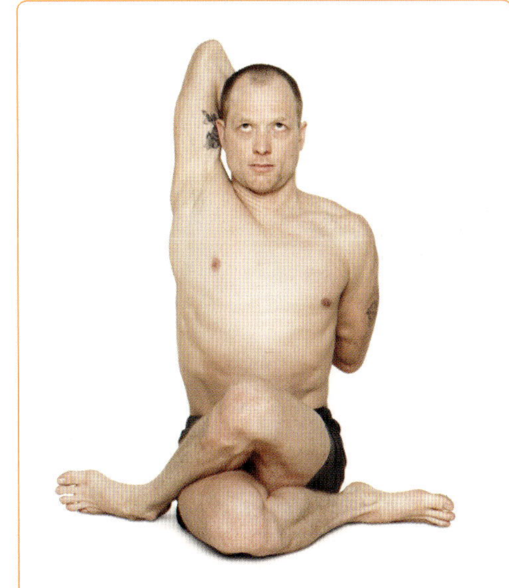

safety (strength) pose
- Press outer edges of feet down, squeeze heels into hips.
- Tone abdomen, move ribs back.
- Lift shoulders up, back. Both shoulders must feel stable and strong.

refinement (stretch) pose
- Lift chest, stretch spine.
- Look between eyebrows.

Repeat on the second side.

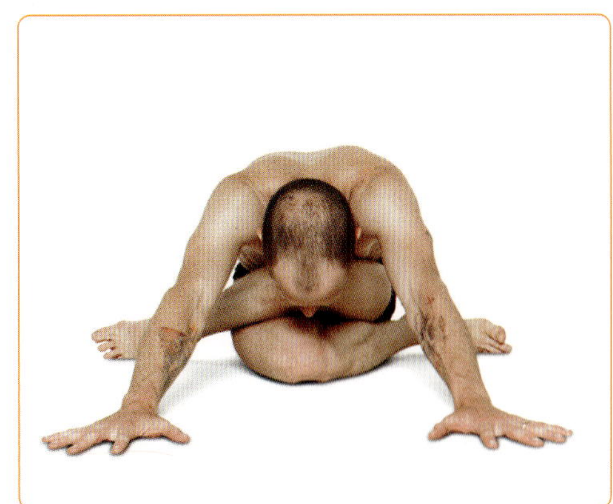

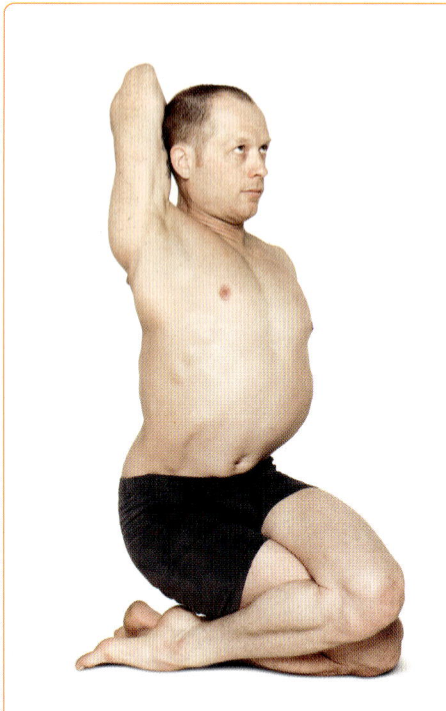

cowface 2
gomukhasana 2

shape prep
■ Come onto hands and knees.
■ Lift left leg up and back, parallel to floor.
■ Take left knee to outer edge of right knee. Place outer shins, ankles together.
■ Keeping ankles together, turn feet out like kick stands.
■ Have a seat on feet, lift torso upright (more doable: keep hips well above feet, hands on floor).

shape pose
■ Take right arm out to side, parallel to floor. Point right thumb down. Place back of right hand behind left shoulder blade. Lift left arm up overhead. Bend left elbow. Clasp hands (more doable: use strap to bind).

safety (strength) prep
■ Squeeze ankles in, heels up.

safety (strength) pose
■ Tone abdomen, move ribs back.

refinement (stretch) pose
■ Curve low back in. Lift chest, stretch spine.

Repeat on the second side.

Once the hips rest firmly on feet, balance in this pose becomes child's play.

seated pigeon
hindolasana

shape prep (from staff)
- Hold right ankle with right hand in front of chest—point knee out.
- Lean back slightly. Bend left knee and swing left heel to right hip.
- Place right foot in crease of left elbow, flex foot.

shape pose
- Wrap right elbow around right knee, interlace fingers in front of shin (more doable: hold right foot with left hand, right knee with right hand).
- Square hips to left with shin parallel to floor (more doable: turn torso slightly to right).
- Lift chin slightly, look straight ahead.

safety (strength) prep
- Flare toes (press inner edge of foot into biceps).

safety (strength) pose
- Squeeze elbows in like a vice.
- Press right heel down.
- Minimize rounding in low back.

refinement (stretch) pose
- Lift low back, lift chest, stretch spine.

Repeat on the second side.

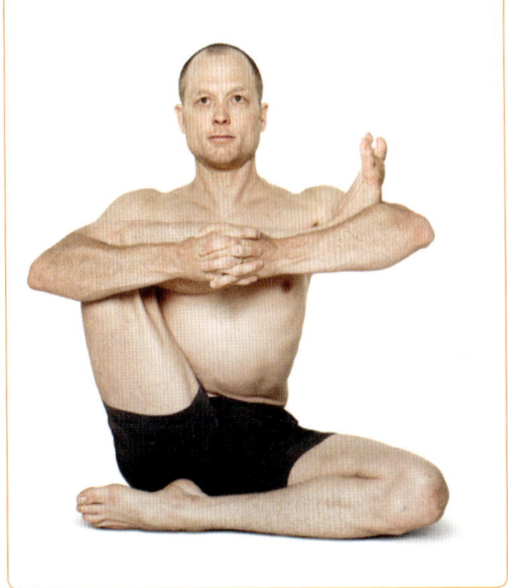

Seated pigeon is a good asana alternative to elevated pigeon.

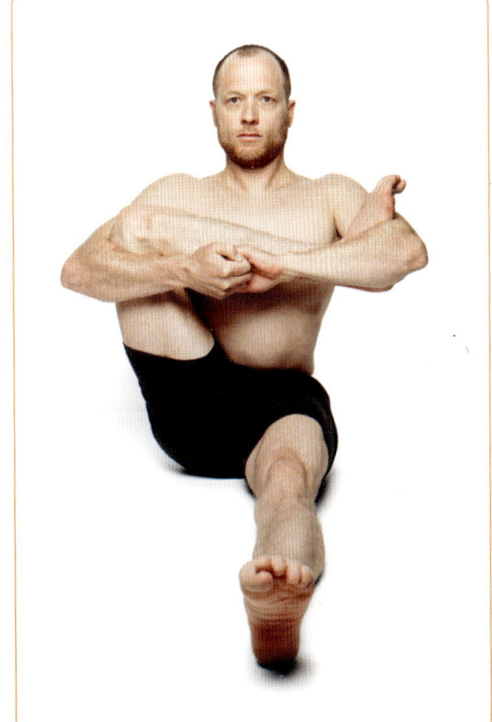

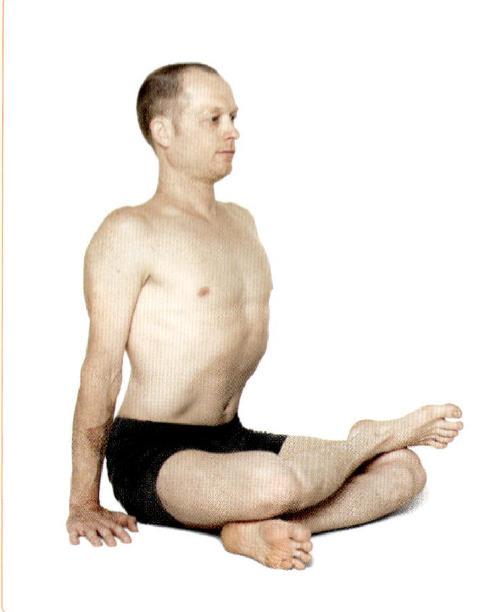

fire logs
agnistambhasana

shape prep (from staff)
- Stack shins—right ankle on left knee; flex feet (more doable: slide bottom heel to right hip).
- Place hands next to hips; curve low back in.

shape pose
- Stay here or fold forward, place hands on floor like in down dog.
- Rest forehead on floor.
- Round back evenly.

safety (strength) prep
- Press outer edges of feet down, lift ankles up, and squeeze heels toward hips.

safety (strength) pose
- Tone abdomen.
- Lift shoulders up.

refinement (stretch) pose
- Press hands down, forward.
- Extend knees out.

Repeat on the second side—change cross of legs.

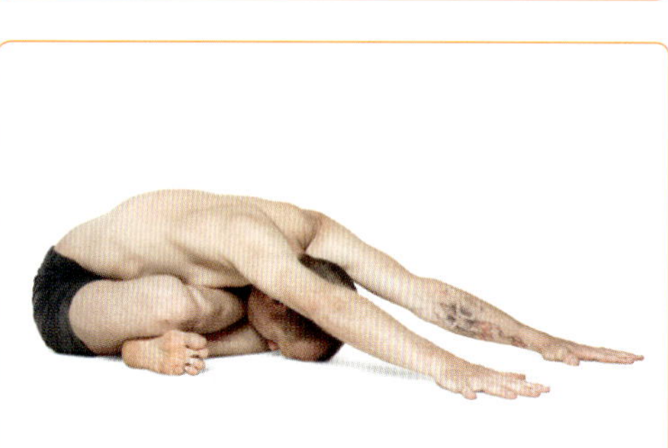

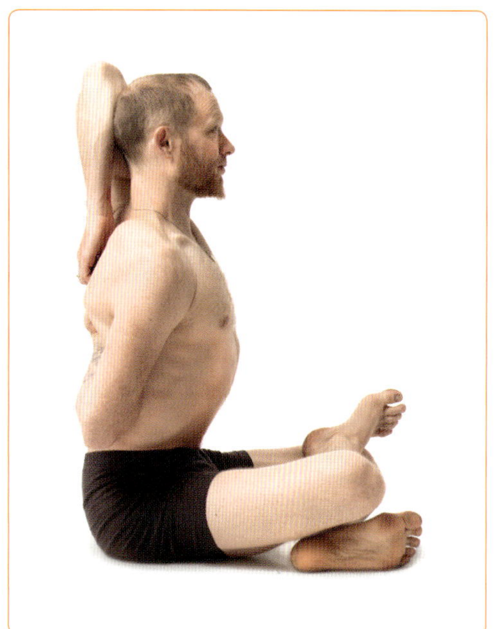

twisted sage
bharadvajasana 1

shape prep (from staff)

▨ Swing feet to right side of hips.
▨ Place right ankle on top of left foot—point top foot back, bottom foot out.
▨ Bring knees to floor—knees as close together as is optimal.

shape pose

▨ Twist torso to left, place right palm on floor under left thigh; close fingers, including thumb—back of hand against thigh (more doable: hold left knee with right hand).
▨ Swing left arm around back, place back of hand against right rib cage; close fingers (more doable: place fingertips on floor behind hips; more difficult: clasp upper right arm with left hand).
▨ Look over front/back shoulder.
▨ Move knees closer together.

safety (strength) pose

▨ Press right fingertips into floor, tone right triceps, biceps.
▨ Press back of left hand into right ribcage (if palm on floor: press hand down).
▨ Lift shoulders up, back.
▨ Tone, turn abdomen to left.

refinement (stretch) pose

▨ Lift low back, chest. Stretch spine.

Repeat on the second side.

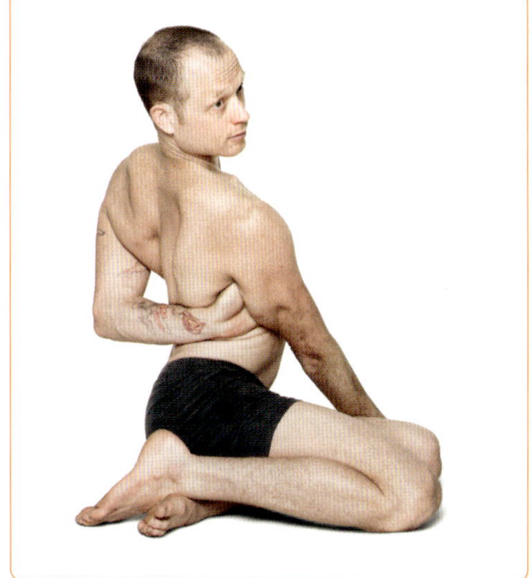

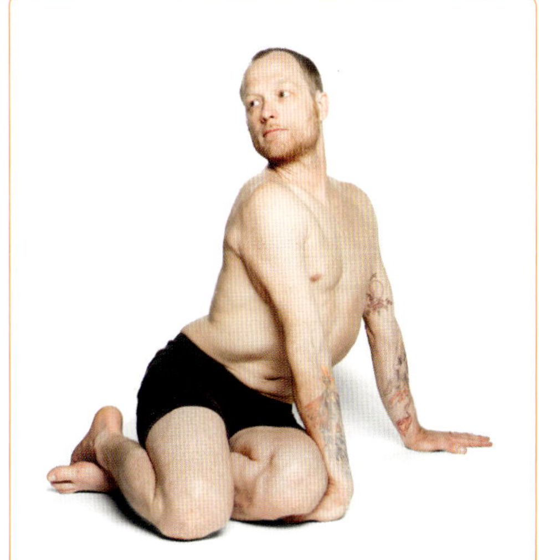

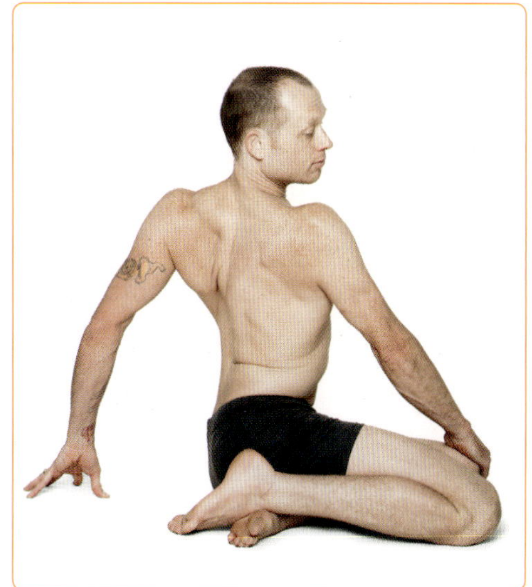

Some poses require certain proportions. If you have long arms and a short torso like me, for example, the classical form of this pose can be a piece of cake. If not, it's possibly impossible. Not to worry, you are not missing out on anything. My dad often says, "Missing out is a divine impossibility." Notice, I wrote above, "classical form" instead of "full form." Full form of the pose can suggest there is such a thing as a partial pose. As long as you find the right modification, I firmly believe you will access all the benefits of this and any pose. Modifications are often a must!

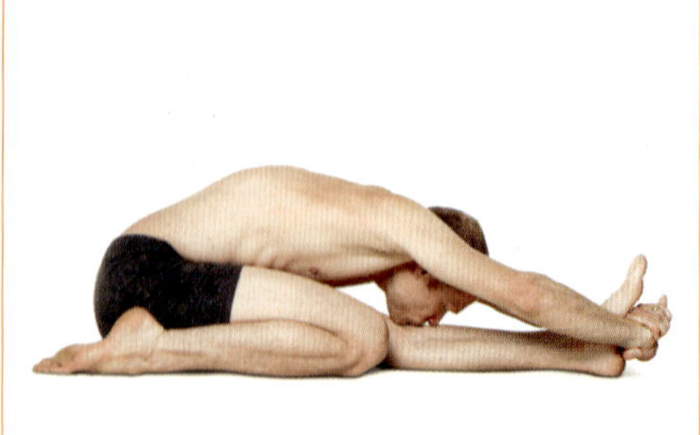

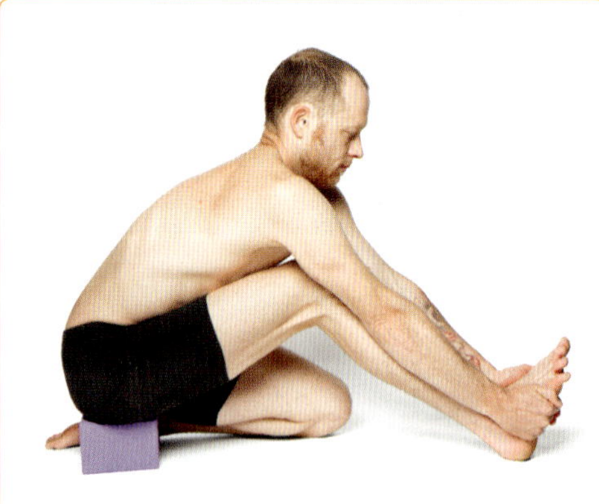

triad
triang mukhaikapada paschimottanasana

shape prep (from staff)
▐ Lean to left hip, bend right knee and hold right ankle with right hand. Place inner right heel against outer right hip. Point right foot and place top of right foot and shin on floor. Point right knee straight ahead (more doable: sit up on a block with inner edge of foot against block).
▐ Bring hands to floor next to hips, torso upright.
▐ Flex left foot.

shape pose
▐ Stay here, or hold left foot with both hands; straighten arms, look straight ahead (more doable: bend left knee, bring thigh and torso together).
▐ Stay here, or bring chin, tip of nose to shin; point elbows out (more difficult: hold back of one hand with the other—point palms out).
▐ Round back evenly.

safety (strength) prep
▐ Tone left thigh, tighten kneecap, firm hamstrings.
▐ Press straight leg down; make thigh heaviest part of pose.
▐ Before folding forward, the low back must curve in. If the low back is rounding even slightly, keep torso upright; do not fold forward.

safety (strength) pose
▐ Press hands, foot together.
▐ Tone abdomen.

refinement (stretch) pose
▐ Extend elbows out.
▐ Stretch spine.

Repeat on the second side.

Poses are not designed to be learned in isolation; one pose informs and leads to another. Each pose exists individually and is also intricately related to the full gamut of asana. Triad pose, for example, is a mix of hero pose and intense west stretch. Is the classical name of this pose really triad? No. It's asana actually three limbs face to one leg back stretched out pose. That's a mouthful! Yogahour often gives poses nicknames to make them more accessible and user friendly (and like any nickname, it's also a sign of affection).

heron
krounchasana

shape prep (from triad pose: hips on floor or block)
- Bend left knee, slide left foot just in front of left hip, well within reach—point knee up.
- Clasp left foot with hands—arms inside leg.

shape pose
- Lift and straighten left leg (more doable: bring shin parallel to floor).
- Straighten arms, look up (more difficult: bring chin, tip of nose to shin—left leg vertical).

safety (strength) pose
- Minimize rounding in low back.
- Tone left thigh, tighten kneecap, firm hamstrings.
- Press hands, foot together.

refinement (stretch) prep
- Lift low back, chest. Stretch spine.

refinement (stretch) pose
- Lift shoulders, extend elbows up, out.

Repeat on the second side.

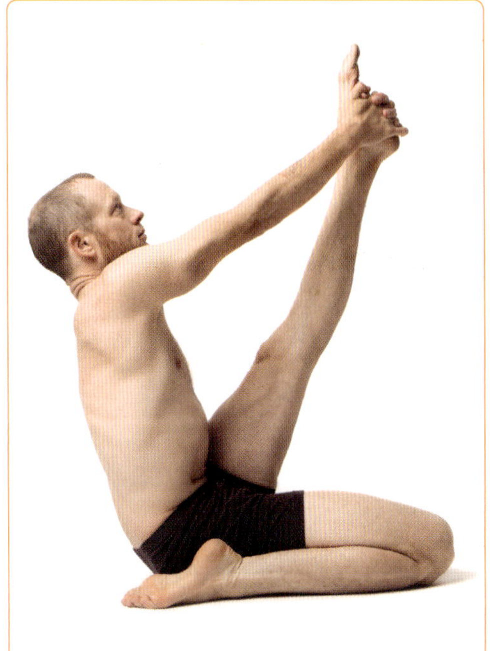

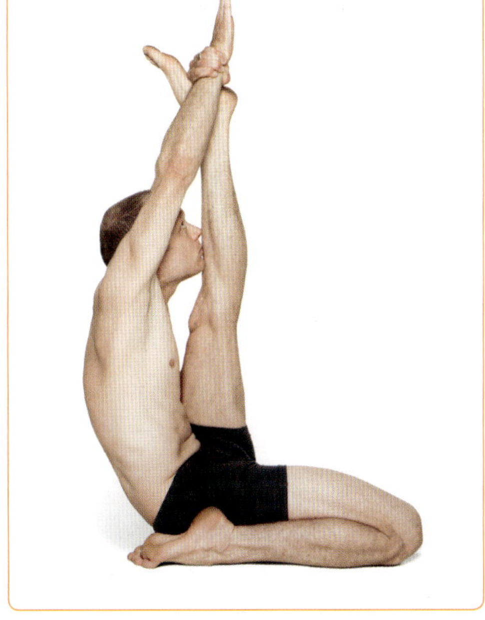

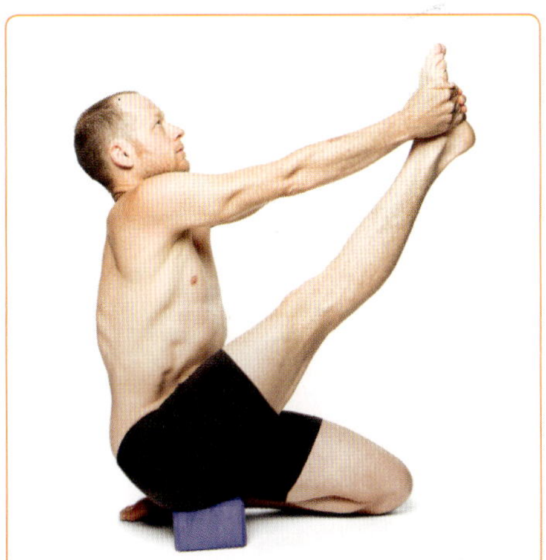

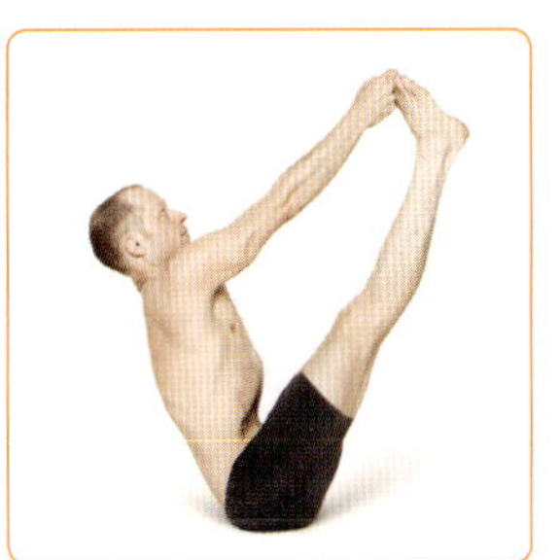

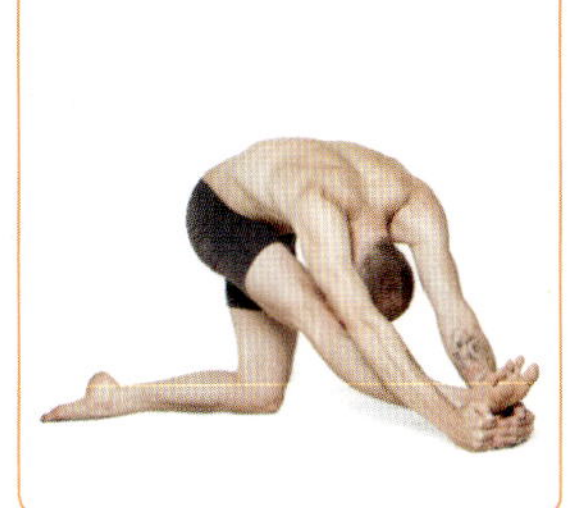

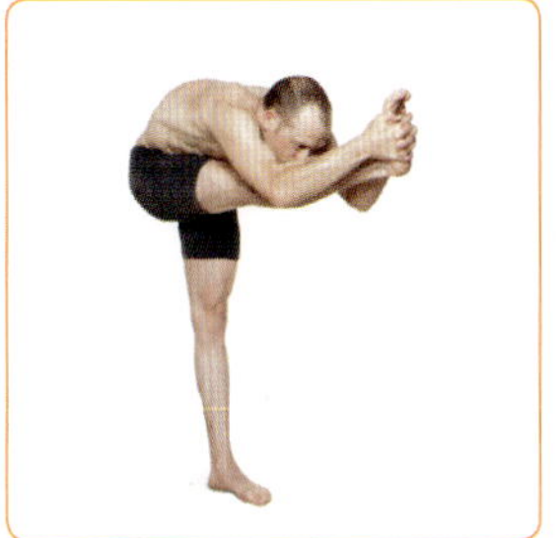

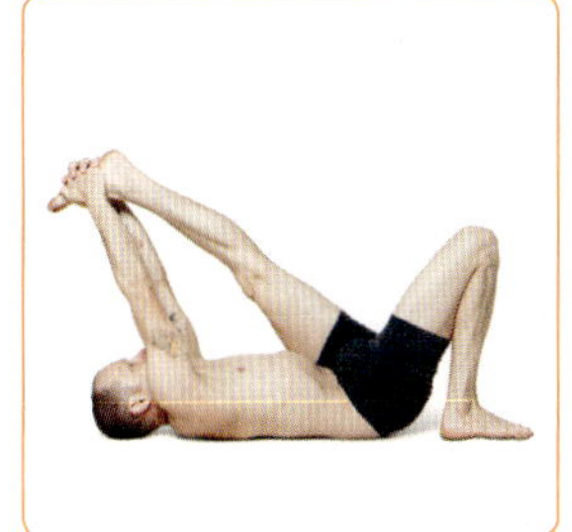

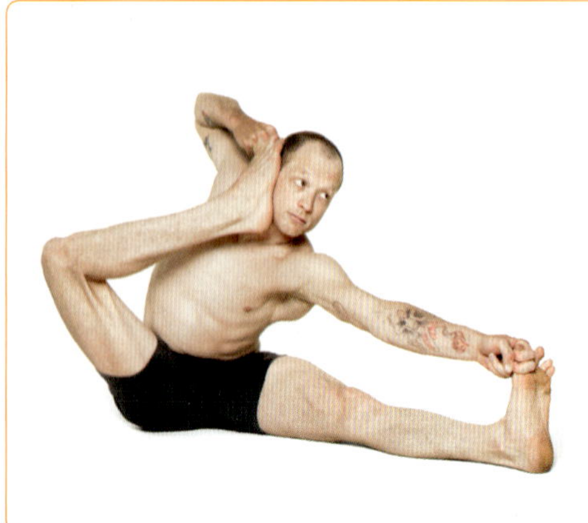

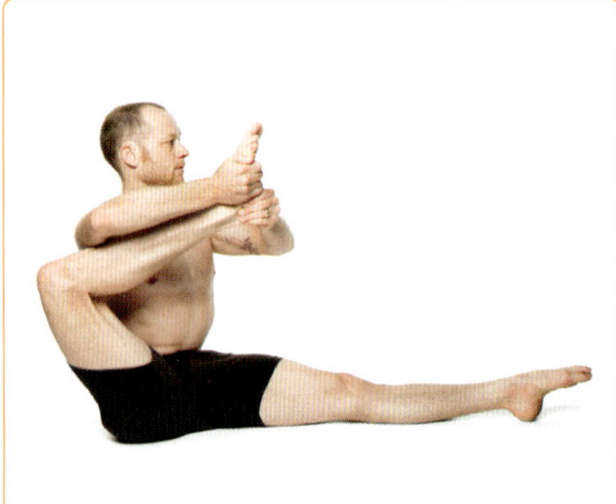

archer's pose 1
akarna dhanurasana 1

shape prep (from staff pose)
▨ Lean forward, hold big toes with first two fingers, thumbs of each hand; straighten arms, legs.
▨ Keeping legs, arms straight, lift right foot as high as optimal (more doable: hold foot with both hands—shin parallel to floor).

shape pose
▨ Bend right knee, move knee out, place sole of foot against ear; point right elbow back.
▨ Look straight ahead.

safety (strength) prep
▨ Tone left thigh, tighten kneecap, firm hamstrings, press thigh/heel down.
▨ Press big toes, fingers together. Flare toes.

safety (strength) pose
▨ Move right leg back with leg (not just arm strength).
▨ Minimize rounding in low back.

refinement (stretch) pose
▨ Lift low back, chest. Stretch spine.

Repeat on the second side.

In the classical form of this pose the ankle takes the shape of a sickle. It's not uncommon for practitioners to associate a sickled ankle with a collapsed ankle/knee. A sickled ankle can be both a versatile and strong ankle. Ideally the foot should be able to take a wide variety of shapes and be strong in all of those positions. If, however, sickling the ankle proves to be too much, flex the foot instead and point sole of foot straight ahead.

archer's pose 2
akarna dhanurasana 2

shape prep (from archer's pose 1)
▮ Lean onto left hip, straighten right leg.

shape pose
▮ Bring right calf and ear together (more doable: move right leg out to side, straighten arm and leg; more doable still: place left hand on floor outside hips—lean onto hand).
▮ Look forward (as in, look forward to coming out of this pose).

safety (strength) prep
▮ Minimize rounding in low back.
▮ Tone quads, tighten kneecaps, firm hamstrings.
▮ Press big toes, fingers together.

safety (strength) pose
▮ Tighten glutes, tone abdomen.

refinement (stretch) pose
▮ Lift low back, lift chest. Stretch spine.

Repeat on the second side.

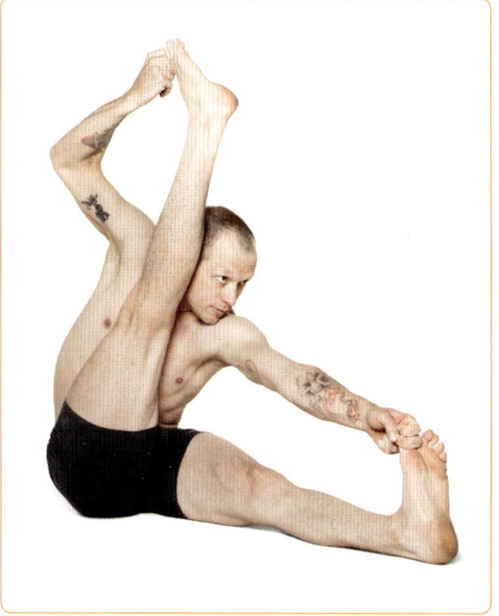

Archer 1 and 2 symbolize the point of asana for me; it's all about having and moving towards an aim. When it comes to asana, aim is the only guru and the only game in town, at least for me. In Light On Yoga, B. K. S. Iyengar says akarna dhanurasana 2 is "full of grace," as is aim. After all, "aim" recalibrated = I AM.

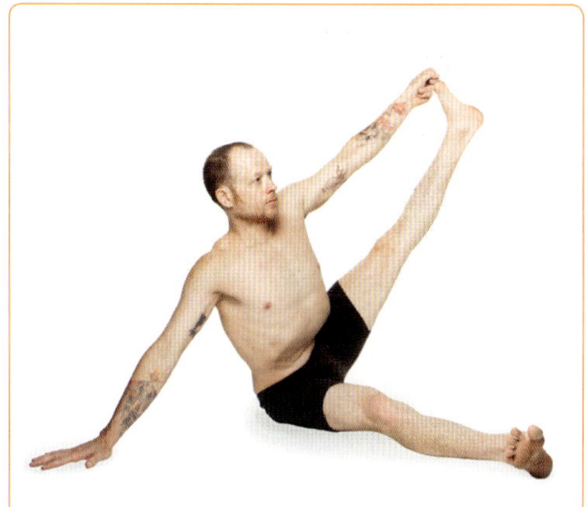

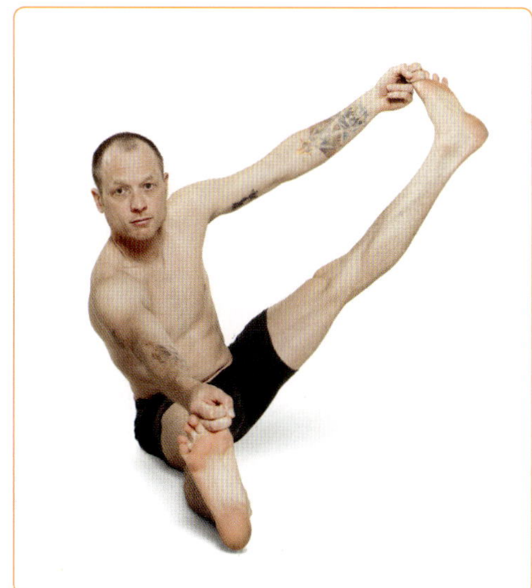

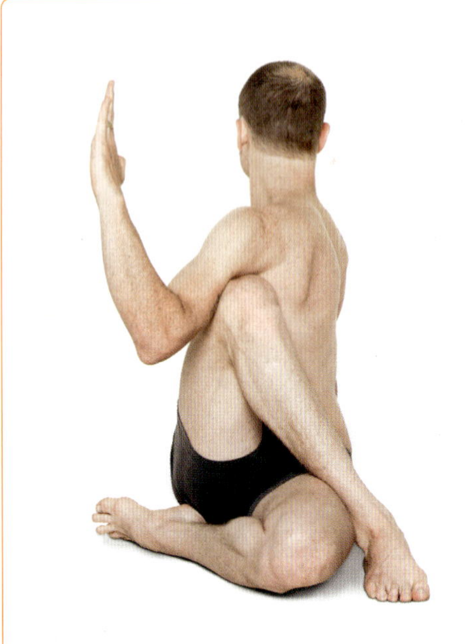

half lord of the fishes *elbow bent*

ardha matsyendrasana 1 prep

shape prep (from staff pose)

- Place hands a foot and half behind hips.
- Point feet.
- Bend knees, bring shins parallel to floor.
- Swing right heel to outer left hip—lower knee to floor.
- Place left foot on floor outside right knee—toes flush with knee (more doable: ankle flush with knee, or do this pose with right leg straight).

shape pose

- Lift right arm vertical, curve low back in, and bring right shoulder/ upper arm to outer left knee—bend elbow, point palm out.
- Look over front/back shoulder.

safety (strength) prep

- Squeeze feet into hips.

safety (strength) pose

- Tone, turn abdomen to left.
- Press front shoulder, top knee together.

refinement (stretch) prep

- Lift low back, lift chest. Stretch spine.

Repeat on the second side.

half lord of the fishes
ardha matsyendrasana 1

shape prep
▓ Come onto hands and knees.
▓ Turn right foot in so that big toe points at left foot.
▓ Step left foot forward, have a seat on inner edge of right foot—right hip to right heel, left hip to big toe mound (more doable: sit up on a block).
▓ Place left foot on floor outside right knee—toes flush with knee (more doable: ankle flush with knee).
▓ Lift right arm vertical, curve low back in, bring right shoulder/upper arm to outer left knee—bend elbow, point palm out.

shape pose
▓ Look at front foot. Clasp inner edge of foot with right hand, place thumb between big toe and second toe; make fist with hand.
▓ Swing left arm behind back, place back of hand against right rib cage—close fingers (more doable: keep hand on floor).
▓ Look over front/back shoulder.

safety (strength) prep
▓ Squeeze feet in.
▓ Press front arm, leg together.
▓ Press shoulder into knee, knee into shoulder.

safety (strength) pose
▓ Press front hand, foot together.
▓ Tone forearm, biceps, triceps of front arm.
▓ Press back hand into rib cage—tone biceps, triceps.
▓ Tone, turn abdomen to left.
▓ Lift left shoulder up, back.

refinement (stretch) pose
▓ Lift chest, stretch spine.
▓ Breathe as deeply and evenly as possible.

Repeat on the second side.

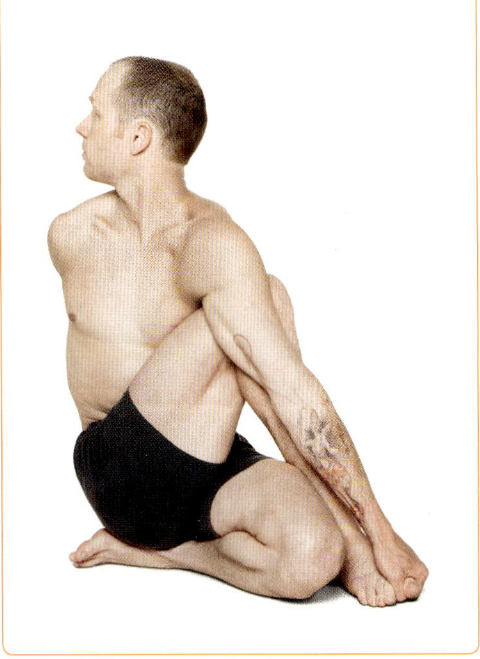

This is among my favorite poses to teach and practice. Who knows, maybe it's because Sage Matsyendra is regarded as one of the founding fathers of hatha yoga, and therefore the essence of the practice is contained in this pose. Although that sounds good, I doubt that's the reason. One thing for sure: we all have our pose preferences. About 20 years ago I told my mom that I didn't like revolved triangle. She said, "Take that as a sign that it has something essential to offer you." And sure enough, I now regard this pose as a hatha treasure that keeps on giving. Another thing for sure: pose preferences have a penchant for changing via practice, please practice.

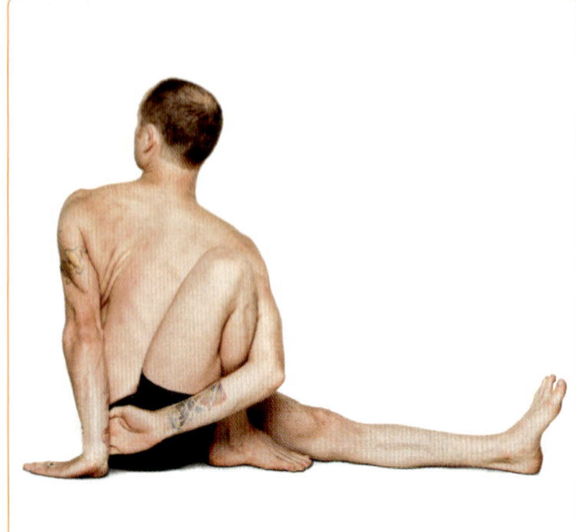

revolved m sage 1 *clasp wrist*
parivrtta marichyasana 1

shape prep (from staff pose)
- Move hands back one foot.
- Bend left knee, bring heel in front of left hip, point knee up.
- Bring left ankle against inner thigh. Slide hips forward, bring left heel to left hip.
- Lift left arm up, curve low back in (more doable: sit up on block).
- Place left shoulder or elbow against inner left knee. Bend elbow.
- Bring left thigh, left ribcage together.
- Twist to right.
- Stay here or hold outer edge of right foot with left hand.
- Stay here or wrap left arm around left leg, place back of wrist just above hip.

shape pose
- Clasp wrist with hand (more doable clasp hands or use strap to bind).
- Stay here or straighten right arm, place palm flat on floor.
- Look over front/back shoulder.

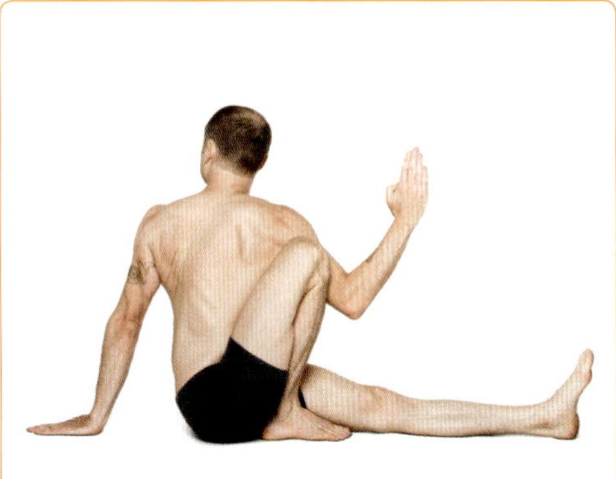

safety (strength) prep
- Straight leg: tone thigh, tighten kneecap, firm hamstrings, press thigh down.

safcty (strength) pose
- Squeeze shoulders towards spine.
- Tone, turn abdomen to right.

refinement (stretch) pose
- Lift low back, chest. Stretch spine.

Repeat on the second side.

m sage 1
marichyasana 1

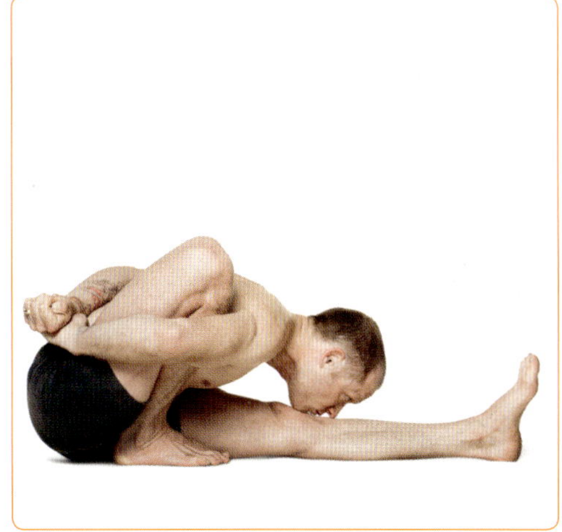

shape prep (from staff pose)
- Move hands back one foot.
- Bend left knee, bring heel in front of left hip; point knee up.
- Bring left ankle against right inner thigh. Slide hips forward, bring left heel to left hip.
- Floint right foot (halfway between flex and point).
- Lift left arm up, curve low back in (more doable: sit up on block).
- Place left shoulder against inner left knee, bend elbow. Bring left thigh, left ribcage together.
- Stay here or hold outer edge of right foot with left hand.
- Stay here or wrap left arm around left leg, place back of wrist just above hip.

shape pose
- Clasp left wrist with right hand (more doable: clasp hands or use strap to bind).
- Stay here or lower chin, tip of nose to shin; allow left hip to lift off floor. Point right kneecap up.
- Round back evenly, bring shoulders equidistant to floor.

safety (strength) prep
- Tone right thigh, tighten kneecap, firm hamstrings, press thigh down.

safety (strength) pose
- Squeeze shoulders towards spine.
- Tone, turn abdomen to right.

refinement (stretch) pose
- Stretch spine.

Repeat on the second side.

In m sage 1, the hands do not hold the foot of the extended leg. To get your forehead to your front knee will, therefore, require core strength. In Light On Yoga, B. K. S. Iyengar says that janu sirsasana, ardha baddha padma paschimottanasana, triang mukhaikapada paschimottanasana, and marichyasana 1 are the four key poses that prepare practitioners for paschimottanasana.[1] As you practice one pose, you can't help but be preparing for another.

1 B. K. S. Iyengar, *Light on Yoga*
   (New York: Schocken Books, 1977) p. 161.

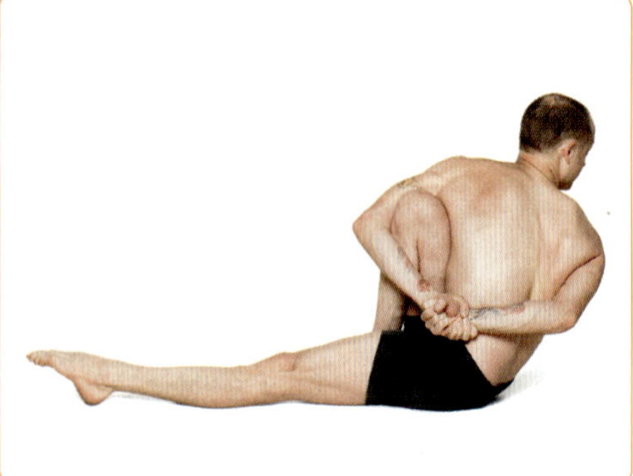

m sage 3
marichyasana 3

shape prep (from staff pose)
- Move hands back one foot or so.
- Bend left knee, bring heel in front of left hip, point knee up.
- Bring left ankle against right inner thigh. Slide hips forward, bring left heel to left hip.
- Move left leg to right—line up knees.
- Lift right arm up, curve low back in (more doable: sit up on block).
- Place right shoulder against outer left knee. Bend elbow.
- Look at front foot.

shape pose
- Stay here or place right hand outside front shin—straighten arm.
- Stay here, or wrap right arm around left leg, place wrist just above hip.
- Clasp wrist with hand (more doable: clasp hands or use strap to bind).
- Look over front or back shoulder.

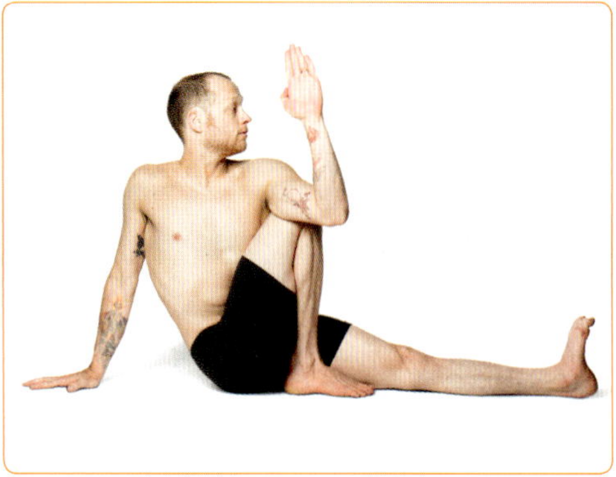

safety (strength) pose
- Straight leg: tone thigh, tighten kneecap, firm hamstrings, press thigh down.
- Press arm, leg together.
- Tone, turn abdomen to left.

refinement (stretch) pose
- Lift low back, lift chest. Stretch spine.

Repeat on the second side.

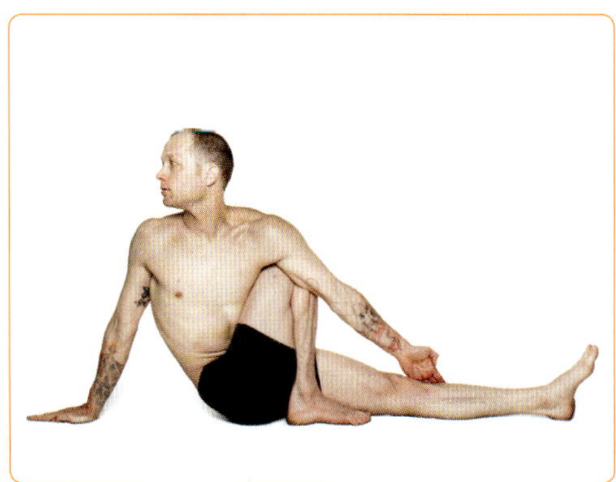

noose *elbow bent*

pasasana prep

shape prep
- Come into a squat position; bring ankles, knees together.
- Lower heels to floor (more doable: lower heels onto a rolled up mat or blankets).
- Place hands on floor behind hips.
- Lift left arm, curve low back in.

shape pose
- Place left shoulder outside right knee—keep knees flush.
- Bend elbow, close fingers.
- Look straight ahead.
- Bring head directly above hips—spine straight up and down.

safety (strength) prep
- Squeeze legs together.

safety (strength) pose
- Press arm, knee together.
- Tone, turn abdomen to right.

refinement (stretch) prep
- Lift chest, stretch spine.

Repeat on the second side.

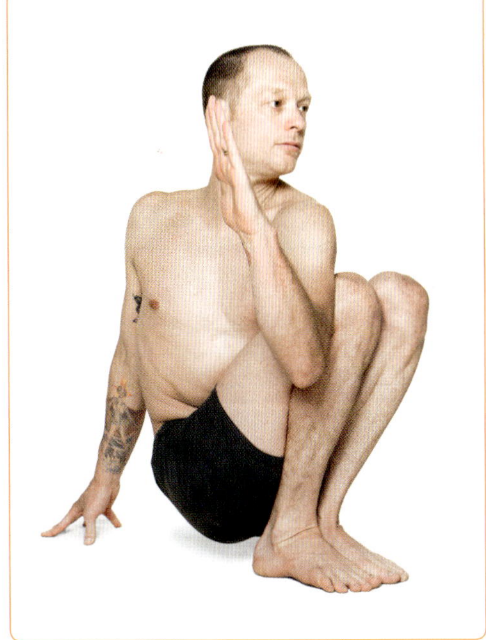

In this pose the breath will likely be quick and shallow. Attempt to breath normally. To do so, requires becoming focused and calm in the midst of discomfort. Again and again, yoga poses put us into stressful situations (seats—asana means seat), and then invite us to become calm and focused. It is an excellent skill to develop.

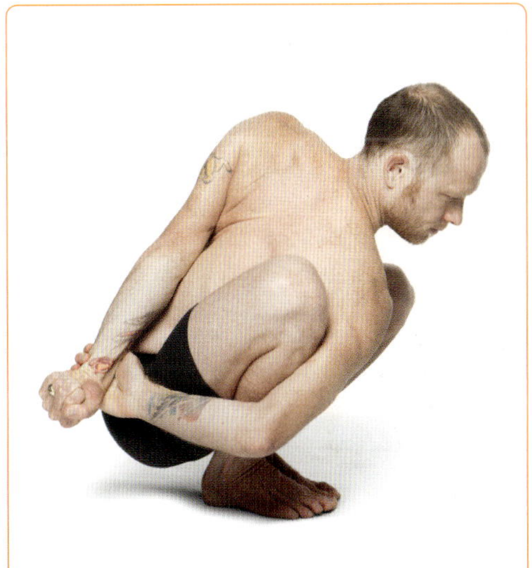

one leg noose

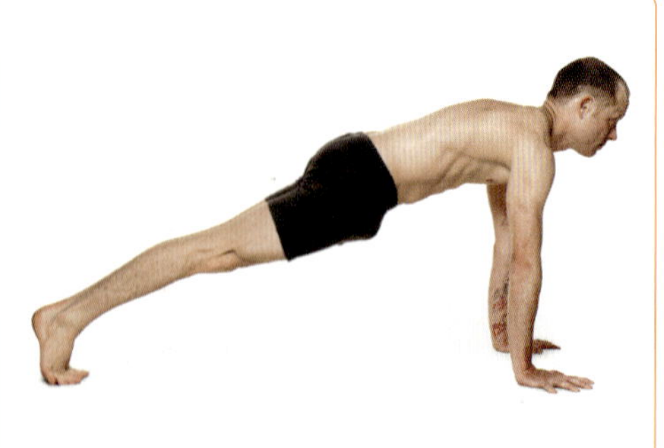

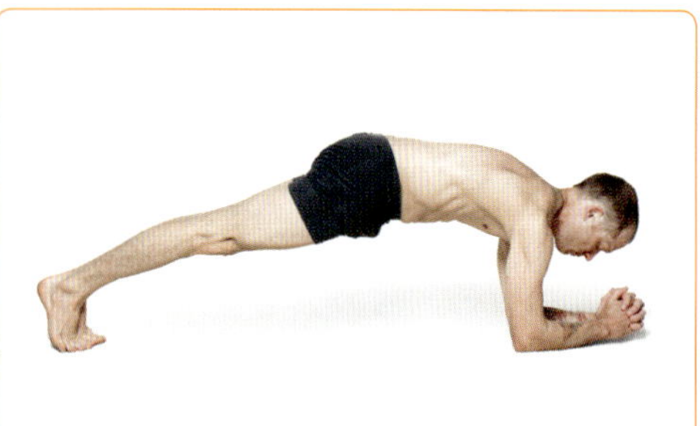

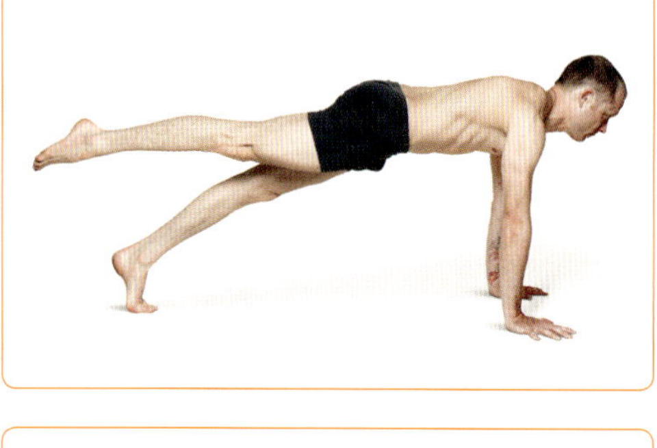

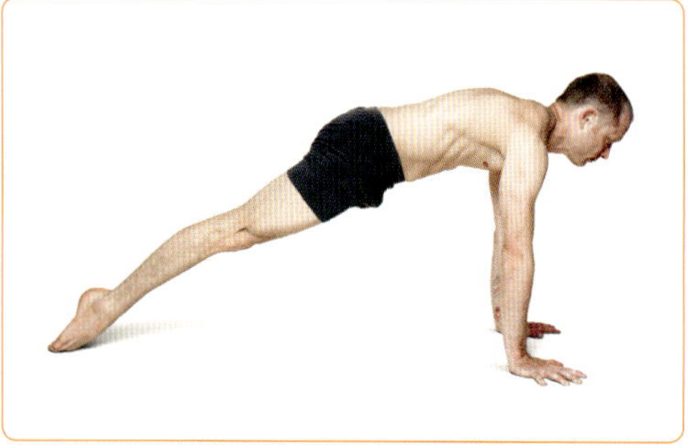

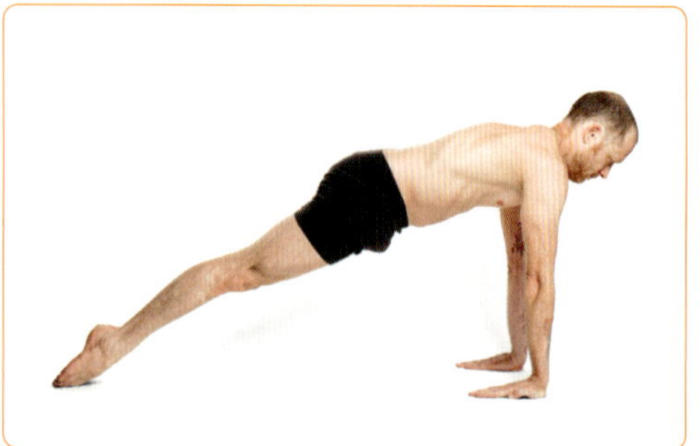

plank pose
phalankasana

shape prep
(from downward facing dog ankles together)
■ Look at hands, check to make they are slightly wider than shoulders, fingers are separated, and index fingers are pointing straight ahead.

shape pose
■ Come into plank—top of a push-up position (more doable: lower knees to floor like in eight angle).
■ Move heels vertical, directly above toe mounds;   straighten legs, arms.
■ Lift chin, look straight ahead.
■ Without lifting hips, round back—low back, mid back, upper back.

safety (strength) prep
■ Grip floor with fingertips—press inner edges of hands down.

safety (strength) pose
■ Tighten glutes, press tailbone down, tone abdomen.

Plank pose is an optimal full body warm-up. It's a good asana alternative for most, if not, all two-handed arm balances, especially the classical form of crane (in my opinion, plank is an arm balance in and of itself).

plank *leg in tree*

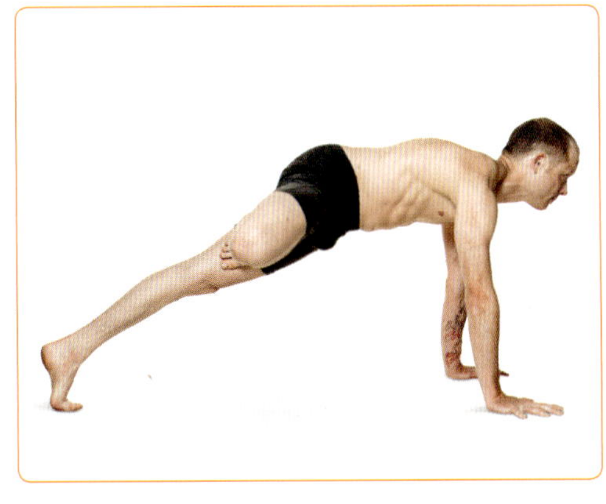

shape pose (from v sage, top leg in tree)
▓ Keep top leg in tree; bring rest of body into plank pose (reminder: in plank, hands are slightly wider than shoulders, fingers are separated, index fingers point straight ahead).
▓ Move back heel vertical—point tree knee directly out.
▓ Lift chin, look forward.
▓ Round back.
▓ More difficult: do 1-5 push-ups in this position.

safety (strength) pose
▓ Grip floor with fingertips—press inner edges of hands down.
▓ Tighten glutes, press tailbone down, tone abdomen.

refinement (stretch) pose
▓ Lift chest, stretch spine.

Repeat on the second side.

four-limbed staff
chaturanga dandasana

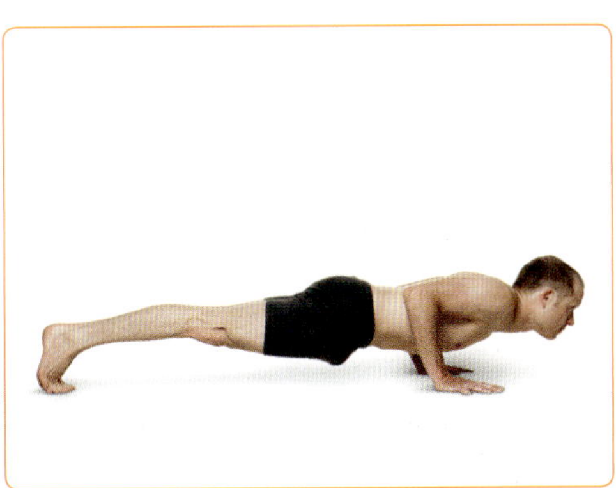

shape pose (from plank pose)
▓ Bend elbows to a 90-degree angle—upper arms parallel to floor, shoulders as high as elbows (more doable: lower knees to floor or stay in plank). Do not point elbows out.
▓ Lift ribs up—do not collapse low back.
▓ Keep heels vertical; keep looking forward.

safety (strength) prep
▓ Grip floor with fingertips—press inner edges of hands down.
▓ Tighten glutes, press tailbone down, tone abdomen.

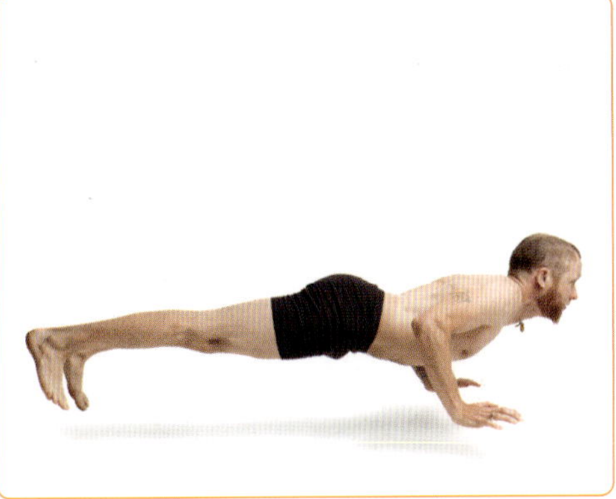

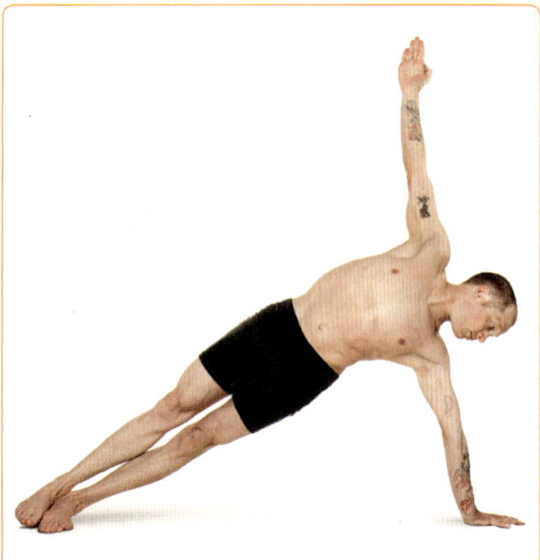

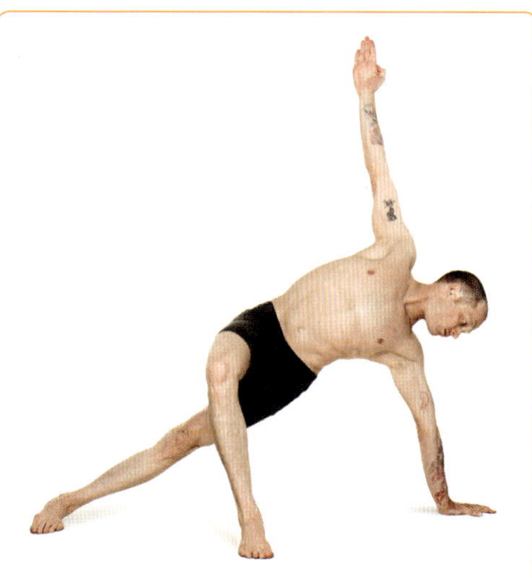

v sage *prep*
vasisthasana prep

shape prep (from downward facing dog)
▌ Look at hands: check to make sure hands are slightly wider than shoulders, separate fingers, point index fingers straight ahead.
▌ Move feet back 2-3 inches.
▌ Come into a sideways plank, balancing on right hand and foot.

shape pose
▌ Stack ankles; lift top arm vertical—close fingers (more doable: lower bottom knee or place top foot on floor in front of bottom leg).
▌ Bring sole of bottom foot flat on floor.
▌ Look down, out, or up.
▌ Point bottom biceps straight ahead.

safety (strength) prep
▌ Grip floor with fingertips, press inner edge of hand down.

safety (strength) pose
▌ Squeeze legs together, tighten glutes, press tailbone in, move ribs back.

refinement (stretch) pose
▌ Press bottom hand down, forward. Move hips up, back.

Repeat on the second side.

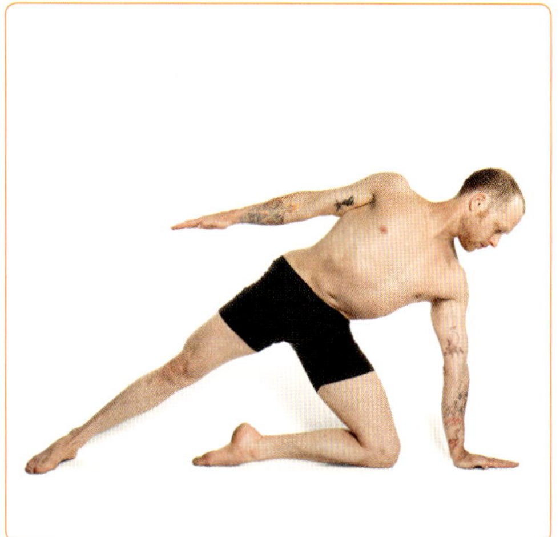

v sage *top leg in tree*
vasisthasana

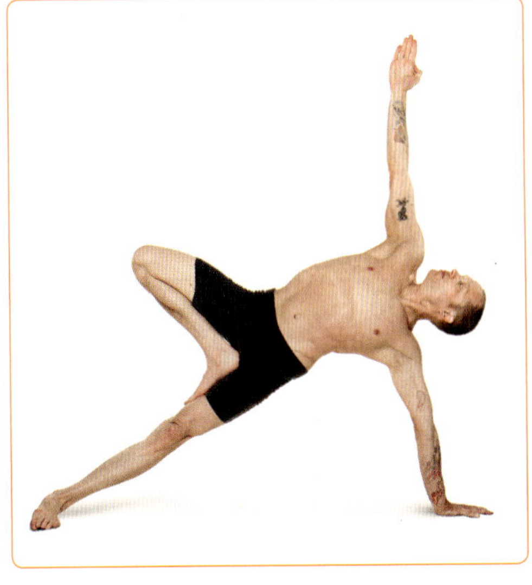

shape prep (from v sage, ankles stacked)
- Hold top ankle with top hand—bring top leg into tree—place sole of foot on right inner thigh well above knee (more doable: place top foot on floor in front of bottom leg).

shape pose
- Point top knee up, lift top arm vertical.
- Point bottom biceps straight ahead.
- Look down, out, or up.

safety (strength) prep
- Grip floor with fingertips, press inner edge of hand down.

safety (strength) pose
- Press top foot into thigh, thigh into foot.
- Tighten glutes, press tailbone in, move ribs back.

refinement (stretch) pose
- Press bottom hand down, forward.
- Lift chest, stretch spine.

Repeat on the second side.

Practice arm balances like standing poses: first side, back to center, directly into second side. Practitioners have a tendency to sit down, take breaks, and even chitchat/chit-ananda-chat between arm balances. Imagine how that would affect the focus and flow of your practice if you did that between the right and left sides of triangle pose? Doing several arm balances in a row, which happens in Barefoot Boot Camp, stokes stamina, and stamina stokes sadhana (practice).

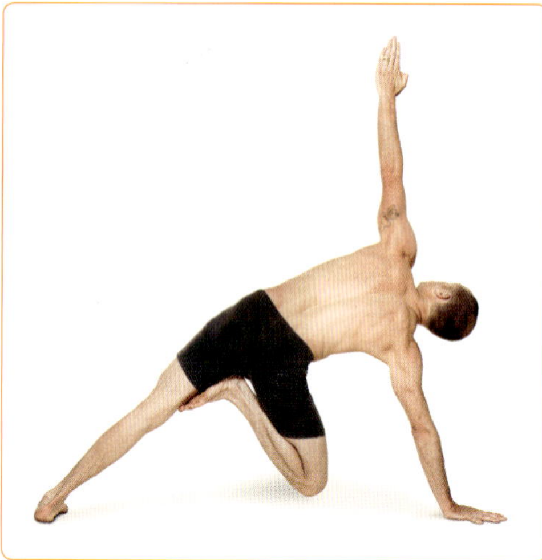

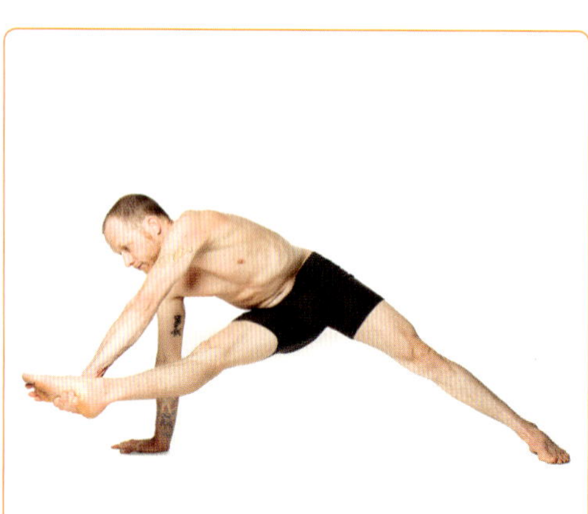

v sage *bottom leg in tree*
vasisthasana

shape pose (from v sage, top leg in tree)
- Keep top leg in tree: lower left hand to floor, point left knee down, lift right arm up (more doable: rest bottom knee on floor).
- Point bottom biceps straight ahead.
- Look down, out, or up.

safety (strength) prep
- Press tree foot into thigh, thigh into foot.

safety (strength) pose
- Grip floor with fingertips, press inner edge of hand and foot down.
- Tighten glutes, press tailbone in, move ribs back.

refinement (stretch) pose
- Press bottom hand down, forward.

Repeat on the second side.

v sage
vasisthasana

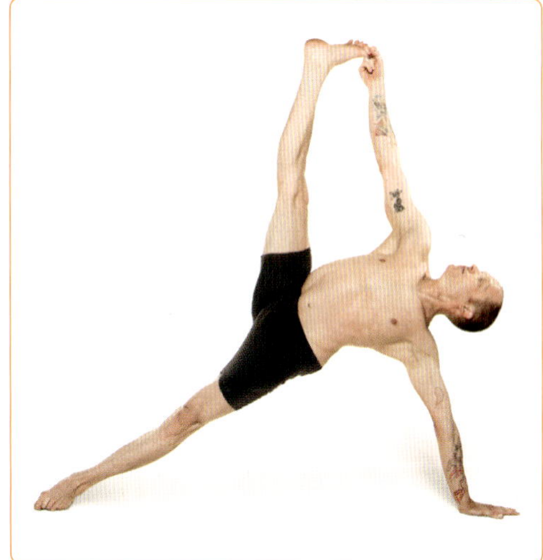

shape prep (from downward facing dog)
- Look at hands: check to make sure hands are slightly wider than shoulders, separate fingers evenly, point index fingers straight ahead.
- Move feet back 2-3 inches.
- Come into a sideways plank pose, balancing on right hand and foot.
- Stack ankles; lift left arm vertical—close fingers (more doable: place top foot on floor behind bottom leg).
- Place sole of bottom foot on floor.
- Point bottom biceps straight ahead.
- Stay here, or bend top knee, hold big toe with first two fingers and thumb—arm inside leg.

shape pose
- Without lifting or lowering hips straighten top leg somewhat or significantly.
- Look down, out, or up.

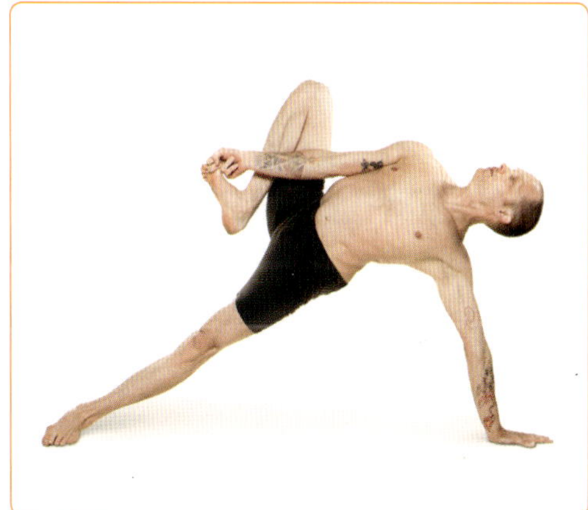

safety (strength) prep
- Grip floor with fingertips, press inner edge of hand and foot down.
- Press big toe, fingers together to help engage top leg.

safety (strength) pose
- Tighten glutes, press tailbone in, move ribs back.
- Tone thighs, tighten kneecaps, firm hamstrings.

refinement (stretch) pose
- Lift chest, stretch spine.

Repeat on the second side.

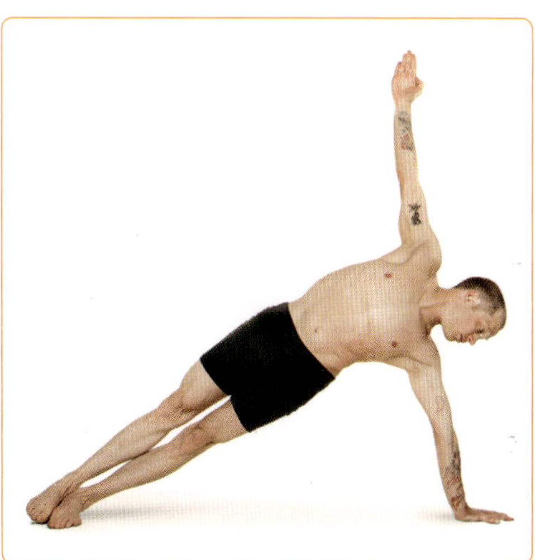

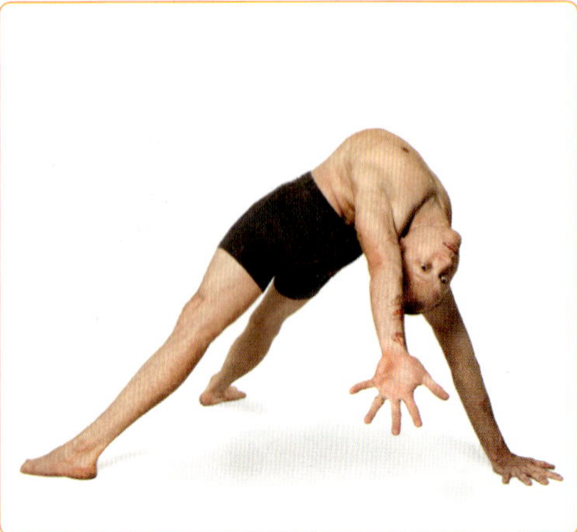

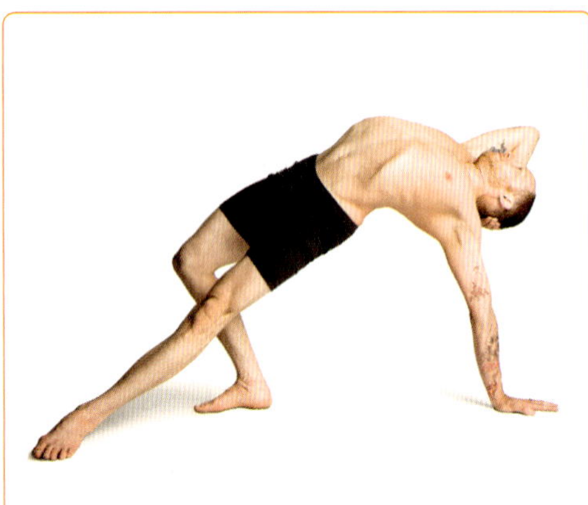

wild thing
camatkarasana

shape prep (from v sage, ankles stacked)
- Place top foot on floor behind bottom leg—shin vertical (more difficult: straighten both legs).
- Place feet flat on floor, top hand on hip.
- Point bottom biceps straight ahead.
- Move hips up, back.
- Turn chest toward ceiling.

shape pose
- Bring left arm across face, point palm up, separate fingers.
- Look up or back.

safety (strength) prep
- Grip floor with fingertips, press inner edge of hand down.

safety (strength) pose
- Press feet down, in.
- Tighten glutes, lift tailbone, tone abdomen.

refinement (stretch) pose
- Press hand down, forward.
- Lift chest, stretch spine.

Repeat on the second side.

baby bird
kapinjalasana prep

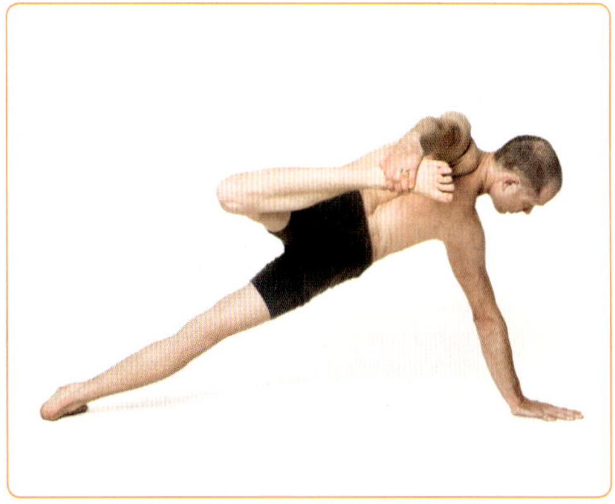

shape pose (from v sage, ankles stacked)
- Hold top foot with top hand behind hip.
- Extend top foot back, hips forward (do not lower or lift hips).
- Point bottom biceps straight ahead.
- Look down.

safety (strength) prep
- Grip floor with fingertips, press inner edge of hand and foot down.

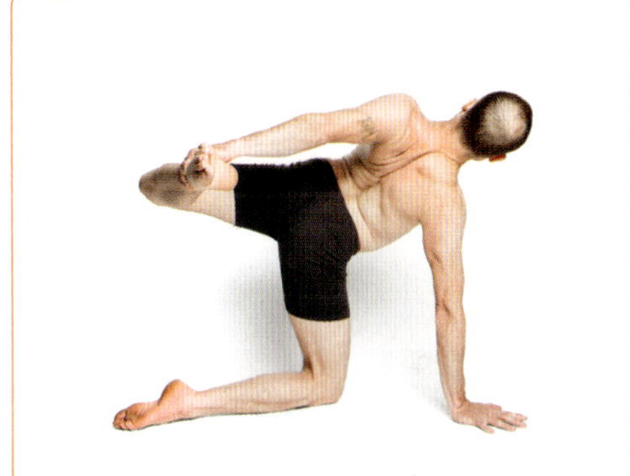

safety (strength) pose
- Tighten glutes, press tailbone in, tone abdomen.

refinement (stretch) pose
- Press hand down, forward.
- Lift chest, stretch spine.

Repeat on the second side.

This a very difficult pose to attain balance in.

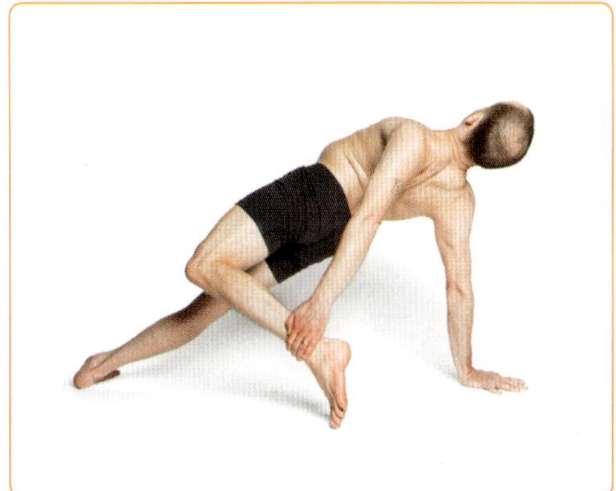

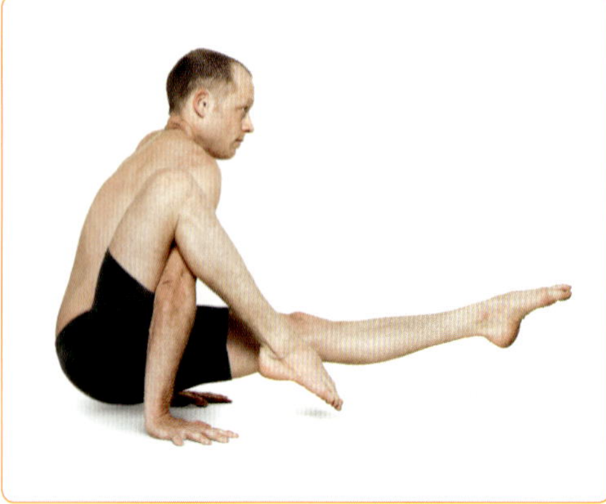

one-hand arm pose
eka hasta bhujasana

shape prep (from staff)

- Bend right knee, hold right foot with hands—arms inside leg.
- Bring shin parallel to floor, straighten arms. Bring shoulder inside knee—minimize rounding in low back.
- Stay here or hold right calf with right hand, place right knee just below right shoulder, above elbow.
- Place right hand on floor in front of hips.
- Place left hand on floor across from right hand—hands slightly wider than shoulder-width apart—separate fingers evenly, point index fingers straight ahead.
- Point feet.

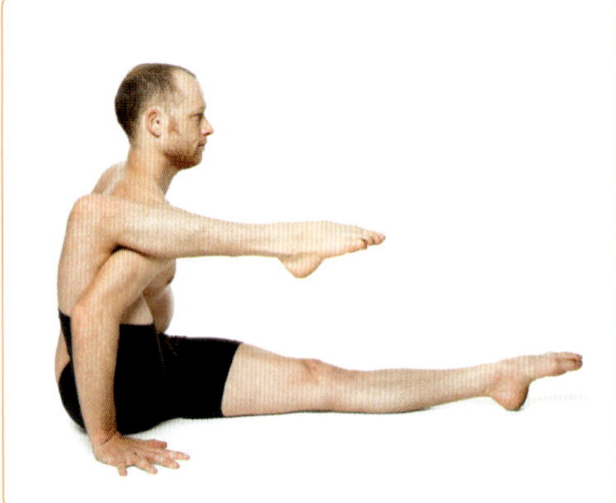

shape pose

- Lean forward, lift everything but hands off floor. Straighten left arm. Bring left leg parallel to floor (more doable: lift only hips or only left leg off floor instead of both).

safety (strength) prep

- Clamp arm with knee.
- Grip floor with fingertips, press inner edges of hands down.
- Move right shoulder back—press right shoulder into leg.

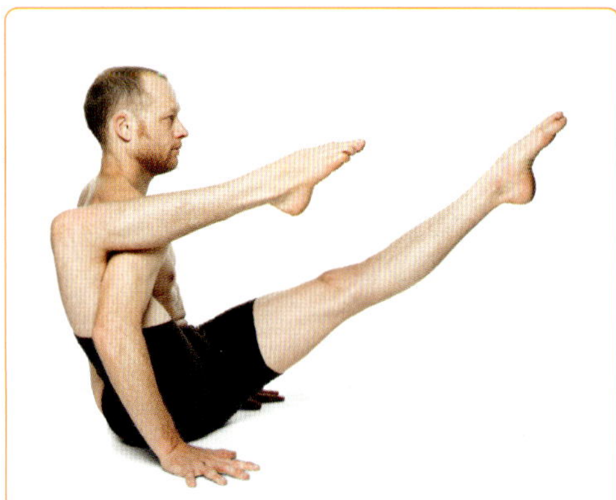

safety (strength) pose

- Squeeze knees in

refinement (stretch) prep

- Press hands down.

refinement (stretch) pose

- Lift chest, stretch spine.

Repeat on the second side.

The pacing of sadhana (practice) is a slowly then suddenly kind of deal. The pose one can't do month after month can become the pose one can suddenly do today. Although the pose is not the point of yogahour, turning can't into can has its place and purpose. It can be one of those the-work-is-always-worth-it kind of moments.

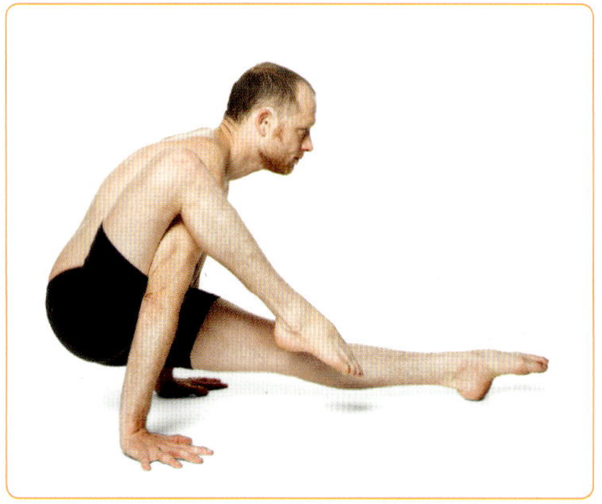

crooked sage
astavakrasana

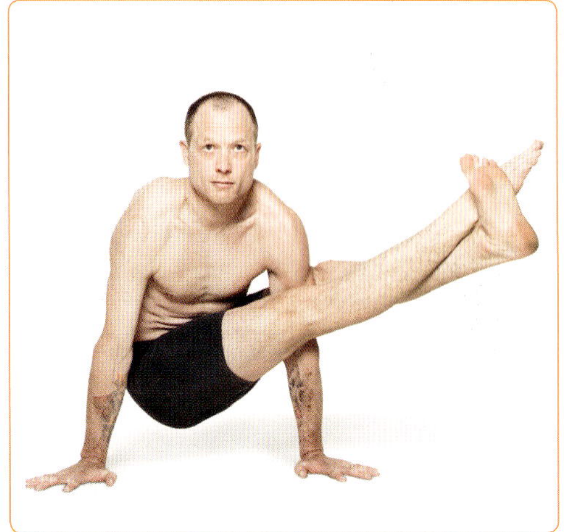

shape prep (from staff)

▪ Bend right knee, hold right foot with hands—arms inside leg.

▪ Bring shin parallel to floor, straighten arms. Bring shoulder inside knee.

▪ Stay here or hold right calf with right hand, place right knee just below right shoulder, above elbow.

▪ Place right hand on floor in front of hips.

▪ Place left hand on floor across from right hand—hands slightly wider than shoulder-width apart, separate fingers, point index fingers straight ahead.

▪ Flex feet.

shape pose

▪ Cross left ankle over right ankle. Lean forward and lift hips off floor. Straighten legs.

▪ Straighten left arm.

▪ Stay here for five seconds and then bend elbows to 90 degrees—upper arms parallel to floor. Stay here for 5 seconds (more difficult: do 5 to 10 push-ups in this position).

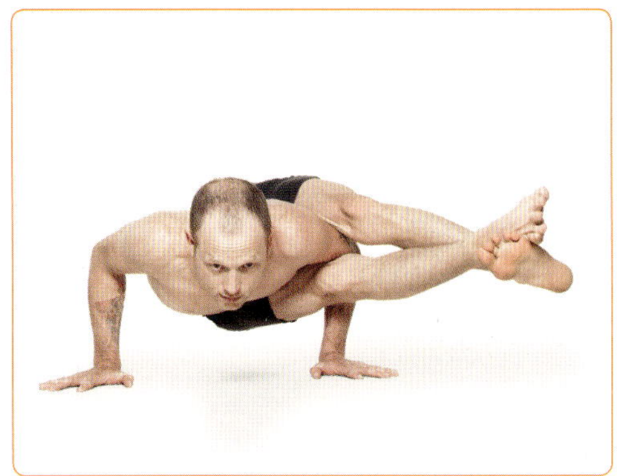

safety (strength) prep

▪ Grip floor with fingertips, press inner edges of hands down.

▪ Clamp arm with legs.

safety (strength) pose

▪ Squeeze legs together.

▪ Lift shoulders.

refinement (stretch) pose

▪ If there is a culprit when it comes to crooked sage it's often con-fusion. The solution = practice + patience.

Repeat on the second side.

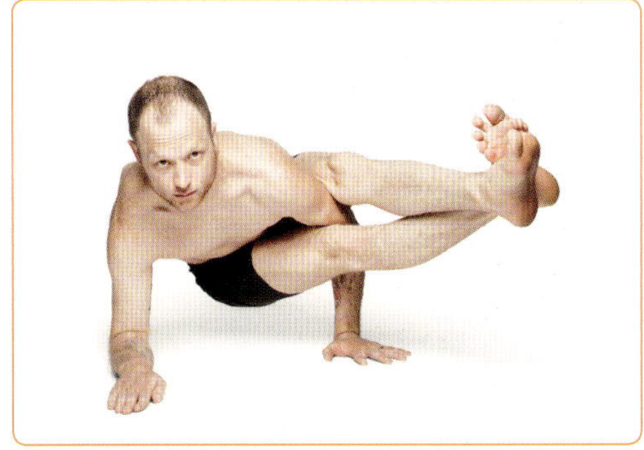

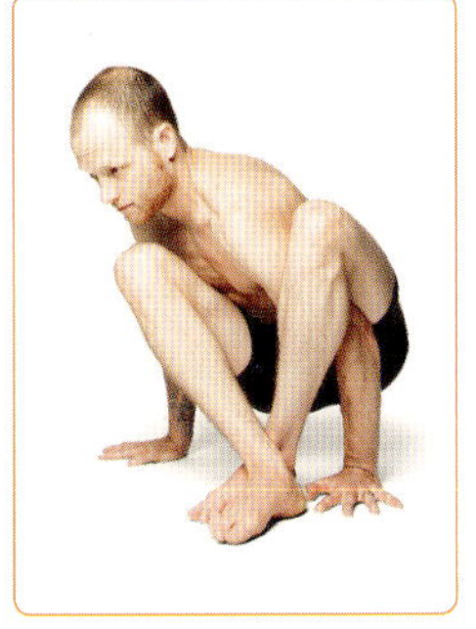

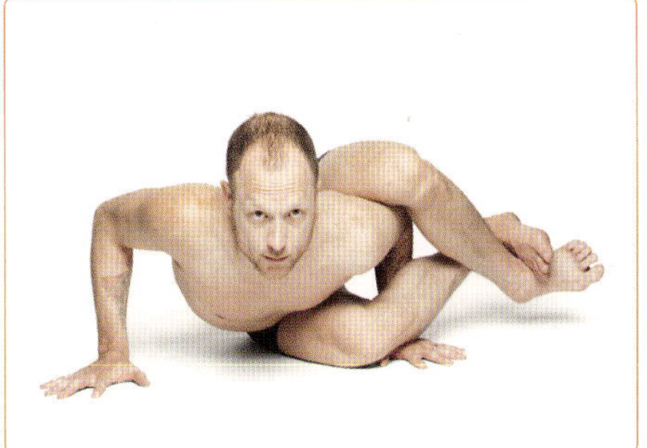

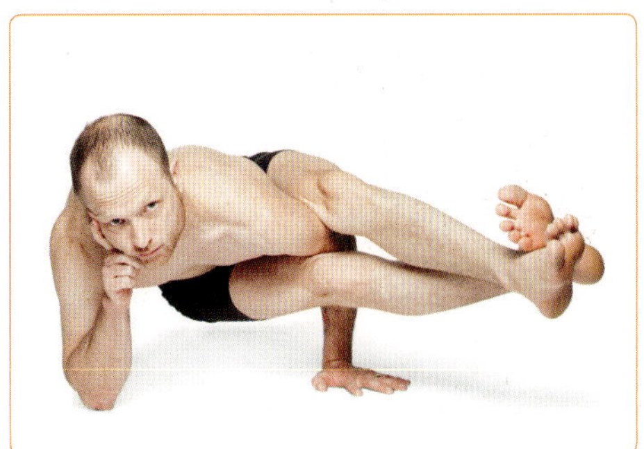

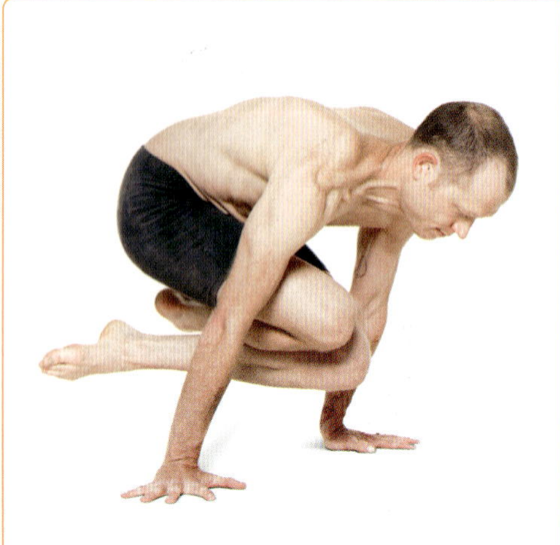

tremulous
lolasana

shape prep
▪ Come onto hands and knees.
▪ Cross shins into the shape of an X (more doable: cross ankles).
▪ Have a seat on feet.
▪ Place hands on floor halfway between knees and hips—hands slightly wider than shoulder-width apart.
▪ Turn hands out, point index fingers straight ahead.

shape pose
▪ Lean forward; lift everything but hands off floor (more doable: keep feet on floor, lift thighs parallel to floor—point feet).
▪ Straighten arms, round back.
▪ Look down.

safety (strength) prep
▪ Grip floor with fingertips, press inner edges of hands down.
▪ Super glue feet to hips.
▪ Tone abdomen.

refinement (stretch) prep
▪ Press hands down.

Repeat on the second side—switch cross of legs.

A friend once told me that she practiced lolasana several times a week for about two years without being able to lift her feet off the floor. Then one random day her feet launched. Now, what if her feet never lifted off the floor and she kept on practicing anyway? I say, all the more impressive! Practice is repetitious, not a broken record.

If tremulous seems more formidable than fun, do lion first to get in the mood and mode of lolasana. After all, lolasana = LOL-asana and LOL = laugh out loud! ☺

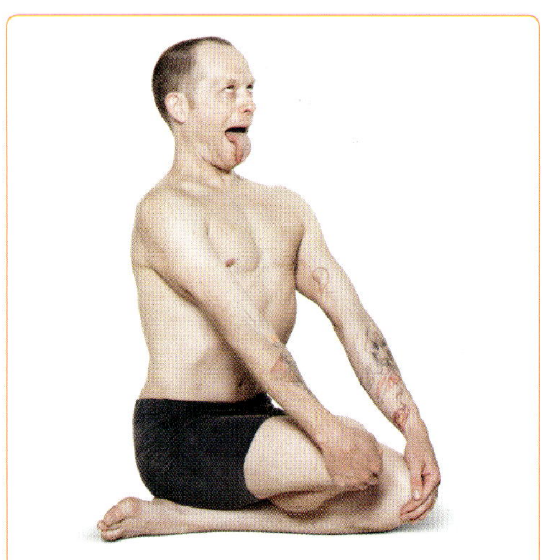

lion's pose

arm pressure pose
bhujapidasana

shape prep (from mountain)
- Separate feet almost as wide as mat.
- Bend knees slightly, bring shins parallel to each other. Place hands just above knees. Straighten arms. Put some weight on hands (for many this is an appropriate prep for arm balances).
- Stay here or fold forward. Bring outer shoulders to inner knees.
- Hold backs of calves with hands.
- Stay here or tiptoe on right foot, bring right shoulder behind right knee. Lower heel to floor. Tiptoe on left foot, bring left shoulder behind left knee. Lower heel to floor.
- Bend knees, lower hips, place hands on floor slightly wider than shoulder-width apart—tip of thumb against back of heel. Separate fingers.

shape pose
- Stay here or lean back, lift feet off floor. Straighten arms (more doable: keep elbows bent). Cross ankles, flex feet.
- Look straight ahead.

safety (strength) prep
- Grip floor with fingertips, press inner edges of hands down. Tone abdomen.
- Press arms and legs together.

refinement (stretch) pose
- Press hands down.

Repeat on the second side—switch cross of legs.

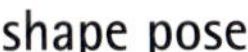

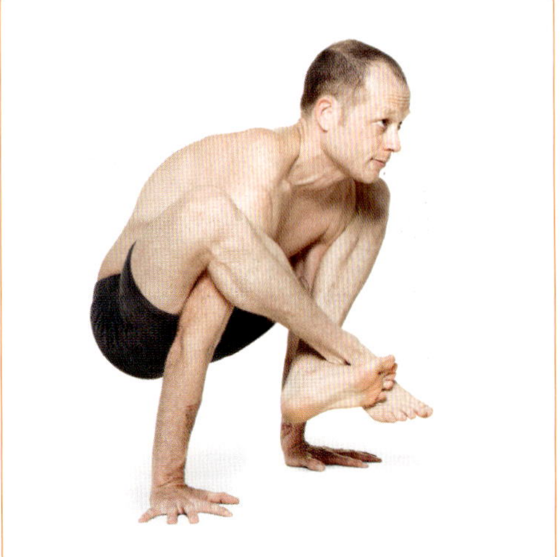

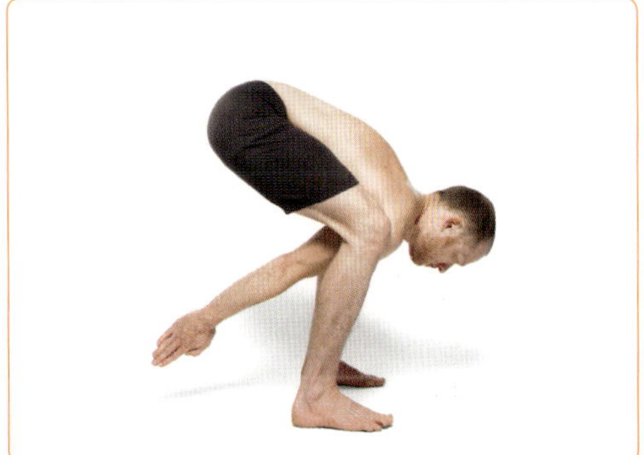

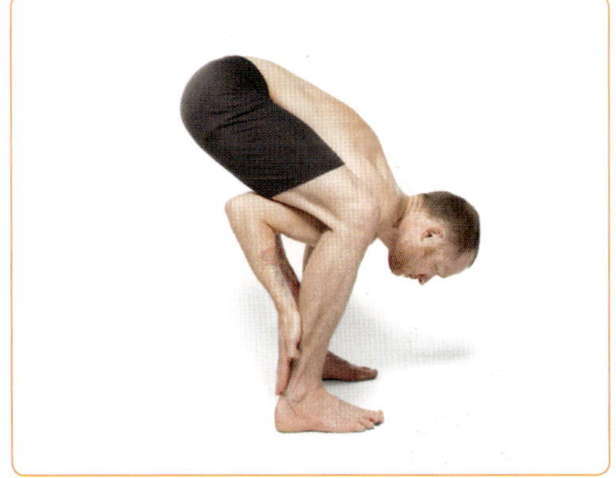

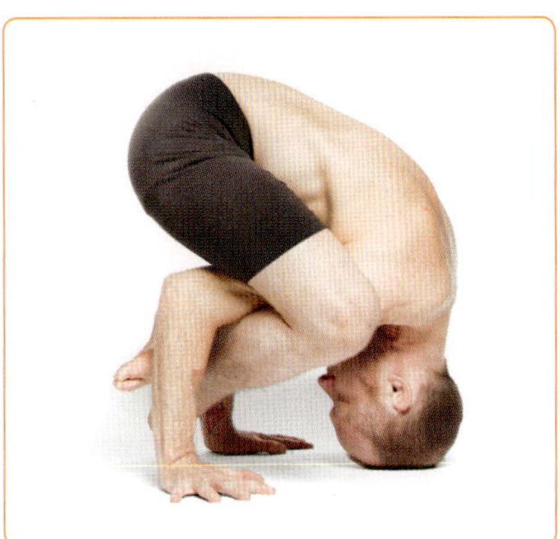

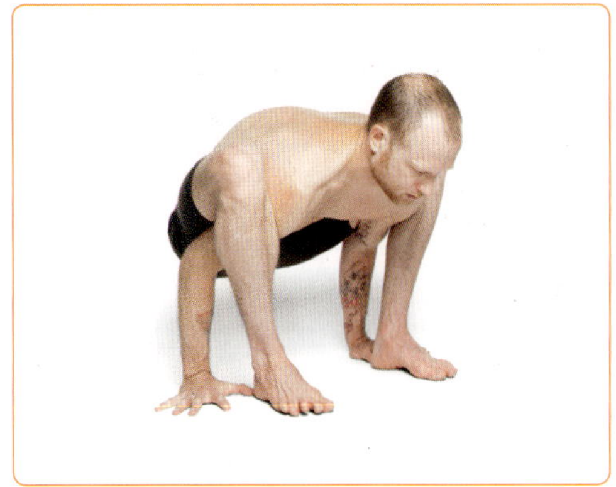

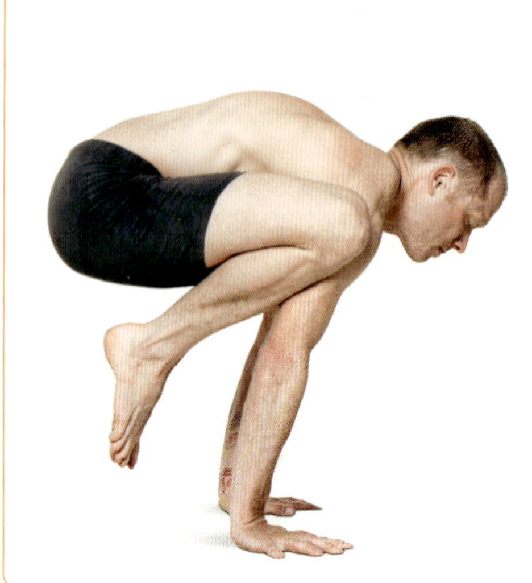

crane
bakasana

shape prep (from mountain)

- Come into a squatting position (more doable: separate feet slightly, turn feet out in line with knees, place heels on a rolled up mat).
- Fold torso inside legs; bring armpits against shins as close to ankles as possible.
- Place hands on floor slightly wider than shoulder-width apart.
- Separate fingers, point index fingers straight ahead.
- Slide hands back to capacity.

shape pose

- Lean forward, lift heels.
- Stay here or lift feet off floor, place inner edges of feet together (more doable: lift one foot, place it back on floor, then lift other foot).
- Straighten arms, round back—bring thighs parallel to floor (more doable: keep elbows bent; more difficult: place knees against triceps, straighten arms, bring shins parallel to floor).

safety (strength) prep

- Grip floor with fingertips, press perimeter of palms into floor with equal pressure (weight tends to go to outer corner of hands).

safety (strength) pose

- Squeeze feet together; squeeze knees in.
- Squeeze elbows in—forearms parallel.
- Lift pelvic floor; tone abdomen.

refinement (stretch) pose

- Press hands down.

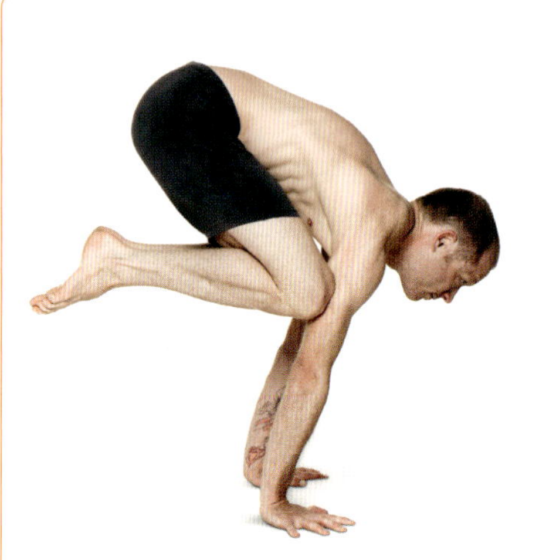

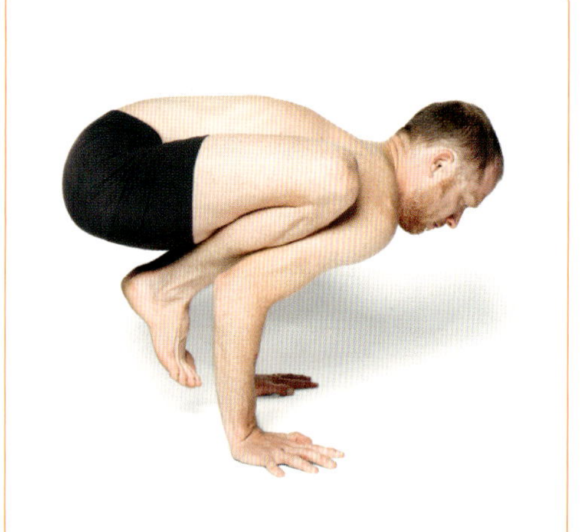

turned crane

parsva bakasana

shape prep
- Come into a squat position.
- Bring ankles, knees together.
- Place fingertips on floor behind hips.
- Lift right arm, twist to left, place right shoulder outside left knee.
- Place hands on floor outside left hip—hands slightly wider than shoulder-width apart. Separate fingers, point index fingers straight ahead.
- Tiptoe, lean to left, transfer weight onto hands.

shape pose
- Stay here or lift hips and feet up (more difficult: straighten left arm).
- Bring hips in line with head—torso parallel to floor.
- Keep knees flush.

safety (strength) prep
- Grip floor with fingertips, press inner edges of hands down.
- Move shoulders back.
- Tone abdomen.
- Squeeze legs together.

refinement (stretch) pose
- Press hands down.
- Lift chest.

Repeat on the second side.

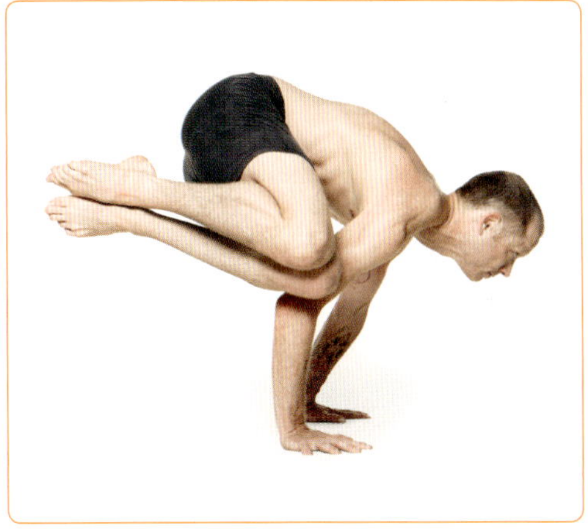

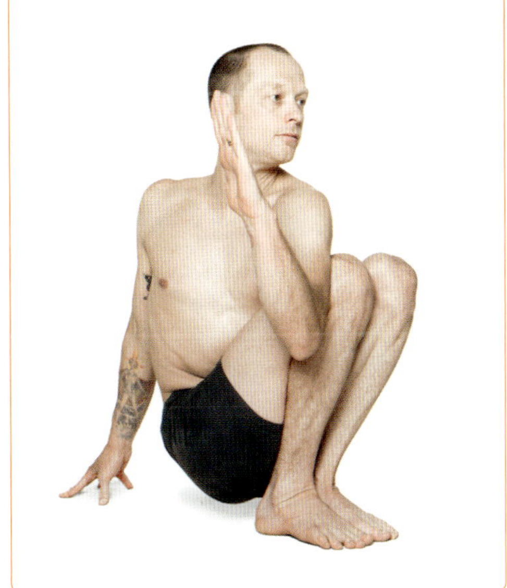

noose prep

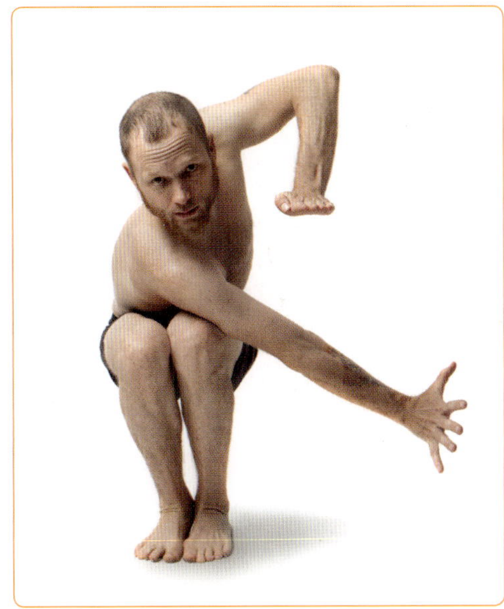

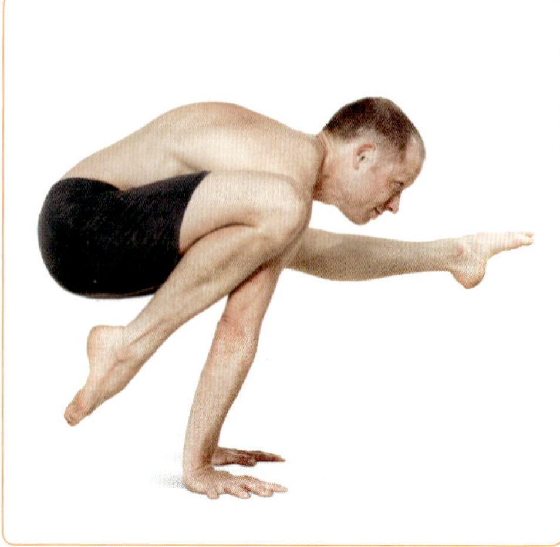

one-leg crane
eka pada bakasana 2

shape prep (from mountain)
▮ Step left foot back about one foot behind right foot.
▮ Turn left foot out slightly—line up left big toe mound with right heel.
▮ Squat: left hip to left heel.
▮ Stay here, or lift hips, hold right calf with right hand, place right shoulder behind knee. Come back into a squat. Place right hand on floor outside right foot.
▮ Stay here, or lift hips again, place left armpit on left shin well below knee. Place left hand on floor across from right hand, hands slightly wider than shoulder-width apart. Separate fingers, point index fingers straight ahead, thumb in line with heel.
▮ Stay here, or lean forward, lift left foot up.

shape pose
▮ Stay here, or lean back and lift right foot off floor with knee bent (more difficult: straighten right leg).
▮ Flex feet (more difficult: point feet).

safety (strength) prep
▮ Grip floor with fingertips, press inner edges of hands down.
▮ Move shoulders back.
▮ Tone abdomen.
▮ Squeeze elbows, legs in.

safety (strength) pose
▮ If right leg is straight: tone thigh, tighten kneecap, firm hamstrings.

refinement (stretch) pose
▮ Press hands down.

Repeat on the second side.

one-leg crane
eka pada bakasana 1

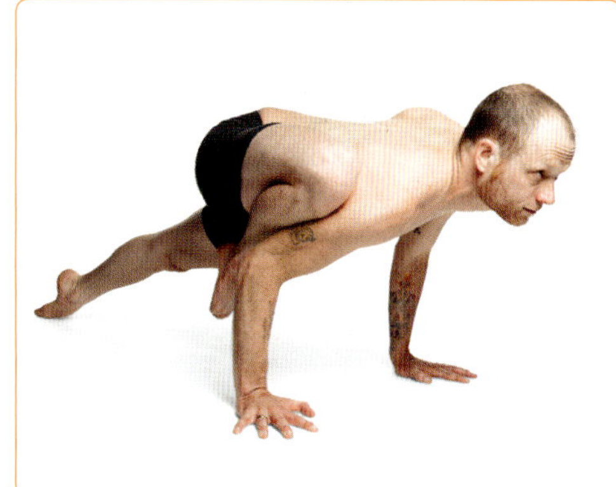

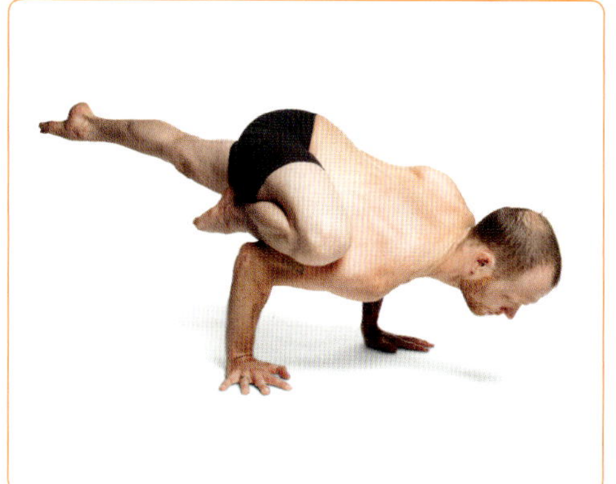

flying pigeon
eka pada galavasana

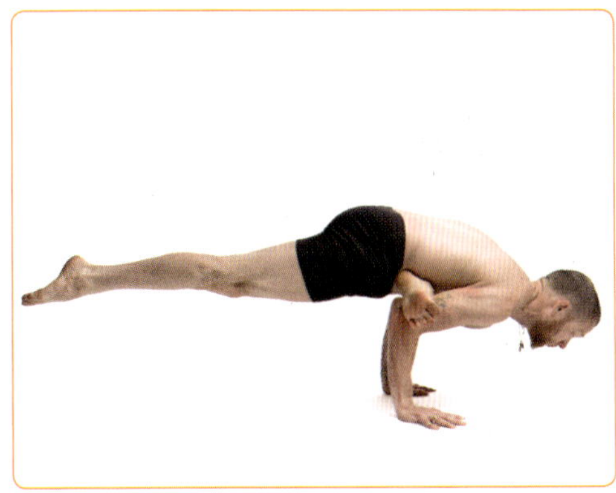

shape prep (from mountain)
Bend knees slightly, place right ankle just above left knee—flex foot.

Place hands or forearms on shin (hands on shin—straighten arms / forearms on shin—place palms together, interlace fingers).

Stay here, or bend left knee more. Place palms flat on floor with hands slightly wider than shoulders—point index fingers straight ahead.

shape pose
Stay here, or place shin above elbows, press right foot into left arm. Lean forward, lift left foot off floor with back knee bent (more difficult: straighten back leg—leg parallel to floor. Point foot, point kneecap straight down).

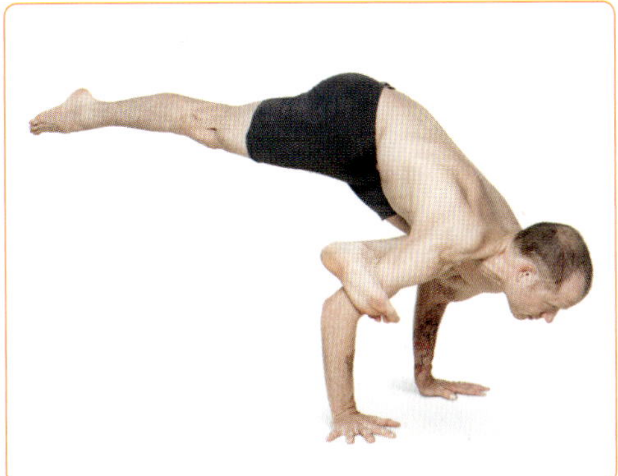

safety (strength) prep
Grip floor with fingertips, press inner edges of hands down.

Squeeze elbows in.

Lift shoulders.

Press right shin down, flare right toes.

Tighten glutes, press tailbone down, tone abdomen.

refinement (stretch) pose
Press hands down.

Repeat on the second side.

If this pose proves to be too difficult, needle's eye or pigeon prep are good alternates. There are instances where substituting one pose for another is optimal.

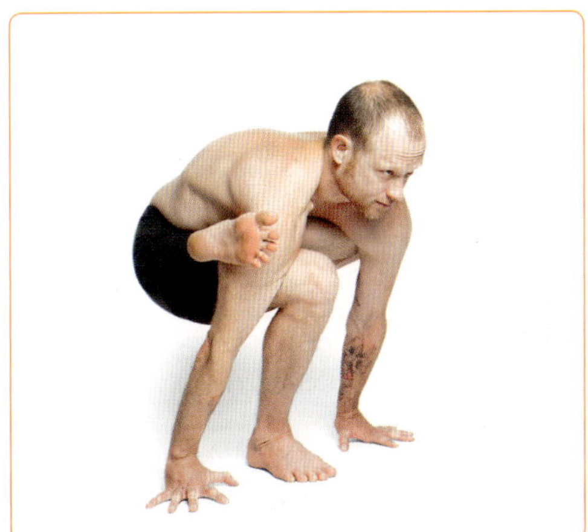

nesting pigeon

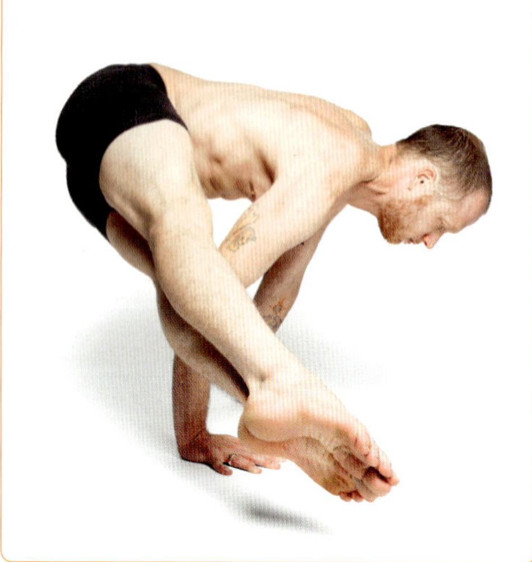

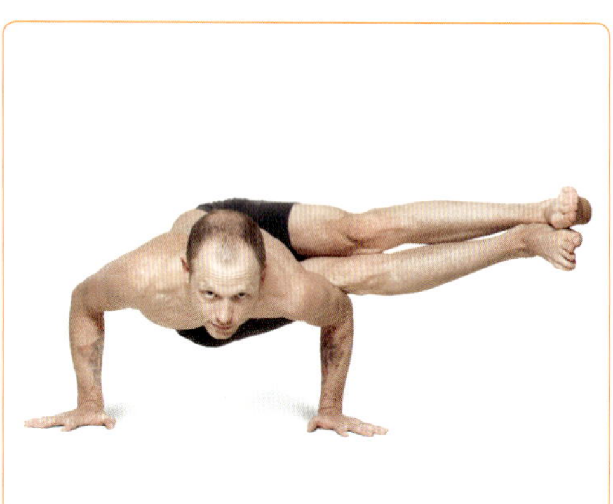

two-leg k sage
dwi pada koundinyasana

shape prep (from mountain)
- Come into a squat position.
- Bring ankles, knees together.
- Place fingertips on floor behind hips.
- Lift right arm, twist to left, place right shoulder outside left knee.
- Place hands on floor outside left hip—hands slightly wider than shoulder-width apart. Separate fingers, point index fingers straight ahead.
- Tiptoe, lean to left, transfer weight onto hands.

shape pose
- Stay here or lift hips and feet up, straighten legs.
- Bend elbows to a 90-degree angle; squeeze elbows in (more difficult: straighten left arm).

safety (strength) prep
- Grip floor with fingertips, press inner edges of hands down.
- Lift shoulders.
- Squeeze legs together.
- Tone, turn abdomen to left.

safety (strength) pose
- Tone thighs, tighten kneecaps, firm hamstrings.

Repeat on the second side.

If two leg k sage practitioner proves too difficult, perform firmly rotated pose instead.

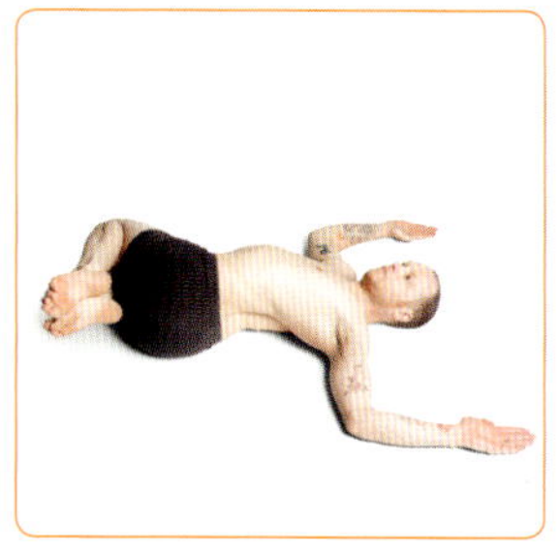

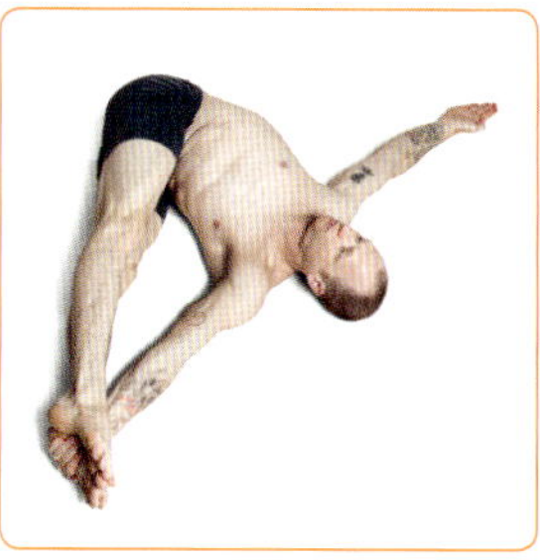

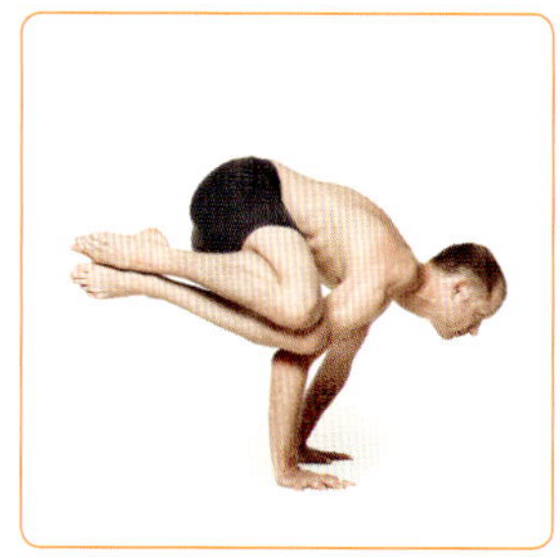

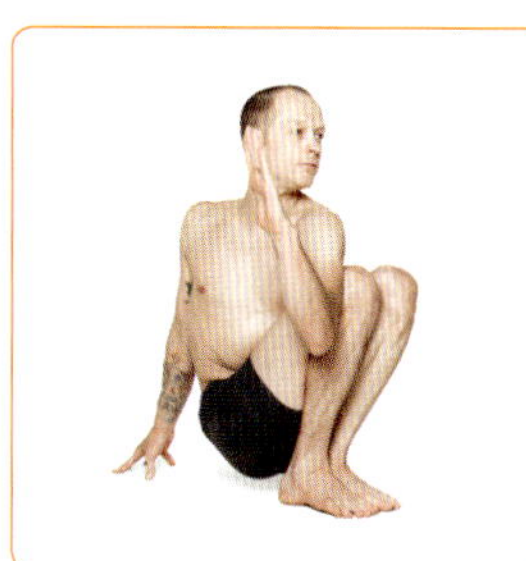

k sage 1
eka pada koundinyasana 1

shape pose (from two leg k sage, elbows bent)

▌ Extend top leg straight back; point kneecap out—parallel to long edge of mat (more difficult: straighten left arm).

▌ Flex feet (more difficult: point feet).

safety (strength) prep

▌ Grip floor with fingertips, press inner edges of hands down.

▌ Lift shoulders.

▌ Tone abdomen.

refinement (stretch) pose

▌ Press hands down.

Repeat on the second side.

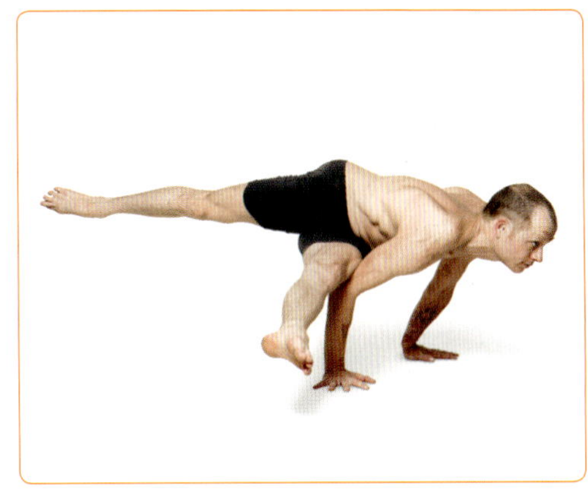

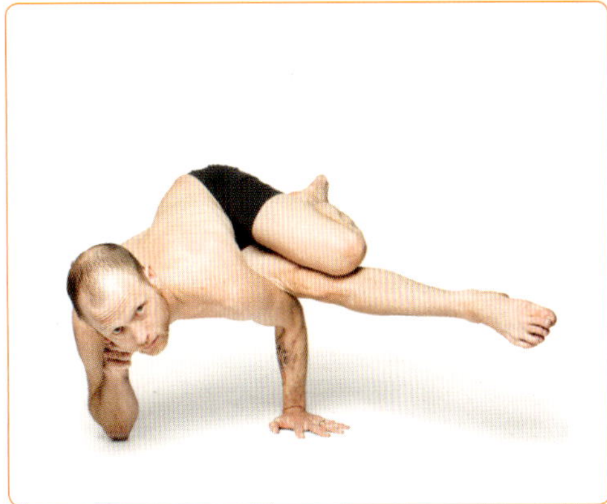

wild card

Like many poses, k sage 1 can be entered into from several different poses. I often teach this pose from down dog:

▢ Separate feet as wide as hands.

▢ Step right foot to floor outside left hand, bend knee, bring shin as vertical as possible.

▢ Slide right hand to right 4-6 inches.

▢ Lift left hand, place left shoulder outside knee, place left hand on floor in line with right hand, hands slightly wider than shoulder-width apart. Separate fingers, point index fingers straight ahead.

▢ Lean to right, transfer weight onto hands.

▢ Stay here, or lift right, then left, foot off floor.

▢ Bend elbows—upper arms parallel to floor, squeeze elbows in (more difficult: straighten right arm).

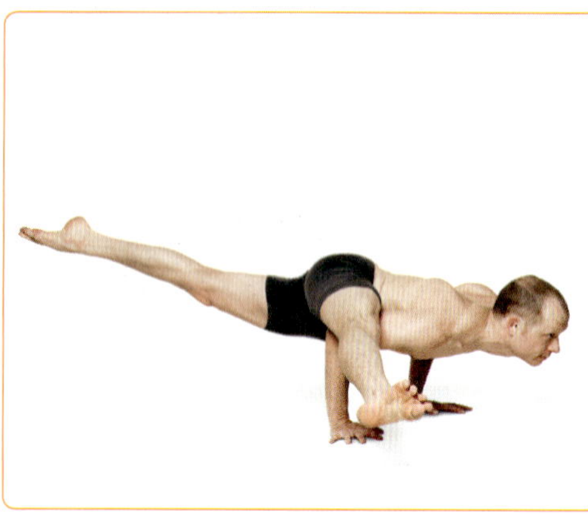

k sage 2
eka pada koundinyasana 2

shape prep (from downward facing dog)
▨ Come into four-limbed staff pose with right knee on upper right arm above elbow, bend right knee.

shape pose
▨ Stay here, or lean forward. Lift back leg up—point back kneecap down.
▨ Keep front knee bent (more difficult: straighten leg).
▨ Point feet.

safety (strength) prep
▨ Grip floor with fingertips, press inner edges of hands down.

safety (strength) prep
▨ Lift shoulders, squeeze elbows in.
▨ Tighten glutes, press tailbone down, tone abdomen.

safety (strength) pose
▨ Tone thighs, tighten kneecaps, firm hamstrings.

refinement (stretch) pose
▨ Press hands down.
▨ Lift chest, stretch spine.

Repeat on the second side.

peacock
mayurasana

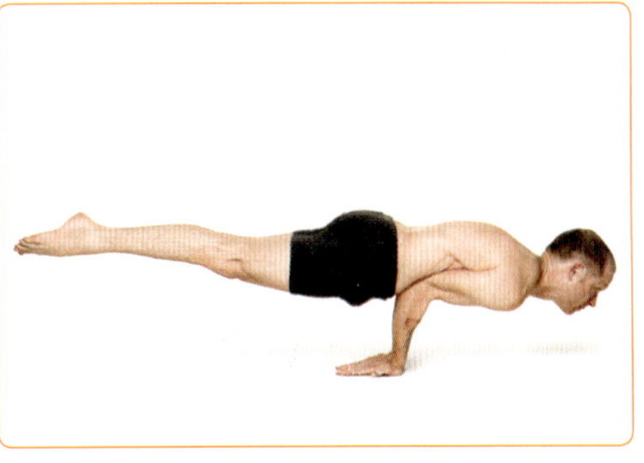

shape prep
▯ Come onto hands and knees. Separate knees slightly wider than hips.
▯ Have a seat on heels with toes curled under.
▯ Bring torso upright.
▯ Bring outer edges of hands together.
▯ Separate fingers (more difficult: close fingers).
▯ Place palms flat on floor under hips with fingers pointing back, pinkies in, thumbs out.
▯ Bend elbows. Rest abdomen on elbows as near to waistline as possible with elbows inside ribs. Place head on floor.
▯ Stay here or one at a time straighten legs—bring ankles together (more difficult: point feet, place tops of feet on floor with heels together).

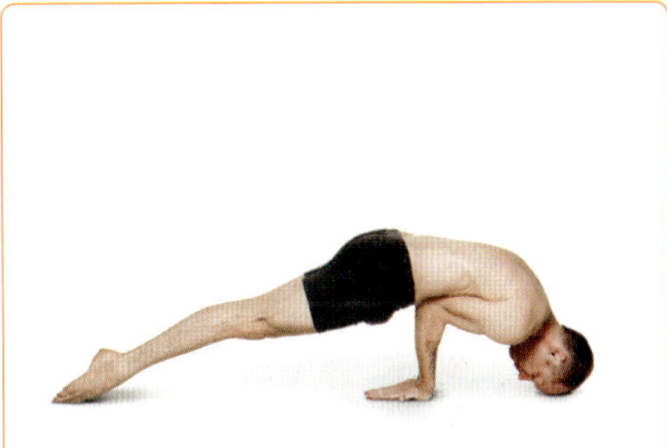

shape pose
▯ Stay here, or straighten arms slightly, lift head then feet off floor.
▯ Point feet.
▯ Lift chin, look forward.

safety (strength) prep
▯ Grip floor with fingertips, press palms down evenly.
▯ Lift shoulders.
▯ Tighten glutes, press tailbone down, tone abdomen, firm hamstrings.
▯ Do not attempt the classical form of this pose until you can hold peacock prep (feet and head on floor) for 30 plus seconds.

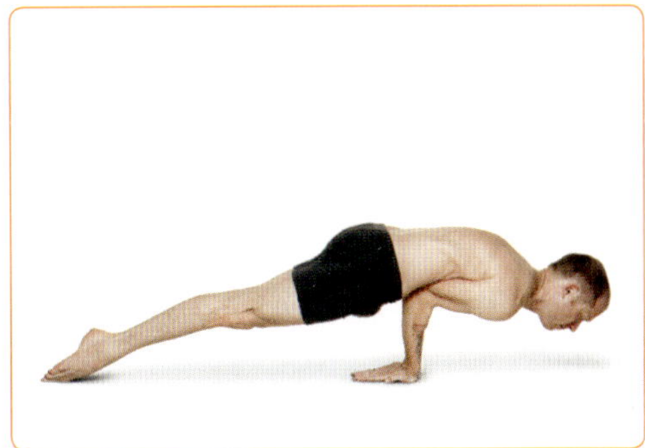

refinement (stretch) pose
▯ Hold pose, not breath.

This pose is very yogahour, in that it puts and keeps the pressure on.

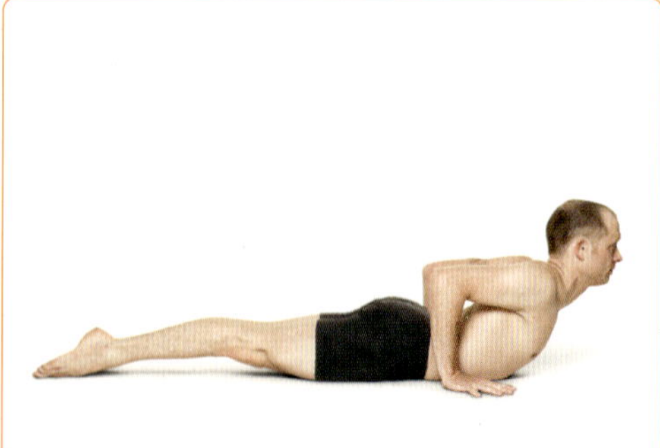

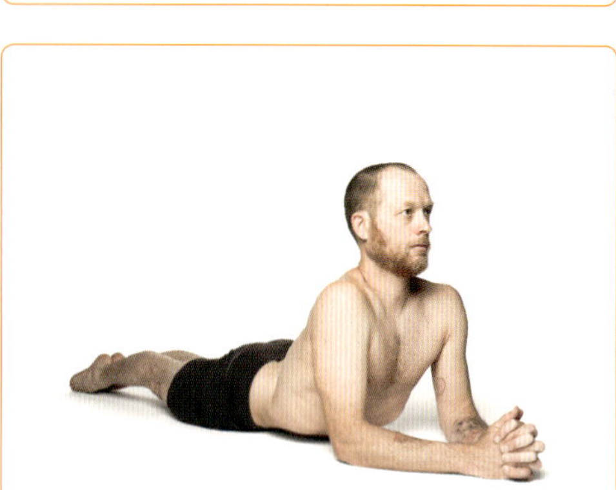

cobra *torso on floor*
bhujangasana prep

shape prep
- Bring front body to floor.
- Lift chin, look straight ahead.
- Place hands in a push-up position—forearms straight up and down. Separate hands slightly wider than shoulders. Separate fingers, point index fingers straight ahead.

shape pose
- Lift shoulders up to capacity.
- Point feet, bring inner heels together.
- Straighten legs.

safety (strength) prep
- Grip floor with fingertips, press inner edges of hands down.

safety (strength) pose
- Press heels together.
- Tighten glutes, press tailbone down, tone abdomen, firm hamstrings.

refinement (stretch) pose
- Press hands down, back.
- Stretch chest forward.

Cobra prep is an excellent warm-up and teaches the key alignment for four limbed staff pose, cobra, and up dog.

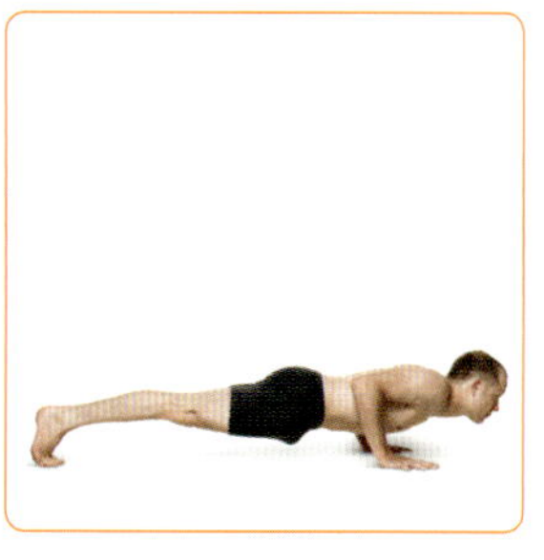

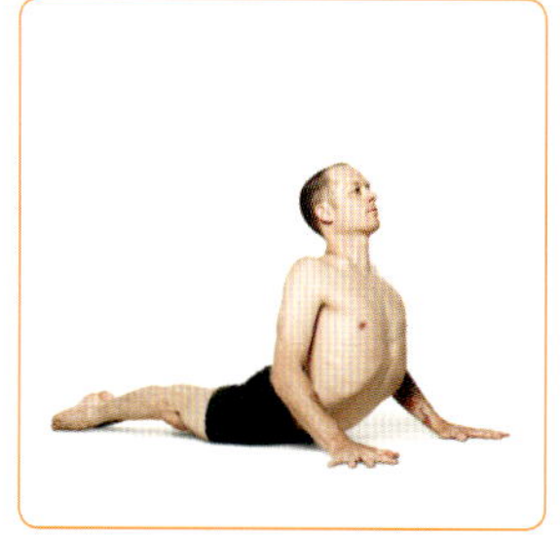

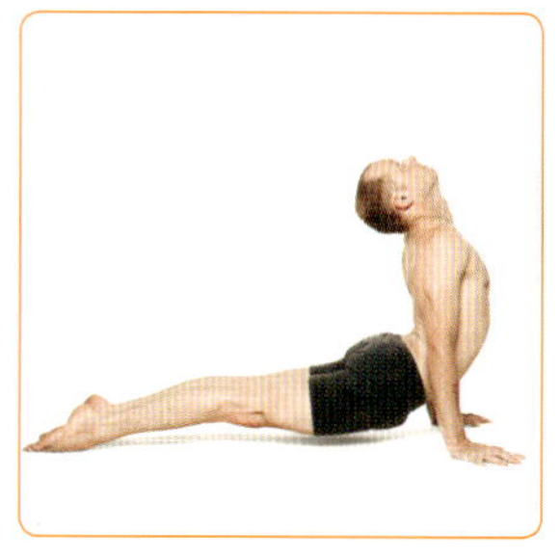

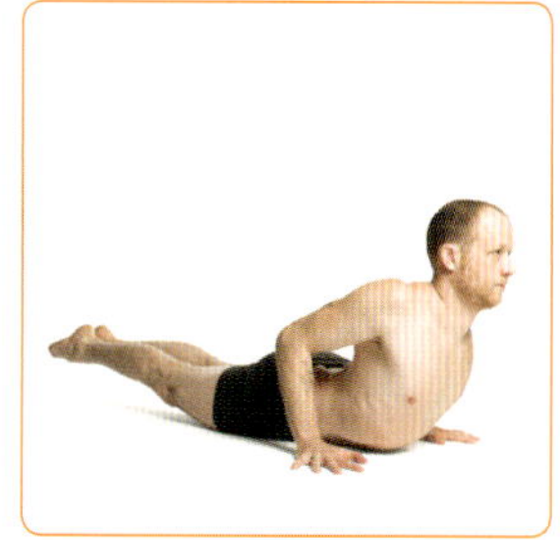

cobra *elbows bent*
bhujangasana prep

shape prep
- Bring front body to floor.
- Point feet, bring inner edges of heels together.
- Straighten legs.
- Lift chin, look straight ahead.
- Place hands by chest with forearms straight up and down.
- Separate hands slightly wider than shoulders. Separate fingers, point index fingers straight ahead.
- Lift shoulders up to capacity.
- Move elbows in.

shape pose
- Lift torso, elbows slightly bent.
- Look straight ahead (more difficult: look up or back).

safety (strength) prep
- Grip floor with fingertips, press inner edges of hands down.
- Engage upper back muscles. Move shoulders up, back and in.
- Press heels together.
- Press feet down, lift knees up.
- Tighten glutes, press tailbone down, tone abdomen, firm hamstrings.

safety (strength) pose
- If looking up or back, tone neck, relax jaw.

refinement (stretch) pose
- Press hands down, back; lift chest up.
- Stretch spine.

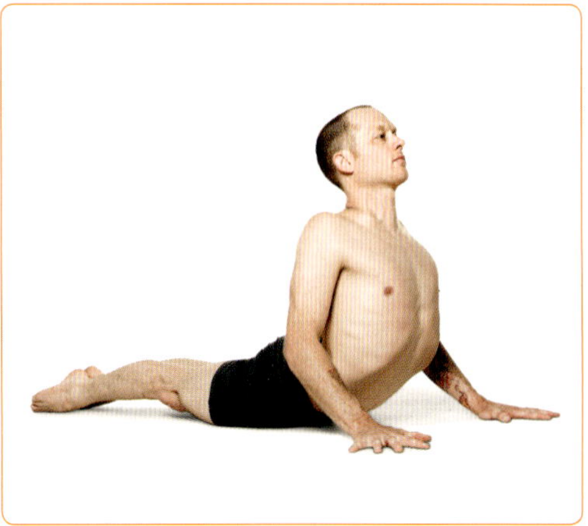

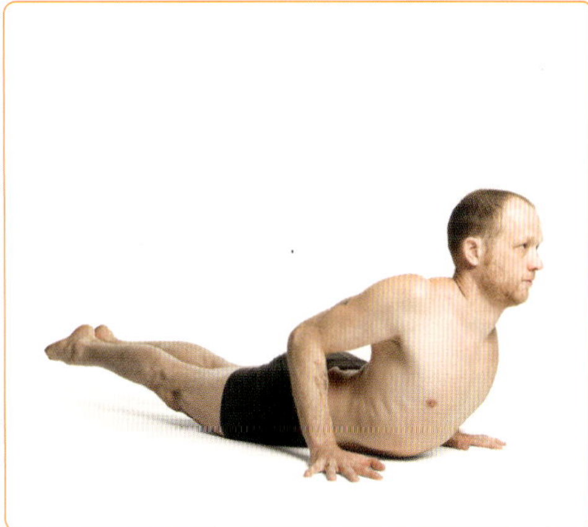

cobra *legs lifted*

upward facing dog

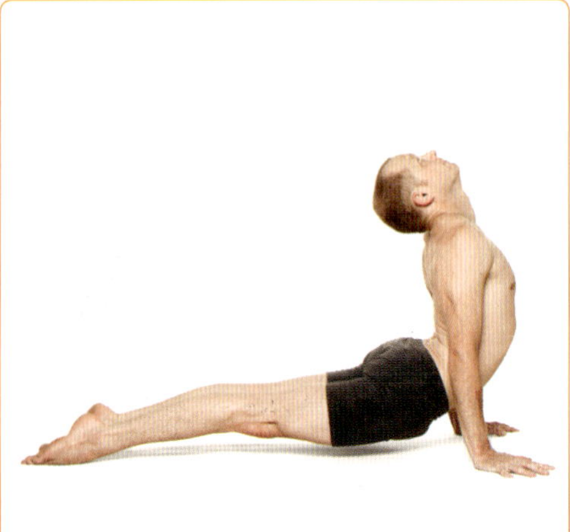

shape prep
- Bring front body to floor.
- Point feet, bring feet outer hip-width apart.
- Straighten legs.
- Lift chin, look straight ahead.
- Place hands by chest with forearms straight up and down.
- Separate hands slightly wider than shoulder-width apart. Separate fingers, point index fingers straight ahead.
- Lift shoulders up to capacity.
- Move elbows in.

shape pose
- Straighten arms—lift hips off floor. In upward facing dog, the hands and feet are the only parts of the body that touch the floor (more doable: come into plank pose with tops of feet on floor).
- Look straight ahead (more difficult: look up or back).

safety (strength) prep
- Grip floor with fingertips, press inner edges of hands down.
- Engage upper back muscles—move shoulders back.
- Press feet down, in.
- Tighten glutes, press tailbone down, tone abdomen, firm hamstrings.

safety (strength) pose
- If looking up or back, tone neck, relax jaw.

refinement (stretch) pose
- Press hands down, back.
- Expand and lift chest up, back.
- Stretch spine.

plank *tops of feet on floor*

locust 2
salabhasana 2

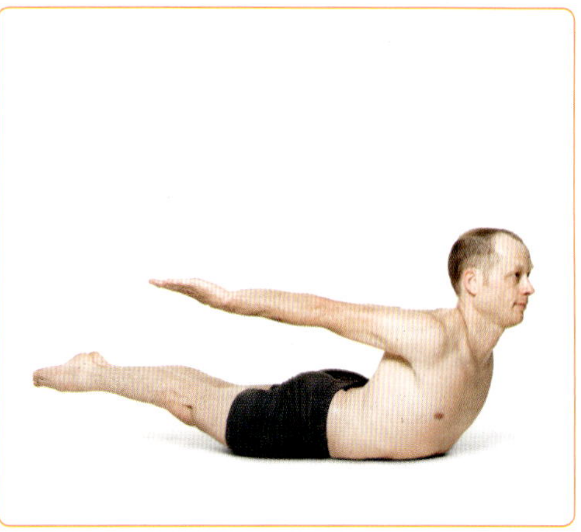

shape prep
- Bring front body to floor.
- Lift chin, look straight ahead.
- Bring arms alongside torso. Close fingers—point palms up.
- Point feet, bring inner edges of feet together—including heels.
- Straighten legs.

shape pose
- Lift everything except hips off floor (more doable: fallen 1—keep feet and hands on floor).
- Straighten arms. Lift hands to capacity—lift inner edges of hands higher than outer edges.
- Bend in upper back as deeply as possible.

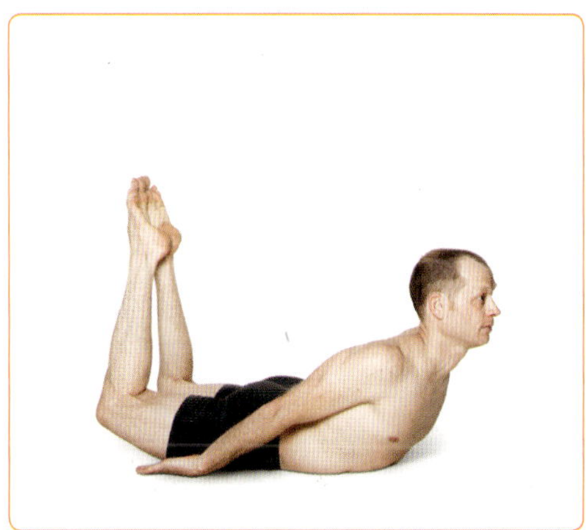

safety (strength) prep
- Squeeze heels together.
- Tighten glutes, press tailbone down, tone abdomen.

safety (strength) pose
- Squeeze shoulders together on back.

refinement (stretch) pose
- Lift chest, stretch spine.

locust 1
salabhasana 1

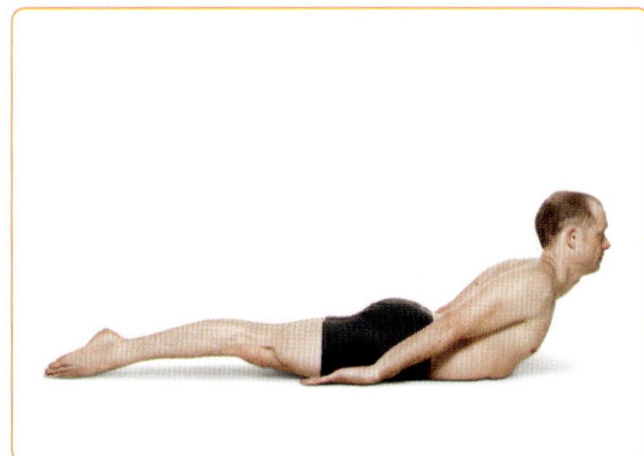

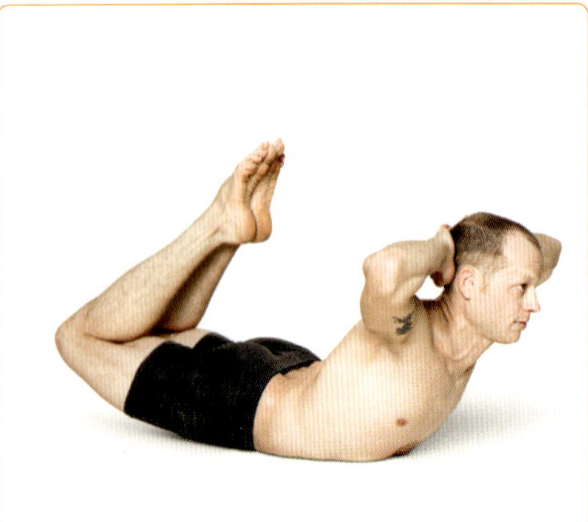

crocodile *knees bent*

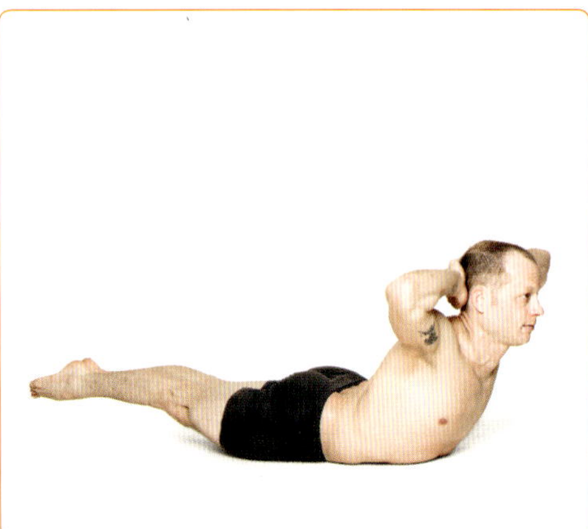

crocodile

crocodile
makarasana

shape prep
■ Place forehead on floor. Interlace fingers behind head—head, not neck. Lift the elbows so arms are parallel to floor.
■ Bend knees to capacity, heels as close to hips as possible.
■ Point feet, bring inner edges of feet together—including heels.

shape pose
■ Lift legs, torso up. Lift chin, look straight ahead.
■ Bend in upper back as deeply as possible.

safety (strength) prep
■ Squeeze feet together.
■ Squeeze knees in slightly—knees outer hip-width apart.
■ Tighten glutes, press tailbone down, tone abdomen.

safety (strength) pose
■ Keeping fingers interlaced, squeeze shoulders in.
■ Press head into hands, with hands lift back of head.

refinement (stretch) pose
■ Lift chest, stretch spine.
■ Extend elbows out.

The prevalence of low back pain can be preventable. Regular practice of makarasana and locust variations is an effective way to strengthen the low back (as I often say when teaching class: "make your spine strong like a crocodile's tail!").

superhero

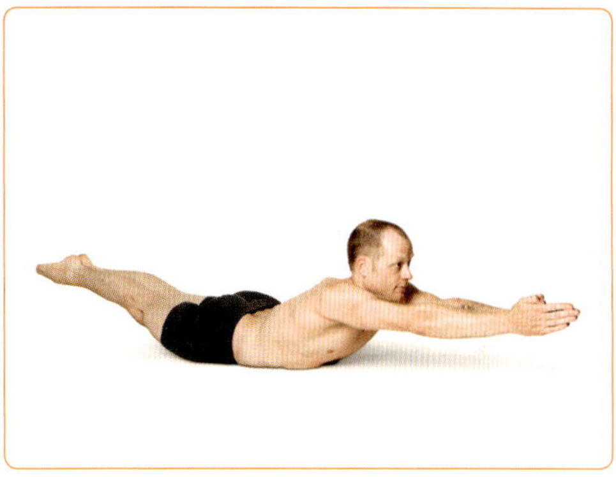

shape prep
- Bring front body to floor.
- Lift chin, look straight ahead.
- Place outer edges of hands on floor in front of torso, straighten arms. Separate hands shoulder-width apart (more difficult: place palms together).
- Keeping hands on floor, lift torso to capacity.
- Separate feet outer hip-width apart.
- Point feet, straighten legs, point kneecaps straight down.

shape pose
- Lift hands, feet off floor—arms parallel to floor.

safety (strength) prep
- Tighten glutes, press tailbone down, tone abdomen, firm hamstrings.

safety (strength) pose
- Lift shoulders—hollow armpits.

refinement (stretch) pose
- Lift chest, stretch spine.

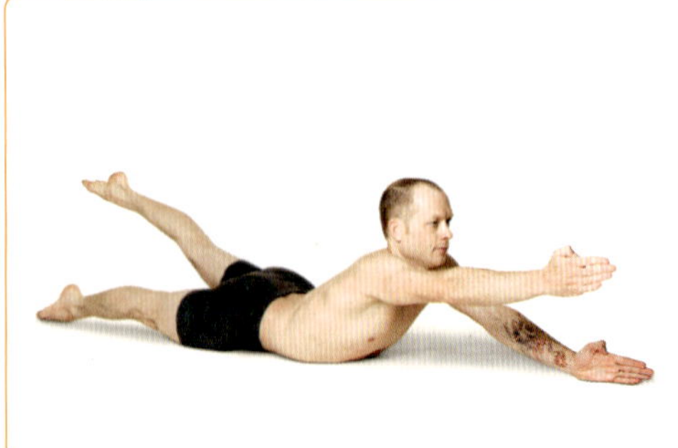

topsy-turvy superhero *opposite arm/leg*

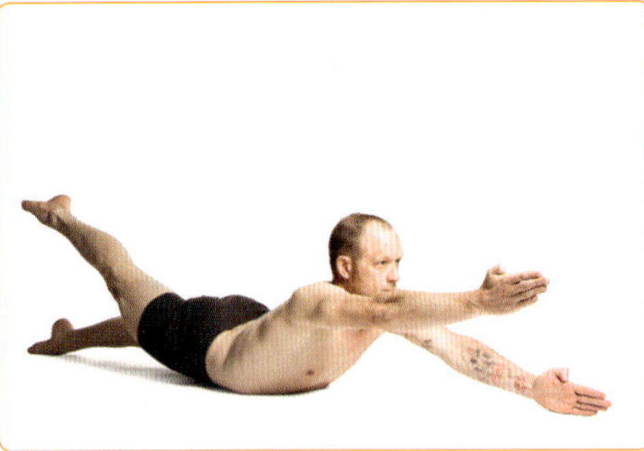

topsy-turvy superhero *same arm/leg*

topsy-turvy superhero

shape prep
- Bring front body to floor.
- Lift chin, look straight ahead.
- Place outer edges of hands on floor in front of torso, straighten arms. Separate hands shoulder-width apart.
- Separate feet outer hip-width apart.
- Point feet, straighten legs, point kneecaps straight down.
- Keeping hands on floor, lift torso to capacity.

shape pose
- Lift right hand, left foot off floor—right arm parallel to floor.

safety (strength) pose
- Push left hand down, lift left shoulder up,
- Press right foot down, lift right knee up.
- Tighten glutes, press tailbone down, tone abdomen, firm hamstrings.

Repeat on the second side.

This asymmetrical pose can be a beneficial exercise for those with scoliosis because it engages the muscles along one side of the spine as it releases the muscles on the other. In doing so, this pose can strengthen the weak side as it releases the strong side, which can reduce back pain. I once had a 40-degree scoliosis C-curve and was in pain on a daily basis. Asana has significantly reduced my C-curve and taken away my back pain.

If you have scoliosis, you will need to learn to practice accordingly in order to shift your curve. For example, the way I twist to the right is different than how I twist to the left. My spine will never be perfectly straight or so-called "normal" —the back of my left ribcage is flat, my right ribcage is overly rounded; the muscles along the right side of my spine are overly developed, the left side underdeveloped. Even so, my back is hatha happy and healthy. I used to be embarrassed about my scoliosis, but yoga has helped me to love my body as it is. The same applies to those of us who were diagnosed with "learning disabilities." Yoga has helped me see that term as a misdiagnosis—"Learning different abilities," thank you very much!

inverted locust
viparita salabhasana prep

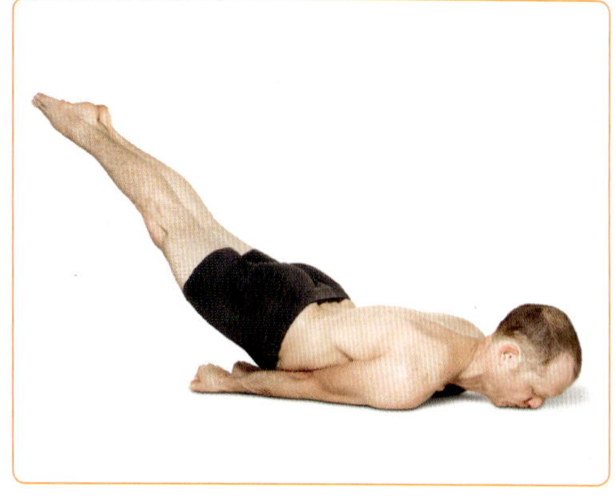

shape prep
- Bring front body to floor.
- One at a time, work arms under torso.
- Point palms down. Make fists with hands. Bring outer edges of hands together (more doable: point palms up).
- Bring face to floor—not chin.
- Point feet. Straighten legs so that knees lift off floor.

shape pose
- Stay here, or lift feet off floor (another variation: lift one foot at a time off floor).

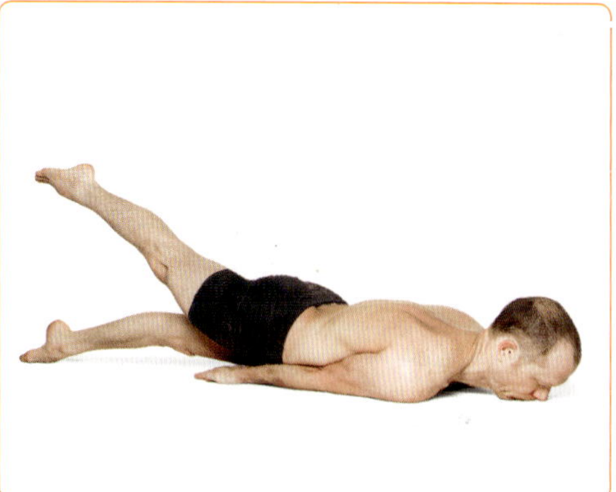

safety (strength) prep
- Press heels together.
- Press feet down, lift knees up.
- Tighten glutes, press tailbone/hips down. Firm hamstrings.
- Tone abdomen.
- Press fists down, lift elbows up (avoid overly stretching elbows or biceps).

refinement (stretch) pose
- Hold pose, not breath.

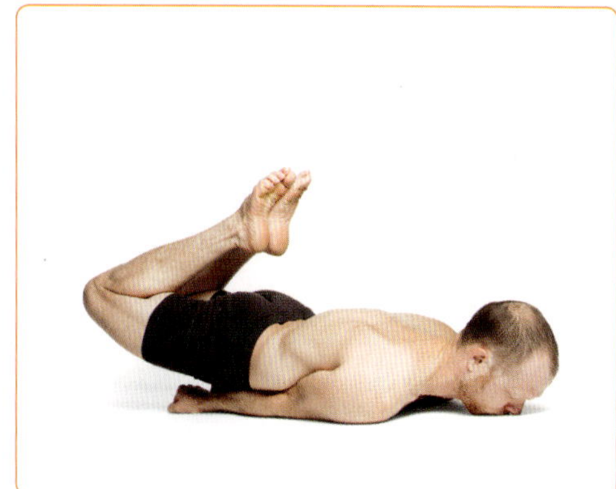

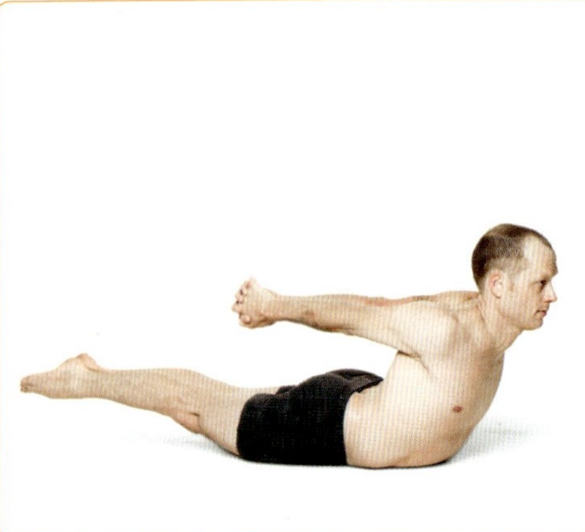

locust *hands bound*
baddha hasta salabhasana

shape prep
- Bring front body to floor.
- Lift chin, look straight ahead.
- Interlace fingers behind hips with elbows slightly bent.
- Bring shoulders together on back, straighten arms.

shape pose
- Lift everything except hips off floor.
- Point feet, bring inner edges of feet together—including heels.
- Straighten legs, arms. Lift hands to capacity.
- Bend in upper back as deeply as possible.

safety (strength) pose
- Squeeze heels together.
- Tighten glutes, press tailbone down, tone abdomen.
- Squeeze shoulders together on back.

refinement (stretch) pose
- Lift chest, stretch spine.

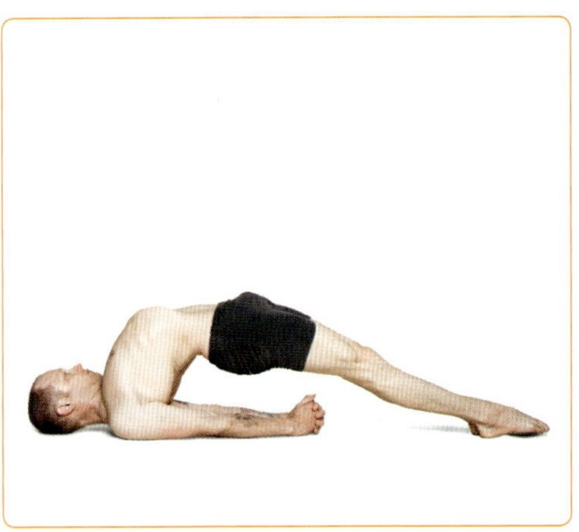

eight-angle pose
astangasana

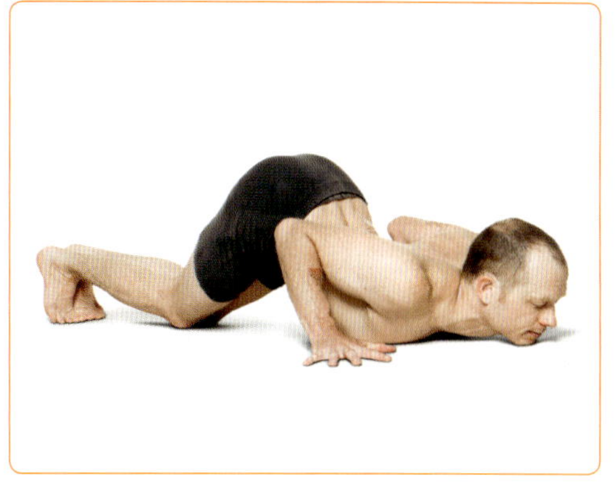

shape prep
- Have a seat on heels with toes curled under at back of mat.
- Bring knees/ankles together.

shape pose
- Keeping toe mounds and knees on floor, lower chest, chin, hands to floor—hips 4–12 inches above floor.
- Place hands by chest, slightly wider than shoulders. Separate fingers, point index fingers straight ahead.
- Move elbows in, lift shoulders up to capacity.
- Look at tip of nose.

safety (strength) pose
- Do not put any weight on chin.
- Grip floor with fingertips, press inner edges of hands down.
- Squeeze ankles, knees together.
- Tone abdomen.

refinement (stretch) pose
- Press hands down, back.

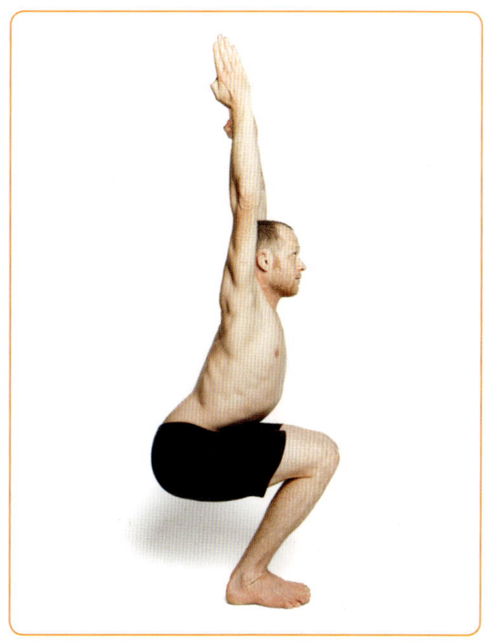

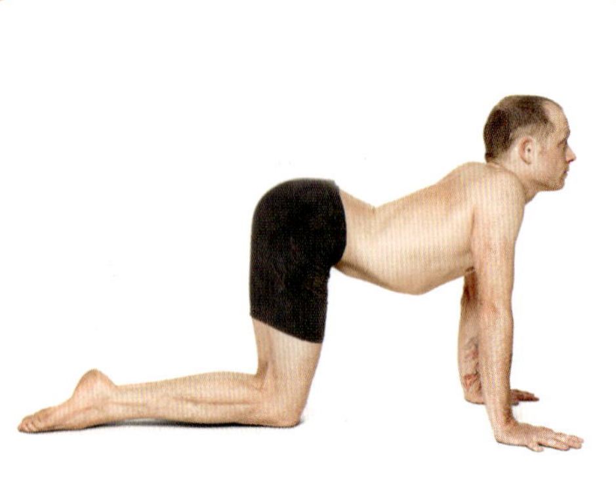

COW
bitilasana

shape prep
- Come onto hands and knees with arms and thighs straight up and down.
- Separate hands slightly wider than shoulder-width apart. Separate fingers, point index fingers straight ahead.
- Bring knees, ankles together. Point feet.

shape pose
- Bring spine into a slight backbend.
- Lift chin, look up.

safety (strength) prep
- Grip floor with fingertips, press inner edges of hands down.
- Tone biceps, triceps.
- Squeeze knees, ankles together.

safety (strength) prep
- Tighten glutes, tone abdomen. Press tailbone down without rounding back.

refinement (stretch) pose
- Lift chest, stretch spine.

Bitilasana—most often done in tandem with cat pose—is an excellent pose in its own right. It's an effective warm-up and intro to backbends.

southpaw tiger
vyaghrasana

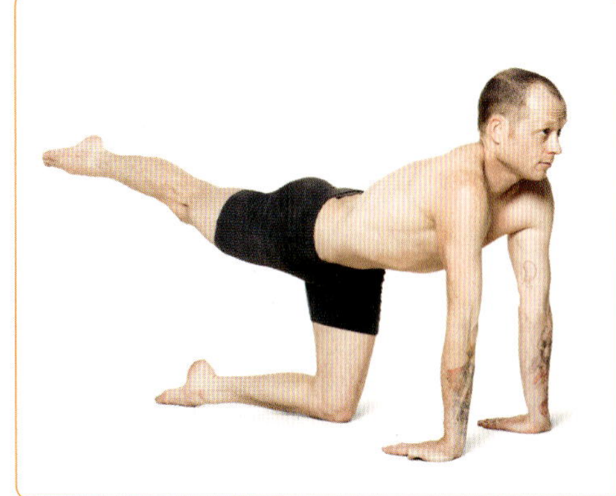

shape prep
- Come onto hands and knees with arms and thighs vertical to floor.
- Separate hands slightly wider than shoulder-width apart.
- Separate knees, feet outer hip-width apart. Point feet.
- Turn hands out 180 degrees so fingers point at knees. Close fingers.

shape pose
- Lift right leg up, back, parallel to floor (more difficult: lift leg to capacity).
- Point right foot, straighten leg. Point kneecap down.
- Lift chin, look straight ahead.
- Round upper back.

safety (strength) prep
- Press fingers down, tone triceps.

safety (strength) pose
- Tighten glutes, press tailbone down, tone abdomen, firm hamstrings.
- Press left foot down, squeeze ankle in.

Southpaw tiger is an optimal warm-up for the forearms, legs, and spine.

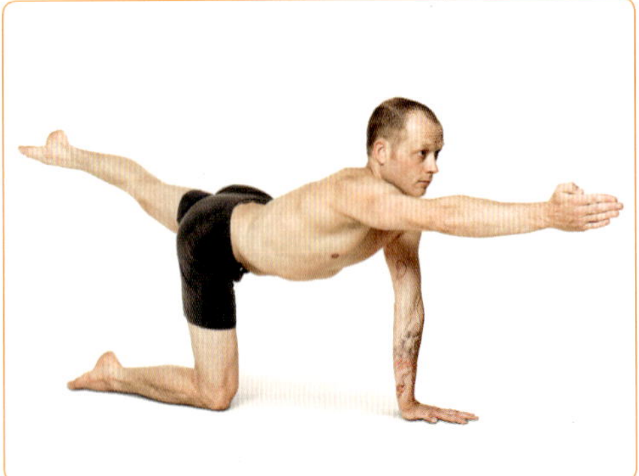

tiger *opposite arm/leg*
vyaghrasana

shape prep
■ Come onto hands and knees with arms and thighs vertical to floor.
■ Separate hands slightly wider than shoulder-width apart. Separate fingers, point index fingers straight ahead.
■ Separate knees, feet outer hip-width apart. Point feet.

shape pose
■ Lift right arm, left leg parallel to floor (more difficult: lift arm, leg to capacity).
■ Point right palm in, close fingers.
■ Point left foot, straighten leg. Point kneecap down.
■ Straighten arms, legs. Square hips.
■ Lift chin, look straight ahead.

safety (strength) pose
■ Grip floor with fingertips, press inner edge of left hand down.
■ Press right foot down, squeeze ankle in.
■ Tighten glutes, press tailbone down, tone abdomen, firm hamstrings.

refinement (stretch) pose
■ Stretch lifted arm, leg.
■ Stretch spine.

Repeat on the second side.

This pose is a good prep for any and all asymmetrical backbends.

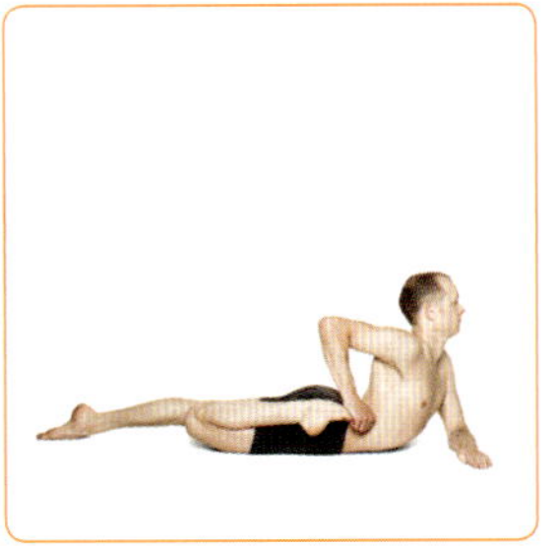
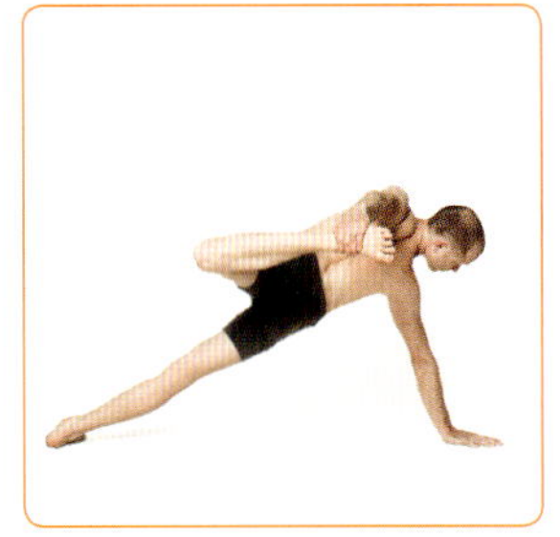
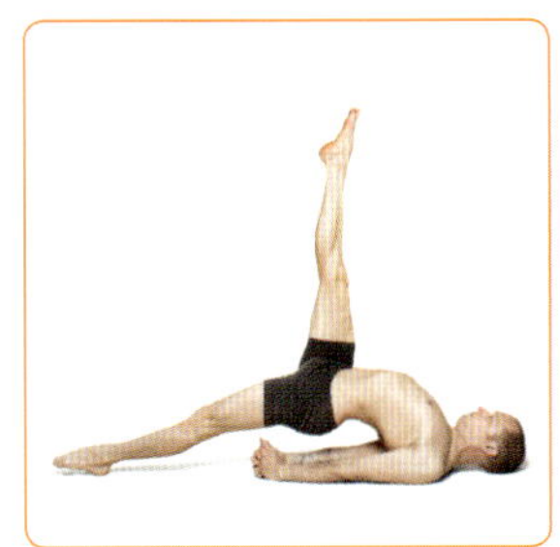
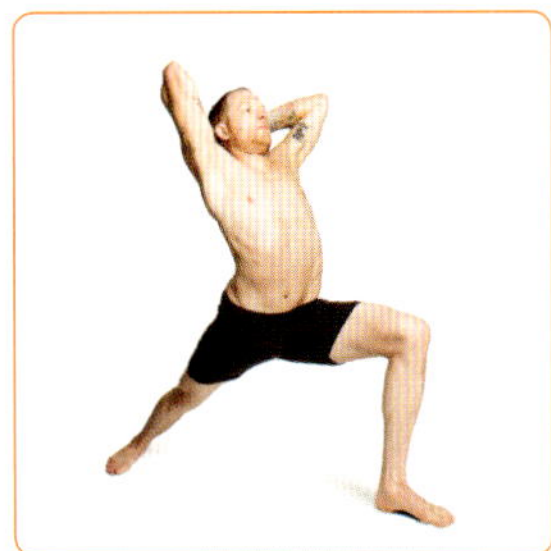

tiger *same arm/leg*
vyaghrasana

shape prep
▮ Come onto hands and knees with arms and thighs vertical to floor.
▮ Separate hands slightly wider than shoulder-width apart. Separate fingers, point index fingers straight ahead.
▮ Separate knees, feet outer hip-width apart. Point feet.

shape pose
▮ Lift right arm, right leg parallel to floor (more difficult: lift arm, leg to capacity).
▮ Point right palm in, close fingers.
▮ Point right foot, point right kneecap down.
▮ Square hips.
▮ Straighten lifted arm, leg.
▮ Lift chin, look straight ahead.

safety (strength) pose
▮ Grip floor with fingertips, press inner edge of left hand down.
▮ Press left foot down, squeeze ankle in.
▮ Tighten glutes, press tailbone down, tone abdomen, firm hamstrings.

refinement (stretch) pose
▮ Stretch lifted arm, leg.
▮ Stretch spine.

Repeat on the second side.

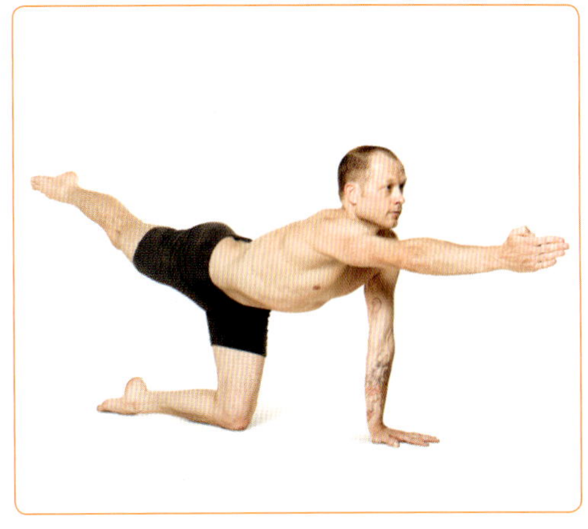

tiger leg lifts

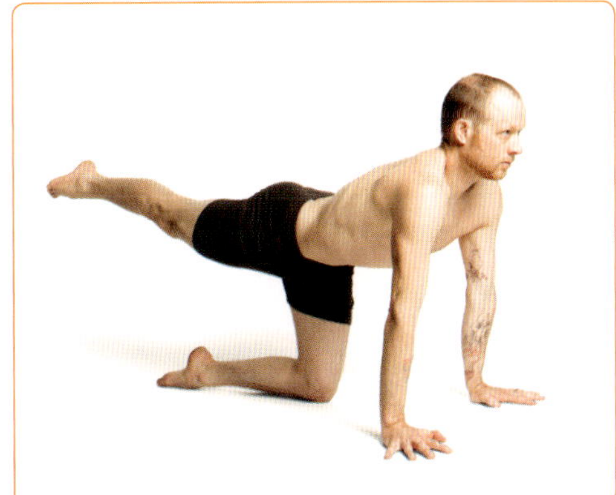

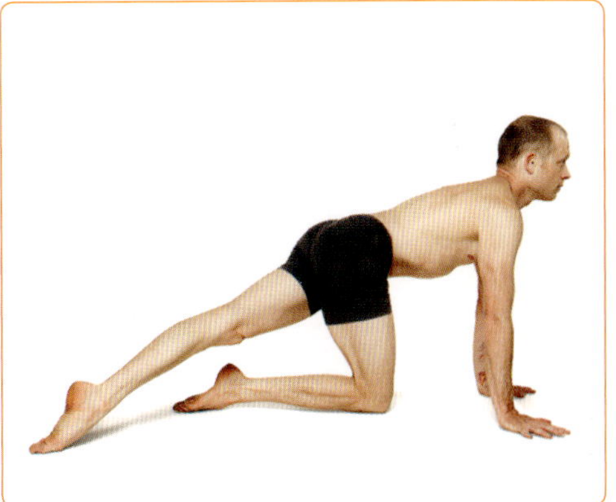

As a high school wrestler I noticed, that unlike many of their opponents, the top wrestlers were comfortable being slightly off balance. They were capable of turning loss-worthy situations into a win. They often spontaneously made up moves on the spot, which their opponent had no counter for. What works and wins in one realm, often works and wins another. As my Dad often told me, "It's all transferable." And as Frank Zappa said, "Without deviation from the norm, progress is not possible." One: know the norm inside and out. Two: dharma deviate.

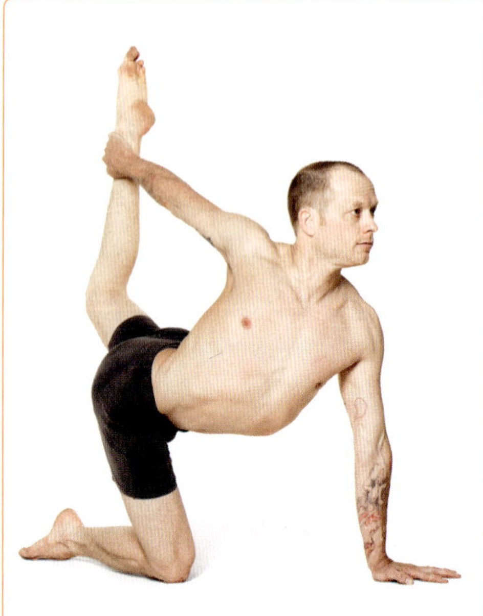

elevated bow 2 *opposite arm/leg*
eka pada dhanurasana

shape prep
- Come onto hands and knees with arms and thighs vertical to floor.
- Separate hands slightly wider than shoulder-width apart. Separate fingers, point index fingers straight ahead.
- Separate knees, feet outer hip-width apart. Point feet.

shape pose
- Lift right leg parallel to floor, bend knee, clasp inner or outer edge of right foot or ankle with left hand; straighten left arm.
- Stay here, or kick top foot back, up.
- Square hips. Look forward.

safety (strength) pose
- Grip floor with fingertips, press inner edge of hand down.
- Press bottom foot down, squeeze ankle in.
- Squeeze top thigh in slightly.
- Tighten glutes, press tailbone down, tone abdomen, firm hamstrings.
- Lift leg with leg.

refinement (stretch) pose
- Lift chest, stretch spine.

Repeat on the second side.

elevated bow 1 *same arm/leg*
eka pada dhanurasana

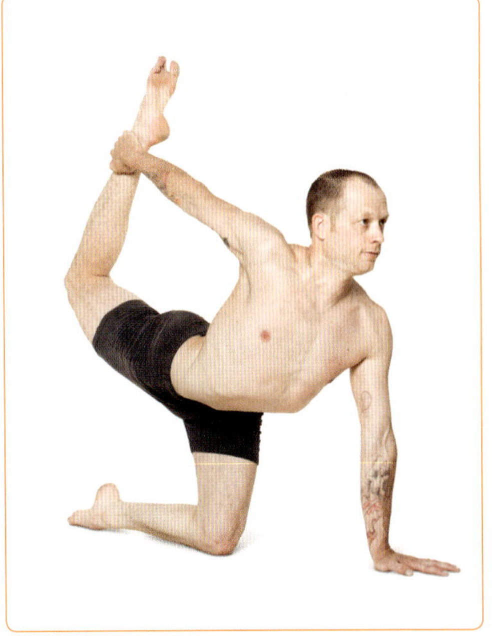

shape prep
■ Come onto hands and knees with arms and thighs vertical to floor.
■ Separate hands slightly wider than shoulder-width apart. Separate fingers, point index fingers straight ahead.
■ Separate knees, feet outer hip-width apart. Point feet.

shape pose
■ Lift right leg parallel to floor, bend knee, clasp outer edge of right foot or ankle with right hand; straighten right arm.
■ Stay here, or kick top foot back, up.
■ Square hips. Look forward.

safety (strength) pose
■ Grip floor with fingertips, press inner edge of hand down.
■ Press bottom foot down, squeeze ankle in.
■ Squeeze top thigh in slightly.
■ Tighten glutes, press tailbone down, tone abdomen, firm hamstrings.
■ Lift leg with leg, not just via kicking foot into hand, which will only work quads.

refinement (stretch) pose
■ Lift chest, stretch spine

Repeat on the second side.

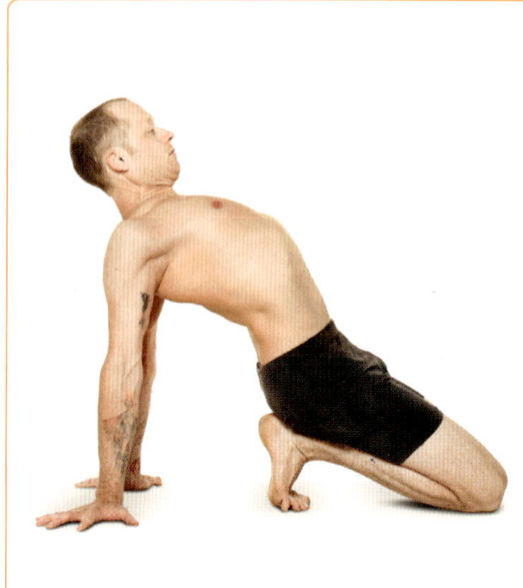

thunderbolt *quad stretch*
vajrasana

shape prep
- Have a seat on heels with toes curled under, bring knees together.

shape pose
- Place hands on floor a foot and a half behind hips; hands slightly wider than shoulders.
- Turn hands out so index fingers point at long edges of mat.
- Straighten arms.
- Look straight ahead (more difficult: look up or back).

safety (strength) pose
- Grip floor with fingertips, press inner edges of hands down.
- Squeeze knees together.
- Tighten glutes, lift tailbone, tone abdomen, move ribs back.
- If looking back, engage throat, relax jaw (do not relax/collapse neck). When in doubt: look forward.

refinement (stretch) pose
- Press hands down, lift chest, stretch spine.

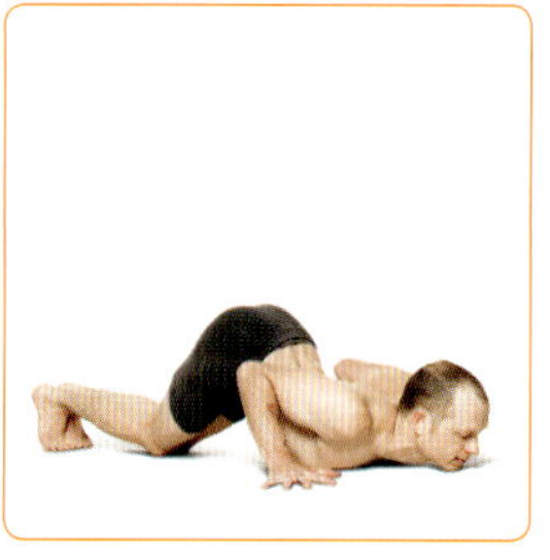
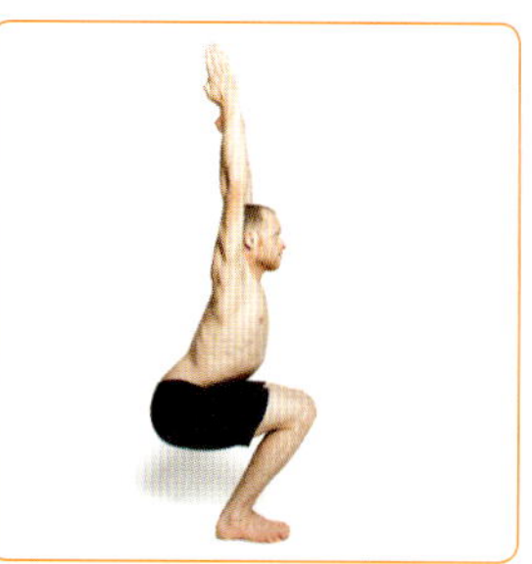
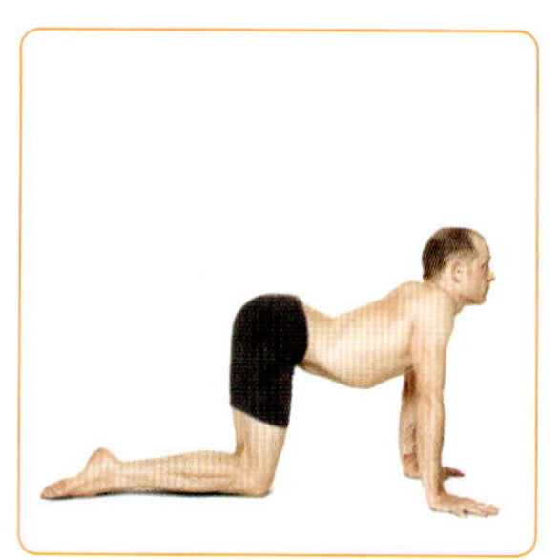
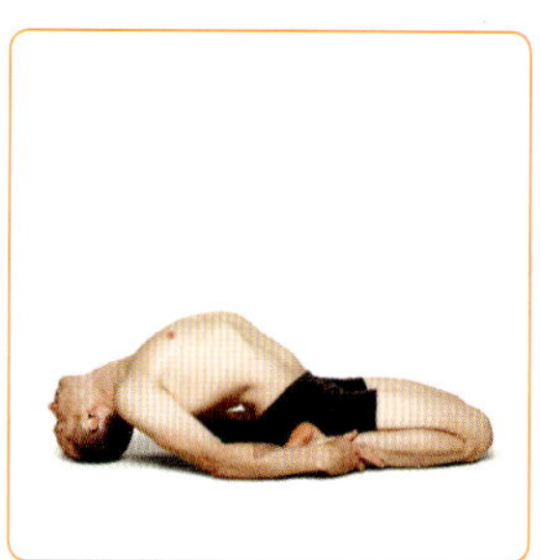

reverse table
purvottanasana prep

shape prep (from staff pose)
Place hands about a foot and a half behind hips with hands slightly wider than shoulders. Turn hands out so that index fingers point toward long edge of mat. Straighten arms.
Bend knees, place feet flat on floor about a foot and a half in front of hips.
Separate feet outer hip-width apart, point big toes straight ahead.

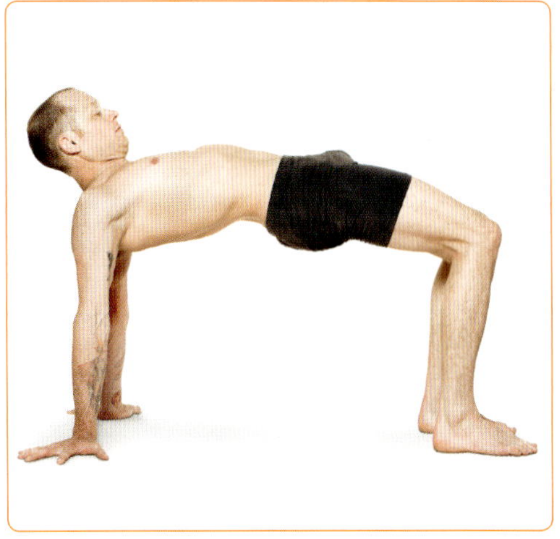

shape pose
Lift hips—thighs parallel to floor and long edge of mat.
Look straight ahead (more difficult: look up or back).

safety (strength) prep
Grip floor with fingertips. Press inner edges of hands down.
Squeeze shoulders onto back.

safety (strength) pose
Tone, turn inner thighs down. Press inner edges of feet down, flare toes. Squeeze feet in.
Tighten glutes, lift tailbone, tone abdomen.
If looking back, tone throat, relax jaw.

refinement (stretch) prep
Lift chest, stretch spine.

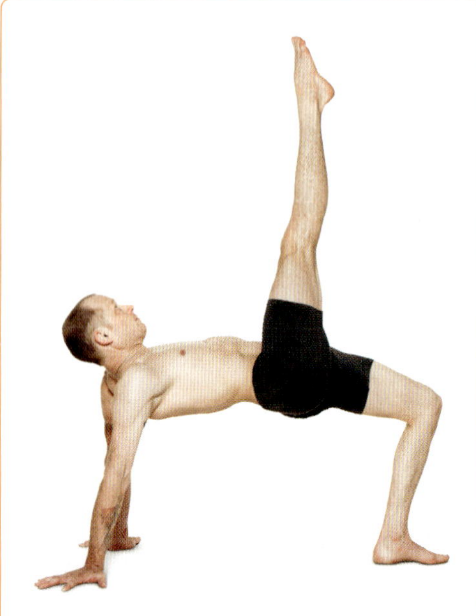

reverse table *leg lifted*
purvottanasana prep

shape pose (from reverse table)
Lift and straighten right leg—leg vertical to floor (more doable: bring right shin parallel to floor or right heel to hip).

safety (strength) prep
Grip floor with fingertips, press inner edges of hands down.

safety (strength) pose
Flare toes, press inner edge of left foot down.
Tone, turn left inner thigh down.
Squeeze right hip, left inner thigh together.
Tighten glutes, lift tailbone, tone abdomen.
If looking back, tone throat, relax jaw (looking forward will tone throat).

refinement (stretch) prep
Lift chest, stretch spine.

Repeat on the second side.

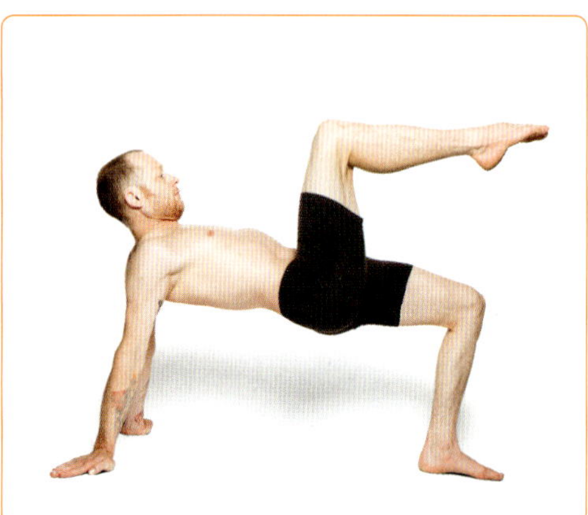

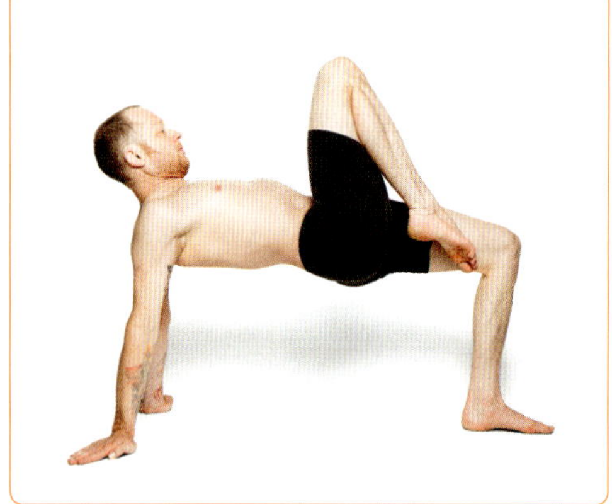

intense east stretch
purvottanasana

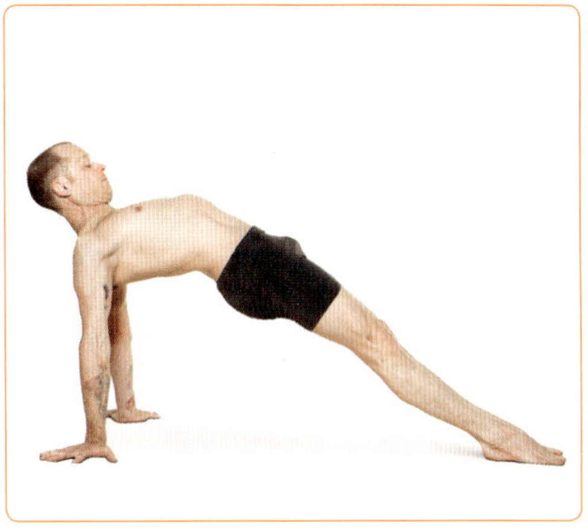

shape prep (from staff pose)
▮ Slide hands back about a foot and a half. Separate hands slightly wider than shoulders. Point index fingers out.
▮ Separate fingers evenly.
▮ Straighten arms.
▮ Point feet.

shape pose
▮ Lift hips—torso parallel to floor (more doable: bend knees to a 90° angle).
▮ Look forward (more difficult: look up or back).

safety (strength) prep
▮ Grip floor with fingertips, press index knuckles down.
▮ Squeeze shoulder blades together on back.

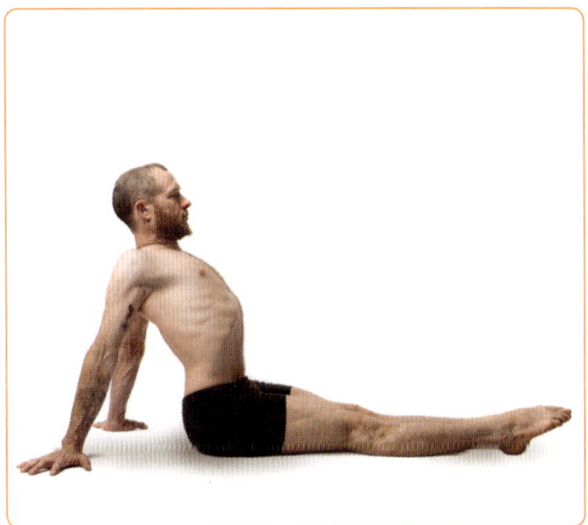

safety (strength) pose
▮ Squeeze ankles together. Press feet down.
▮ Tighten glutes, lift tailbone, tone abdomen.
▮ If looking back, tone throat, relax jaw.

refinement (stretch) prep
▮ Lift chest, stretch spine.

refinement (stretch) pose
▮ Lift hips two inches higher.

Purvottanasana is versatile: a warm-up prior to deep back-bends; a counterbalance post forward folds. It's also the other side of the same coin as intense west stretch.

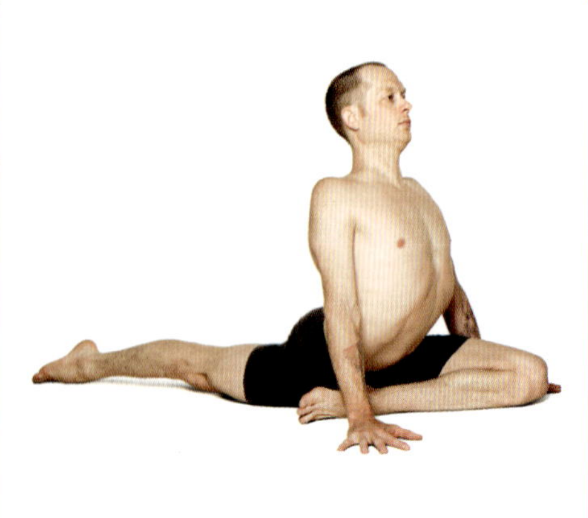

pigeon *torso upright*
eka pada rajakapotasana 1 prep

shape prep (from downward facing dog)
- Place right knee against right wrist.
- Lower hips, left leg to floor.
- Bring right heel against left hip (more doable: lean onto right hip so that right knee, thigh, and hip all touch the floor).
- Point back foot, bring back leg parallel to long edge of mat. Straighten back leg so knee lifts off floor.
- Place hands flat on floor, in front of hips, slightly wider than shoulders.

shape pose
- Lift torso upright.
- Square hips to right.
- Look straight ahead.

safety (strength) prep
- Press outer edge of front foot down, lift ankle up. Press heel into hip.
- Press back foot down, in.
- Squeeze front knee, back foot toward each other, which will create a slight lift in hips.
- Point back knee straight down.
- Tighten glutes, press tailbone down, tone abdomen.

refinement (stretch) pose
- Press hands down, back.
- Lift chest, stretch spine.

Repeat on the second side.

pigeon *quad stretch*
eka pada rajakapotasana 1 prep

shape prep (from downward facing dog)
- Place right knee against right wrist.
- Lower hips, back leg to floor.
- Bring right heel against front of left hip—back leg parallel to long edge of mat. Point back foot.
- Place right hand on floor in front of hips or on right knee.

shape pose
- Bend back knee. Clasp left foot with left hand. Bring heel to hip—inner edge of foot against outer hip.
- Hold top of foot/tips of toes with hand (more doable: hold foot any which way you can).
- Look straight ahead (more difficult: lower hips to floor; more doable: lower right hip to floor so that hip, thigh, and knee are on floor).

safety (strength) prep
- Press outer edge of front foot down. Lift ankle up.
- Press front heel into hip. Squeeze knees toward each other.

safety (strength) pose
- Tone, turn back inner thigh up.
- Tighten glutes, press tailbone down, tone abdomen.
- Lift shoulders up, back.
- Back foot must be in line with left hip, not wider for the sake of knee.
- Point back foot start to finish—don't sickle.

refinement (stretch) pose
- Lift chest, stretch spine.

Repeat on the second side.

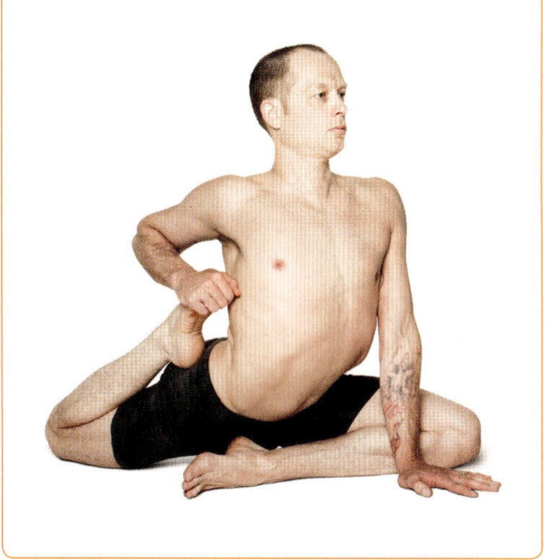

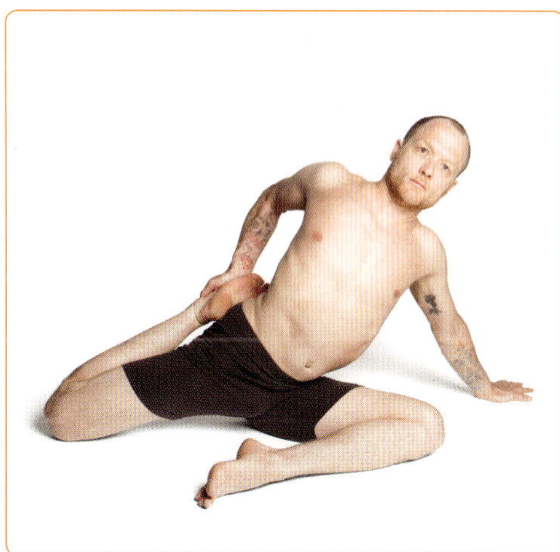

pigeon quad stretch *hip on floor*

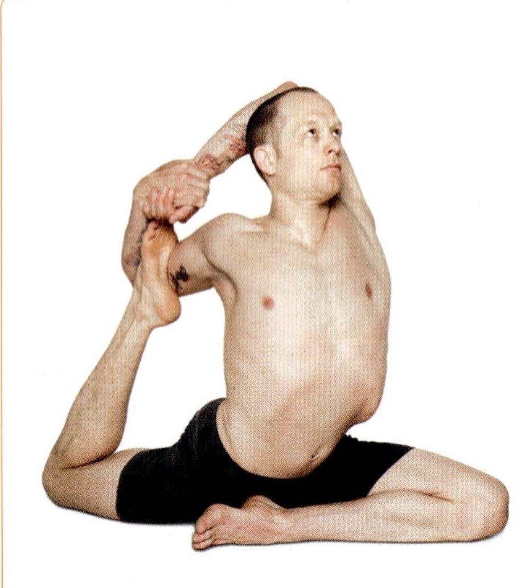

mermaid 1
naginyasana 1

shape prep (from pigeon torso upright)
- Place left foot in left elbow crease. Bend left elbow 100%.

shape pose
- Lift right arm overhead. Clasp hands or use strap to bind).
- Look between eyebrows (more difficult: lower back thigh to floor).

safety (strength) prep
- Press outer edge of front foot down, lift ankle up.
- Press front heel into hip.
- Without lifting hips, squeeze knees toward each other.

safety (strength) pose
- Press back foot, bottom elbow together.
- Press top elbow, head together.
- Tighten glutes, press tailbone down, tone abdomen.
- Lift shoulders up, back.

refinement (stretch) pose
- Lift chest, stretch spine.

Repeat on the second side.

Crescent and gatekeeper are good prep poses for mermaid 1.

mermaid 2
naginyasana 2

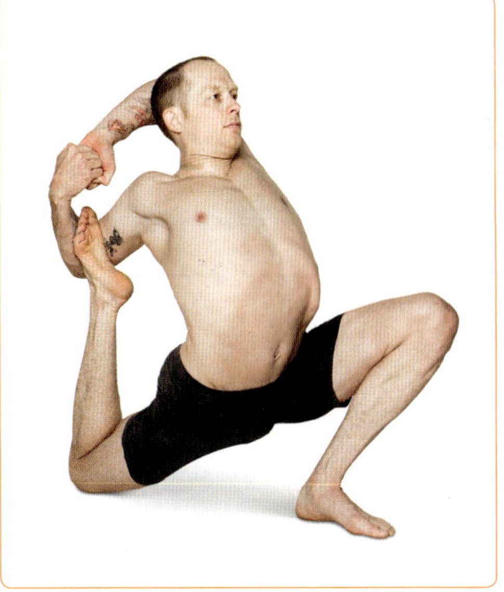

shape prep (from monkey lunge quad stretch)
▪ Place left foot in left elbow crease.

shape pose
▪ Bend left elbow. Lift right arm overhead. Clasp hands or use strap to bind.
▪ Look between eyebrows (more difficult: lower hips down and forward to capacity).

safety (strength) prep
▪ Without lifting hips, press front foot, back knee toward each other.

safety (strength) pose
▪ Press back foot, bottom elbow together.
▪ Press top elbow, head together.
▪ Tighten glutes, press tailbone down, tone abdomen.
▪ Lift shoulders up, back.

refinement (stretch) pose
▪ Lift chest, stretch spine.

Repeat on the second side.

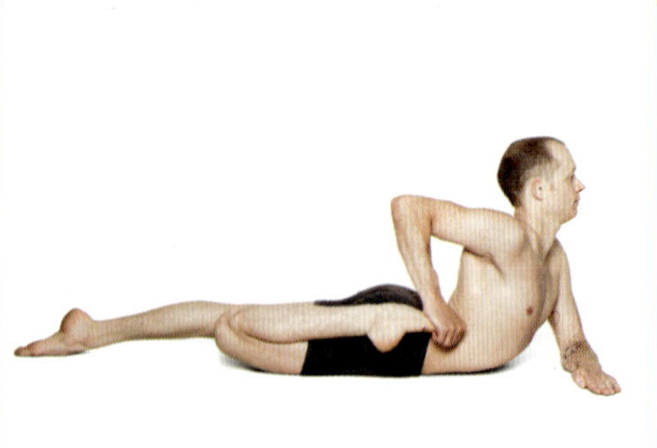

half frog
eka pada bhekasana

shape prep
▌ Bring front body to floor.
▌ Separate feet outer hip-width apart. Point feet, straighten legs.
▌ Place right forearm on floor parallel to top of mat—elbow slightly in front of and wider than shoulder.

shape pose
▌ Bend left knee, hold foot with hand. Bring heel to/toward left hip (more doable: turn to the left, bring hip to heel to close knee joint.
▌ Lower hip to floor, keeping heel connected to hip.
▌ Hold tips of toes with left hand (more doable: hold foot any which way you can).
▌ Point left elbow up.
▌ Look straight ahead.

safety (strength) pose
▌ Press back foot down, in. Squeeze thighs toward each other.
▌ Squeeze back foot, forearm toward each other.
▌ Tighten glutes, press tailbone down, lift low belly.
▌ Lift shoulders up, back.

refinement (stretch) pose
▌ Pull left foot forward, extend bent knee back.
▌ Lift chest, stretch spine.

Repeat on the second side.

elevated half frog
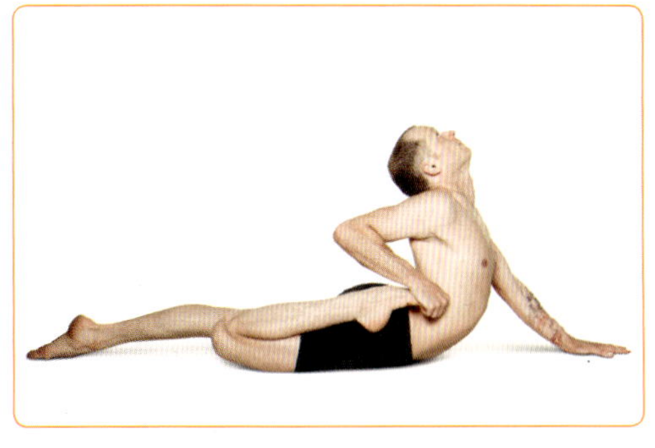

urdhva eka pada bhekasana

shape pose (from half frog)
- Place right hand on floor directly in front of and slightly wider than right shoulder. Straighten right arm (more doable: slide hand forward, well in front of shoulder. The further forward the hand, the more doable the pose).
- Look up (more doable: look straight ahead).

safety (strength) prep
- Press back foot down, in. Lift back knee.
- Squeeze thighs toward each other.
- Tighten glutes, press tailbone down, lift abdomen.

safety (strength) pose
- Lift shoulders up, back.
- If looking up: tone throat, lift back of head.

refinement (stretch) pose
- Lift chest, stretch spine.

Repeat on the second side.

frog
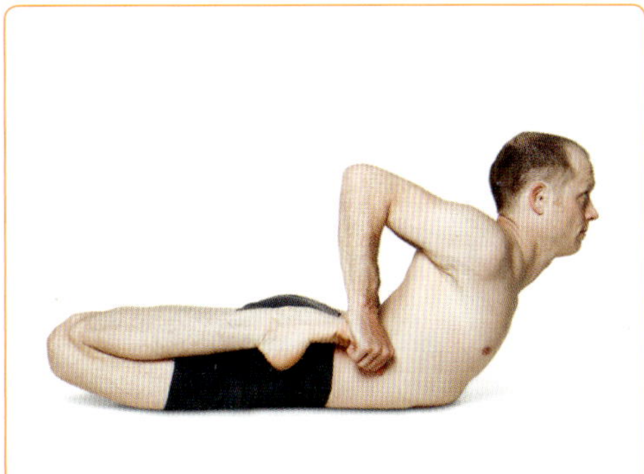

bhekasana

shape prep
- Bring front body to floor with forehead on floor.
- Hold feet with hands. Bring heels to hips—thighs parallel to each other.
- Point feet. Point elbows up—elbows up, not in.
- Climb hands on top of feet with fingers facing knees.
- Stay here, or turn hands out 180 degrees. Wrap fingers around tips of toes.
- Stay here or lift chin, look straight ahead.

shape pose
- Lift torso to capacity.

safety (strength) prep
- Squeeze thighs in.
- Tighten glutes, press tailbone down, tone abdomen.
- Lift shoulders up, in. Squeeze ankles in (more doable: widen knees slightly wider than hip-width apart).

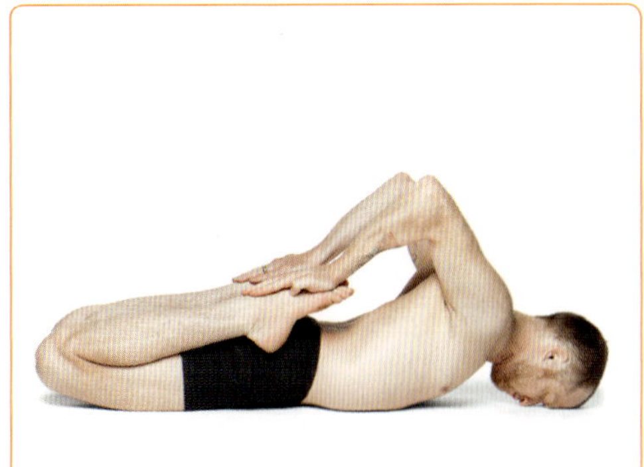

refinement (stretch) pose
- Pull feet forward with hands. Extend knees back.
- Lift chest, stretch spine.

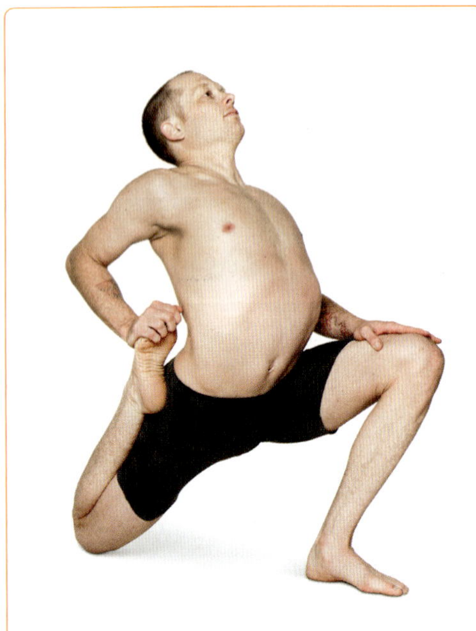

monkey lunge *quad stretch*
eka pada rajakapotasana 2 prep

shape prep (from downward facing dog)
▌ Step right foot forward between hands.
▌ Lower back knee to floor.
▌ Place right hand on right knee. Lift torso upright.
▌ Lift and hold back foot with left hand.

shape pose
▌ Bring heel to/toward hip—inner edge of foot against outer hip.
▌ Hold top of foot/tips of toes with hand (more doable: hold foot any which way you can).
▌ Look straight ahead (more difficult: lower hips down, forward to capacity. Look up).

safety (strength) prep
▌ Squeeze front foot, back knee toward each other.

safety (strength) pose
▌ Tighten glutes, press tailbone down, tone abdomen.
▌ Lift shoulders up, back.
▌ Left foot must be in line with left hip; not wider.
▌ Point back foot start to finish—don't sickle.

refinement (stretch) pose
▌ Lift chest, stretch spine.

Repeat on the second side.

twisted monkey

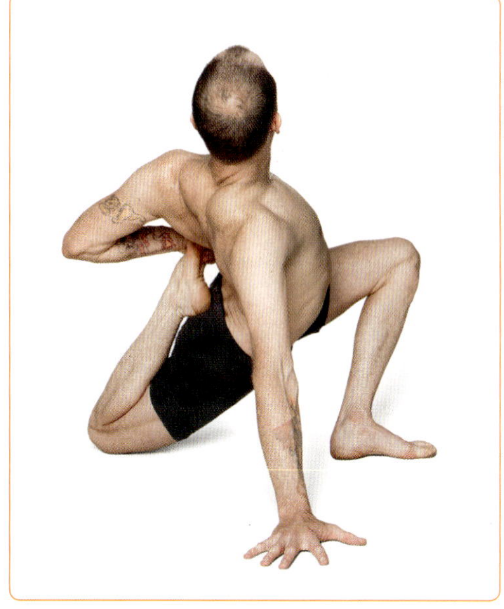

shape prep (from downward facing dog)

- Step right foot forward between hands, lower back knee to floor.
- Turn front foot out 30 degrees. Tilt knee out, in line with front foot.
- Move left hand forward and out six inches. Turn hand out 30 degrees. Line up bottom biceps with bottom hand. Lean onto hand.
- Lift back foot—clasp back foot with right hand. Bring heel to hip.
- Point back foot (more doable: move hip to heel; bring back thigh vertical to floor; more difficult: move hips down, forward to capacity).

shape pose

- Twist to right; look over top shoulder. Bend in upper back.

safety (strength) prep

- Squeeze back knee, front foot toward each other.

safety (strength) pose

- Tone, turn inner thigh back.
- Tighten glutes, press tailbone down.
- Tone, turn abdomen up.

refinement (stretch) pose

- Lift chest, stretch spine.

Repeat on the second side.

Twisted monkey is a quad stretch, twist, and backbend. First things first: focus on the quad stretch. To get a quad stretch, the back heel must press into the hip.

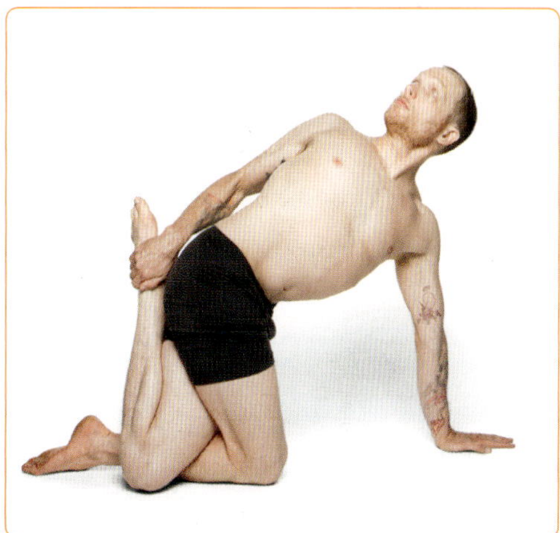

funky monkey

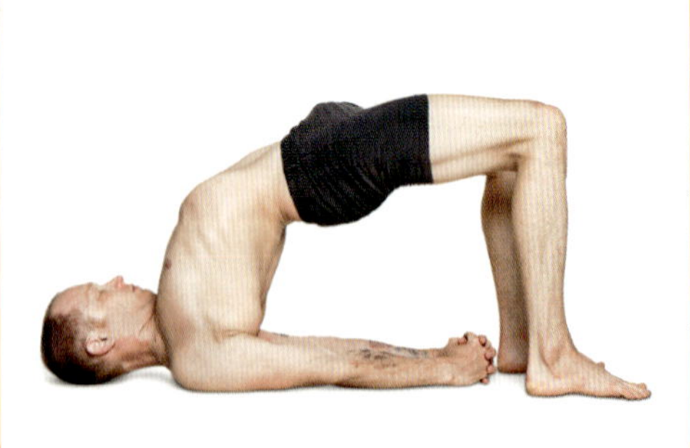

bridge
setu bandha sarvangasana

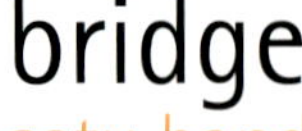

shape prep

- Lie down on back with arms alongside torso.
- Place feet flat on floor just in front of hips.
- Separate feet outer hip-width apart. Point feet straight ahead.
- Interlace fingers under hips (more doable: grab outer edges of mat).
- One at a time, walk shoulders in towards spine.

shape pose

- Lift hips, chest, chin up—thighs parallel to each other.

safety (strength) prep

- Shrug shoulders to minimize neck stretch.
- Press head, shoulders, feet down—press inner edges of feet down, flare toes.

safety (strength) pose

- Tone, turn inner thighs down.
- Tighten glutes, lift tailbone, tone abdomen.

refinement (stretch) pose

- Lift chest, stretch spine.

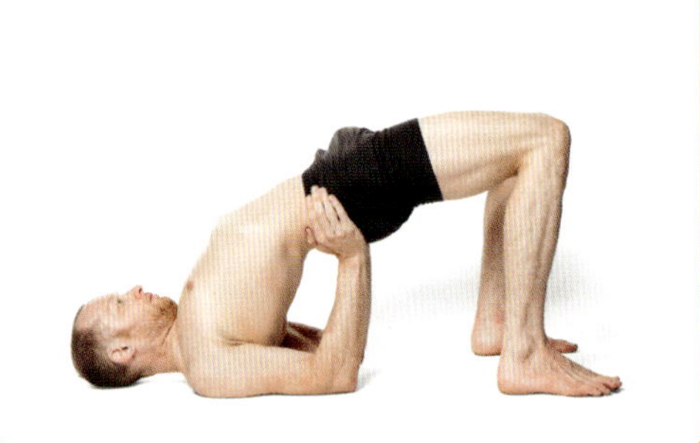

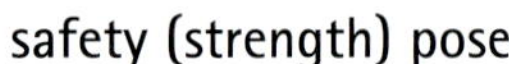

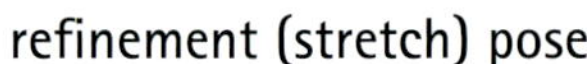

Bridge is unique in that it's a forward folding backbend. It can, therefore, be used to prep for both backbends and/or savasana.

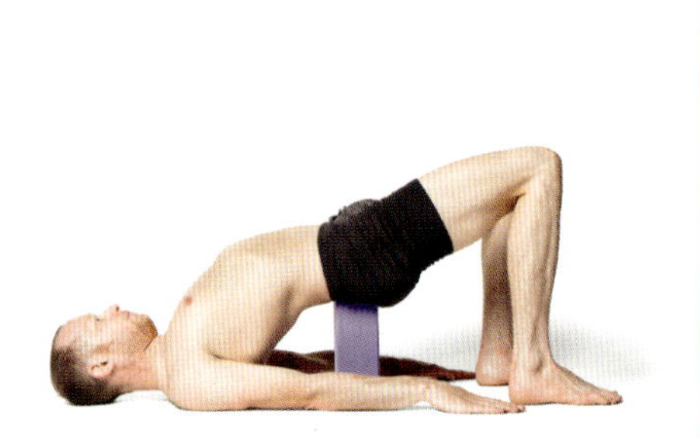

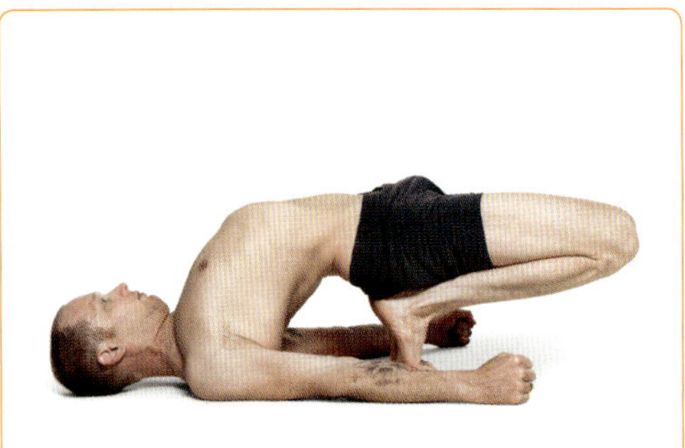

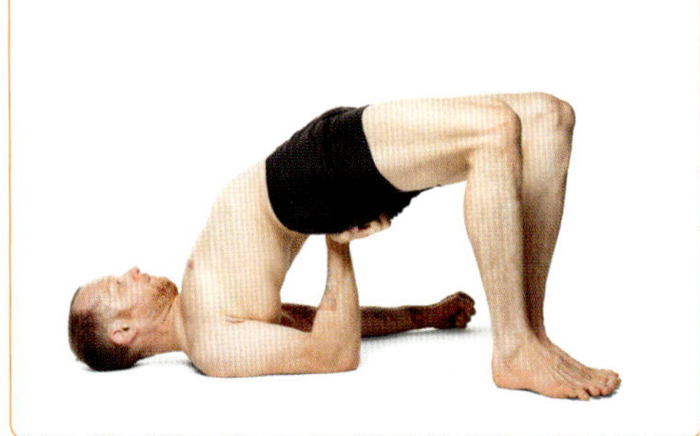

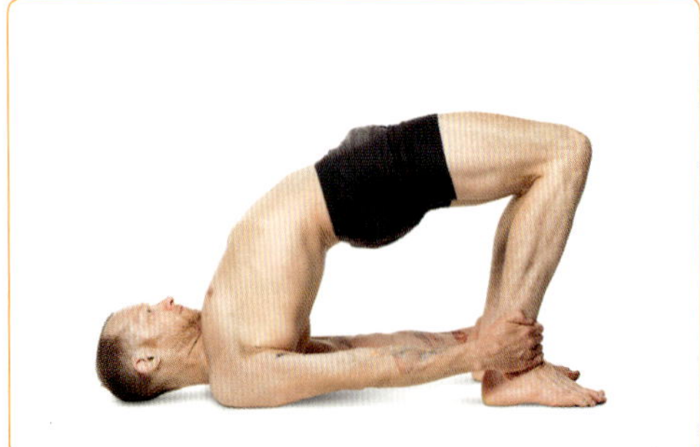

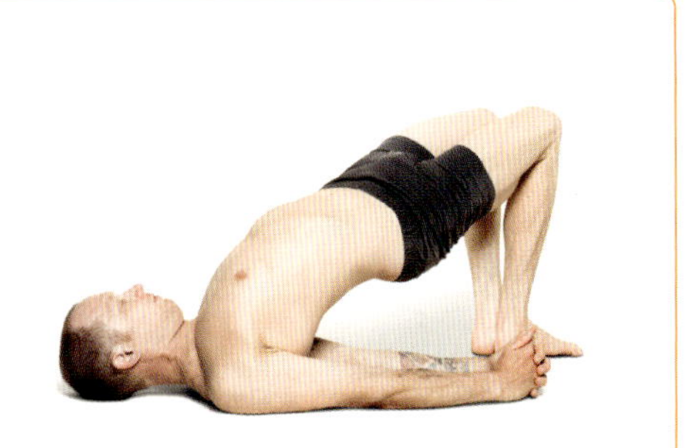

building bridge
uttana mayurasana prep

shape prep (from bridge)
- Bring inner edges of feet together.

shape pose
- Use toes to crawl feet away from hips. Straighten legs, point feet.
- Lift hips, chest, chin.

safety (strength) prep
- Shrug shoulders.
- Press head, shoulders, feet, down.

safety (strength) pose
- Tone thighs, tighten kneecaps, firm hamstrings.
- Tighten glutes, lift tailbone, tone abdomen.

refinement (stretch) pose
- Lift chest, stretch spine.

When going from bridge to building bridge, do not lose any of the bend in upper back.

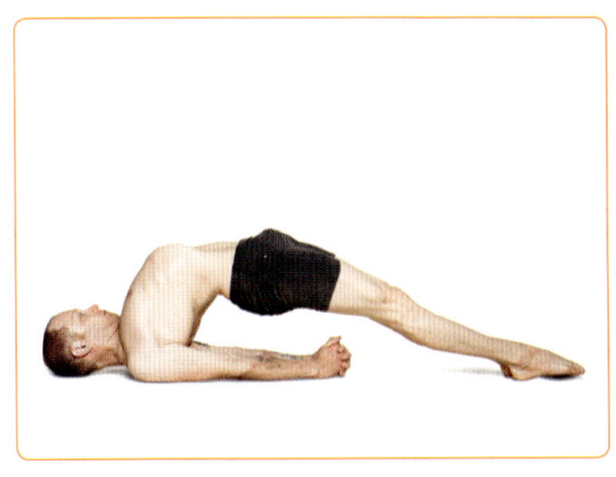

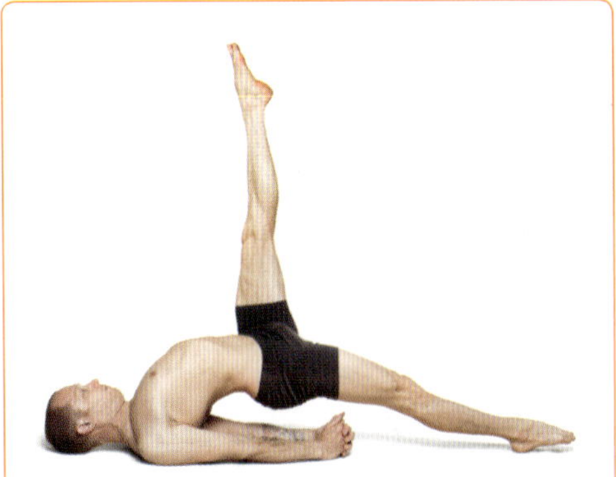

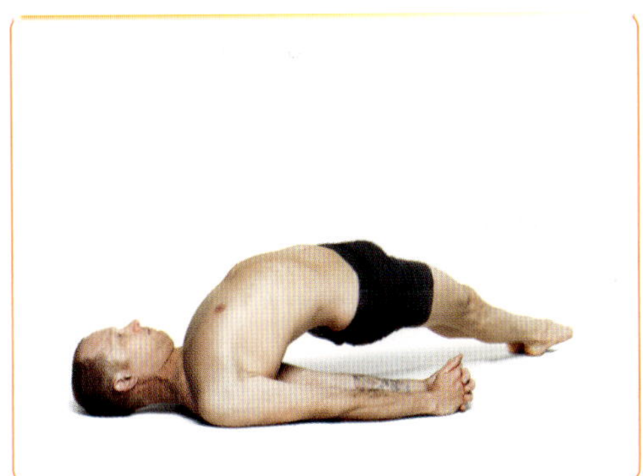

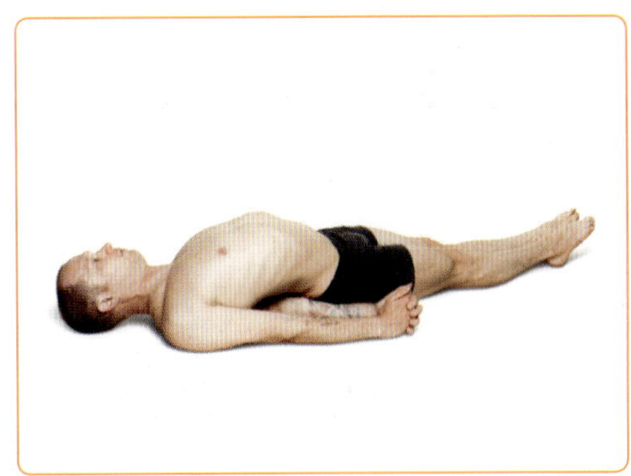

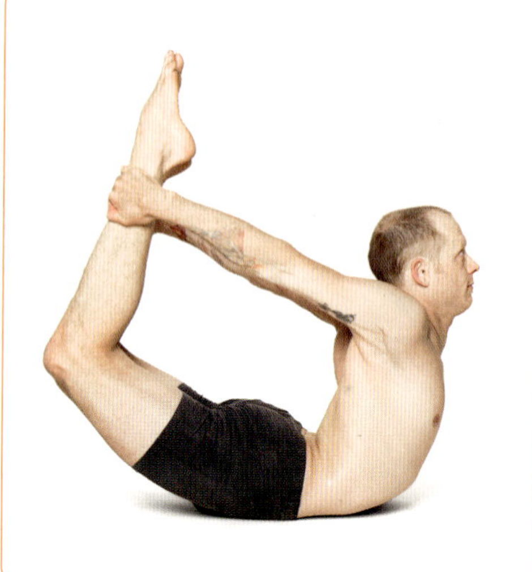

bow

dhanurasana

shape prep

▓ Bring front body to floor.
▓ Bend knees. Clasp outer edges of feet with hands.
▓ Straighten arms. Lift chin, look straight ahead.
▓ Point feet.

shape pose

▓ Kick feet back, up (more difficult: place inner edges of feet together).

safety (strength) prep

▓ Squeeze thighs in—knees outer hip-width apart.
▓ Tighten glutes, press tailbone down. Lift abdomen off floor.
▓ Squeeze shoulders together on back.

safety (strength) pose

▓ Lift legs with legs not just via kicking feet into hands—flare toes.
▓ If there is any discomfort in knees, hold ankles, flex feet.

refinement (stretch) pose

▓ Lift chest, stretch spine.

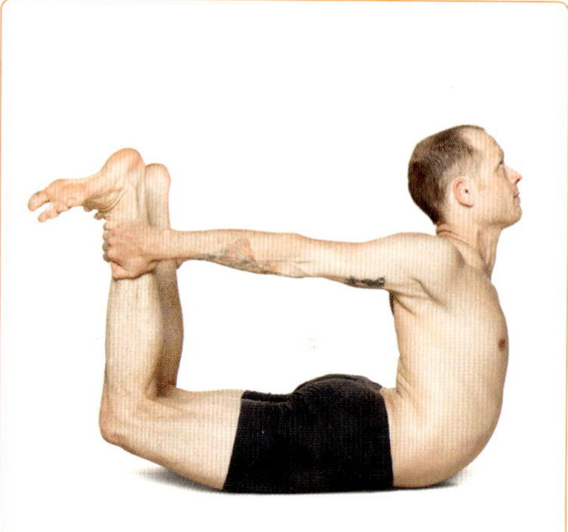

one-leg bow
eka pada dhanurasana

shape prep
- Bring front body to floor.
- Separate feet outer hip-width. Point feet, straighten legs.
- Place right forearm on floor parallel to top of mat—elbow slightly in front of and wider than shoulder.
- Bend left knee. Hold foot with left hand. Point foot—flare toes.
- Straighten left arm.
- Look straight ahead.

shape pose
- Stay here or kick left foot up, back.
- Straighten back leg so knee lifts up off floor.

safety (strength) prep
- Press bottom foot down, in. Squeeze knees in, knees outer hip width apart.
- If there is any discomfort in bent knee, hold ankle, flex foot.
- Pull front forearm, bottom foot toward each other.
- Tighten glutes, press tailbone down, tone abdomen.
- Move shoulders up, in.

safety (strength) pose
- Lift back leg with leg, not just via kicking foot into hand.

refinement (stretch) pose
- Lift chest, stretch spine.

Repeat on the second side.

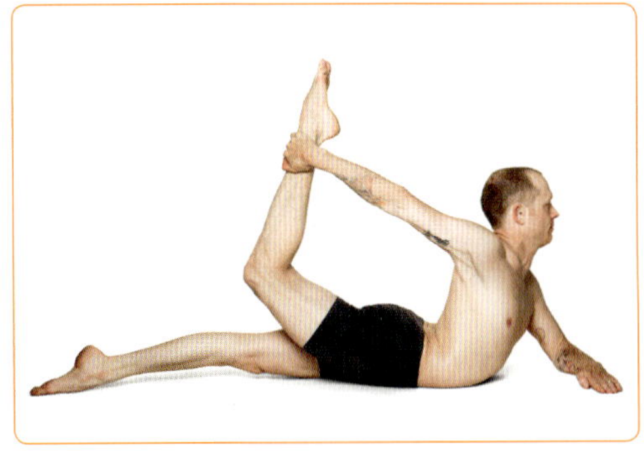

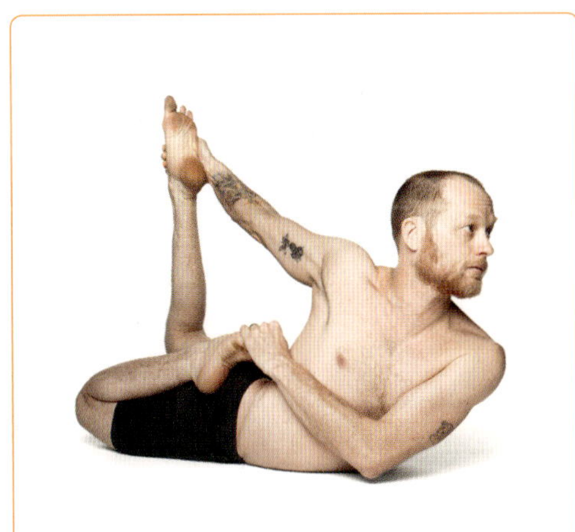

gherandasana II

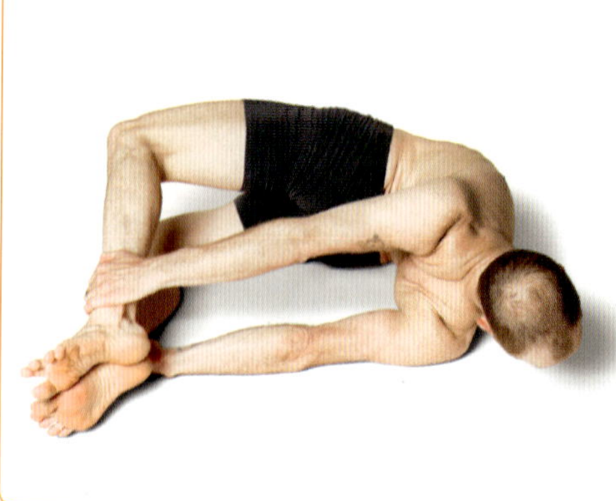

sideweays bow
parsva dhanurasana

shape prep (from bow)
- Bend right elbow slightly.
- Roll to right side of body.
- Straighten right arm.
- Look down, past bottom shoulder.

shape pose
- Move hips forward, kick feet back.
- Move bottom shoulder back so inner shoulder rests on floor (more difficult: place inner edges of feet together).

safety (strength) prep
- Squeeze thighs in—knees outer hip-width apart.
- Tighten glutes, press tailbone in, tone abdomen.
- Squeeze shoulders together on back.

refinement (stretch) pose
- Lift chest, stretch spine.

Repeat on the second side.

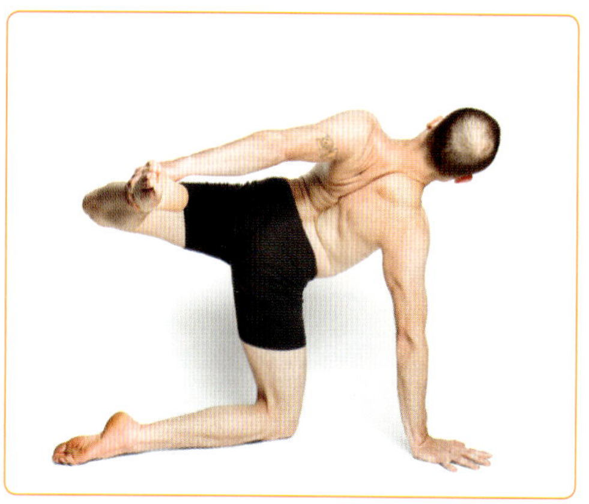

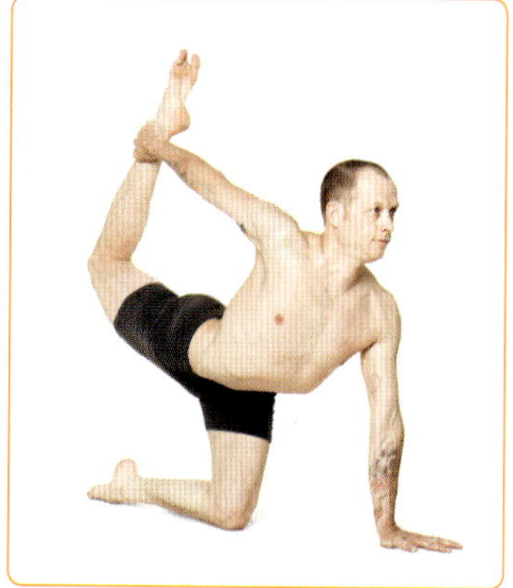

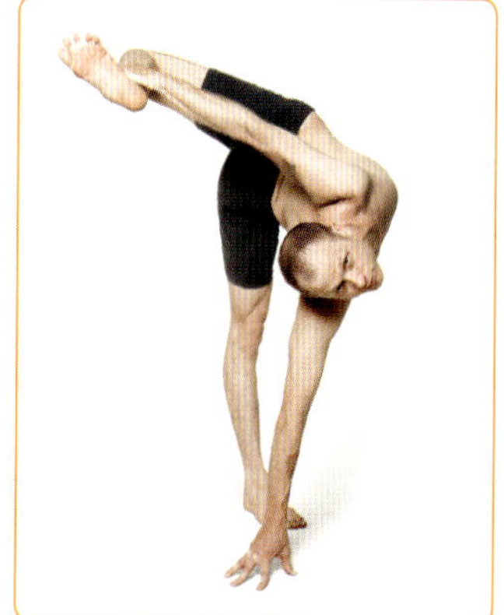

king pigeon *prep*
rajakapotasana prep

shape prep
- Bring front body to floor.
- Point feet. Bring inner edges of feet together.
- Straighten legs.
- Lift chin, look straight ahead.
- Place hands by upper chest—forearms straight up and down.
- Separate hands slightly wider than shoulder-width apart. Separate fingers, point index fingers straight ahead.
- Lift shoulders up to capacity.
- Move elbows in.
- Bend knees—shins vertical to floor.

shape pose
- Straighten arms. Lift torso.
- Bend deeply in upper back (more doable: bend elbows).
- Look straight ahead (more difficult: look up or back).

safety (strength) prep
- Grip floor with fingertips, press inner edges of hands down.
- Engage upper back muscles. Squeeze shoulders onto back.
- Press heels together. Flare toes.
- Squeeze thighs in—knees outer hip-width apart.
- Tighten glutes, press tailbone down, tone abdomen.

safety (strength) pose
- If looking up or back, tone neck, relax jaw.

refinement (stretch) pose
- Press hands down, back.
- Stretch spine.

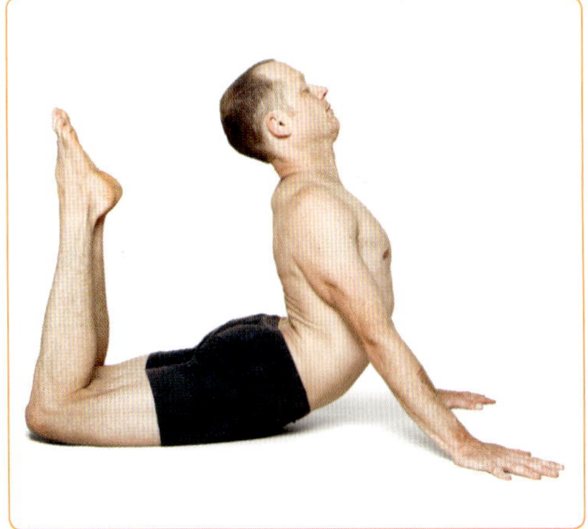

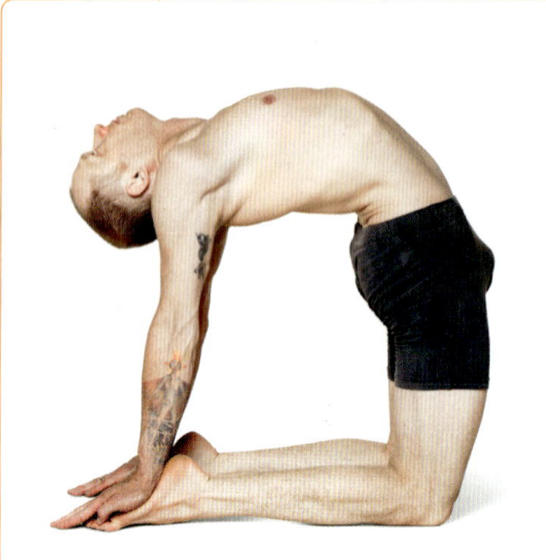

camel
ustrasana

shape prep
■ Come into an upright kneeling position—knees and feet outer hip-width apart. Point feet.
■ Place hands on hips; point elbows back.
■ Look down. Move hips forward slightly.

shape pose
■ Backbend as deeply as is optimal. Keep thighs vertical to floor.
■ Stay here, or if the feet are within easy reach, place palms on soles of feet just below heels. Close fingers.
■ Stay here, or look back.

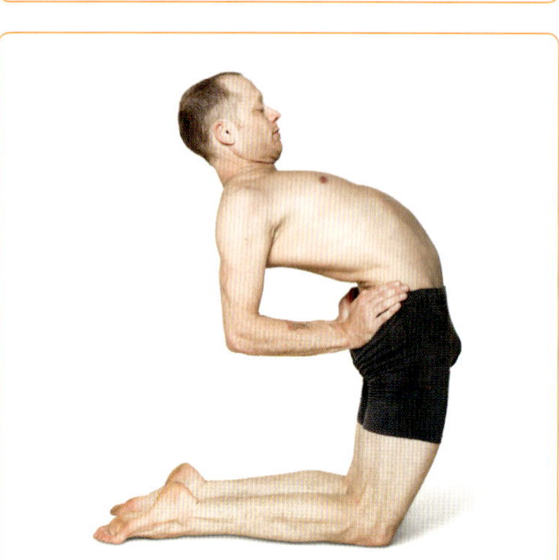

safety (strength) prep
■ Press feet and knees down, in.
■ Squeeze ankles in, flare toes.
■ Squeeze thighs in, lift pelvic floor.
■ Tighten glutes, press tailbone in, tone abdomen.

safety (strength) pose
■ If looking back tone throat, relax jaw.

refinement (stretch) prep
■ Lift chest, stretch spine.

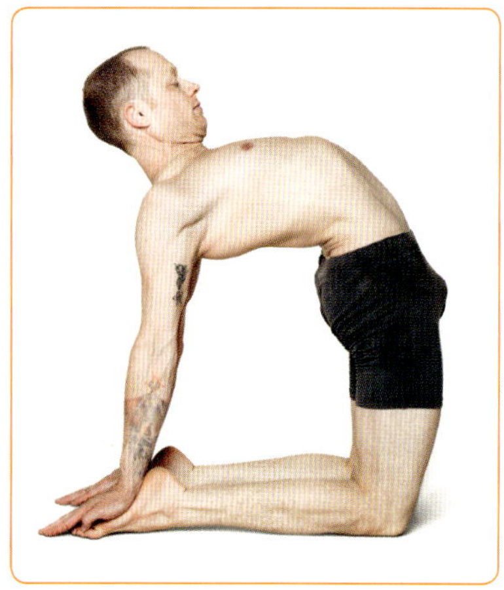
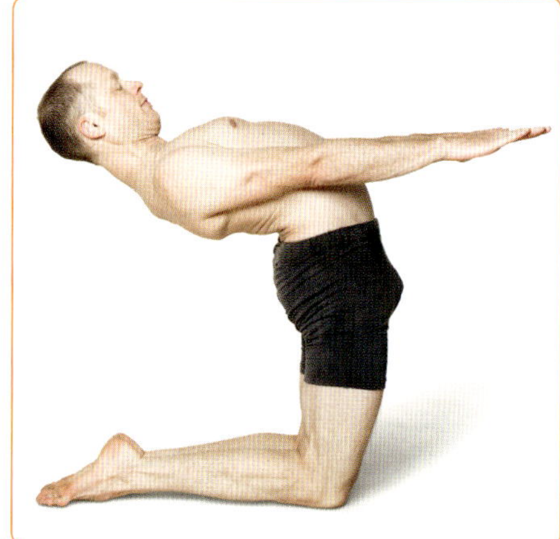
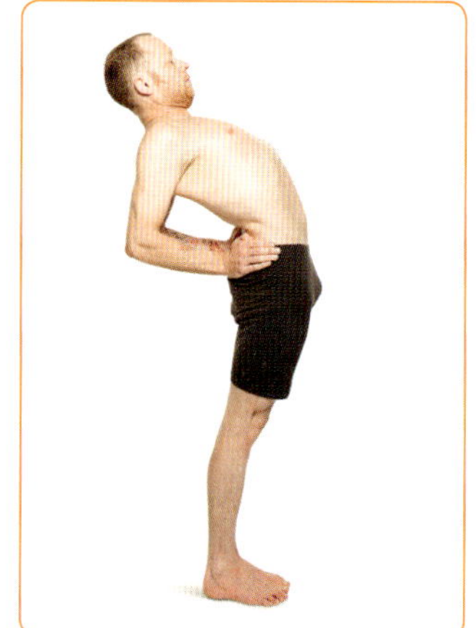

upward bow *head on floor*
urdhva dhanurasana prep

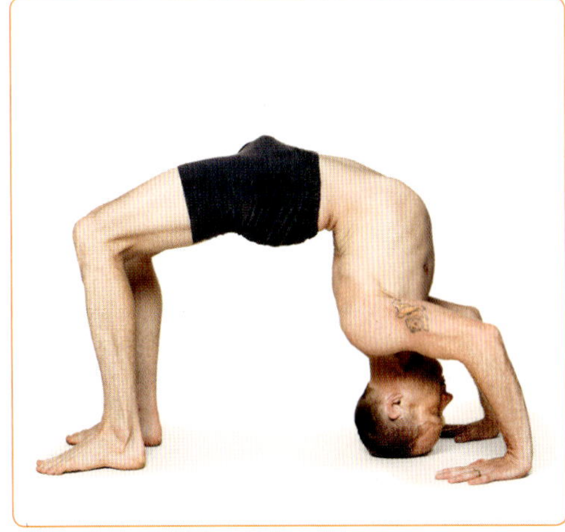

shape prep (from reclined mountain)
- Bend knees, place feet on floor just in front of hips.
- Separate feet outer hip-width apart, point big toes straight ahead.
- Place hands flat on floor beside head—thumbs under shoulders.
- Separate fingers, turn hands out slightly. Point elbows up.

shape pose
- In one movement lift up onto top of head.
- Move hips forward and up (toward head).
- Widen elbows slightly.

safety (strength) prep
- Grip floor with fingertips including pinkies, thumbs.
- Press inner edges of feet down, flare toes.
- Tone, turn inner thighs down—squeeze thighs in.

safety (strength) pose
- Put little to no weight on head.
- Move shoulders down back, chest forward (these two opposing movements help to stabilize the shoulders).
- Tighten glutes, lift tailbone, tone abdomen.

refinement (stretch) pose
- Lift chest, stretch spine.

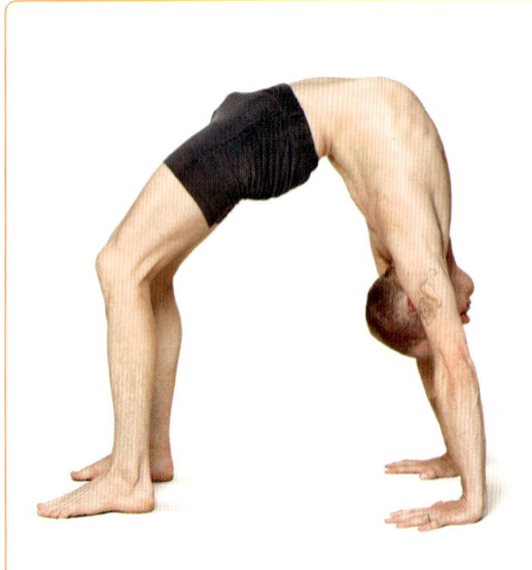

upward bow
urdhva dhanurasana

shape prep (from reclined mountain)
- Bend knees, place feet on floor just in front of hips. Separate feet outer hip-width apart, point big toes straight ahead.
- Place hands flat on floor beside head—thumbs under shoulders.
- Separate fingers, turn hands out slightly. Point elbows up.

shape pose
- In one movement lift hips, chest, head up—straighten arms to capacity. Look between hands (more doable: come into upward bow head on floor first and proceed from there).

safety (strength) prep
- Grip floor with fingertips including pinkies and thumbs. Squeeze elbows in. Move shoulders back, as if to hollow out armpits.
- Press inner edges of feet down, flare toes.
- Tone, turn inner thighs down—squeeze thighs in.

safety (strength) pose
- Tighten glutes, lift tailbone, tone abdomen.

refinement (stretch) pose
- Press hands and feet down.
- Expand chest, stretch spine.

In the classical form of this pose the shins and forearms are vertical (forearms can go even slightly past vertical). There is a horizontal line from the pubic bone to the base of the sternum. If you look at me in this pose you will see I am not in the classical form. There are, however, photos of me doing the classical form like in the Penchant for Practice Poster.

I chose to not do the classical form here because for me it's more balanced and true to my day-to-day practice. It, along with all of the photos in this manual, reflects my 75% to 80% capacity. Jade Beall took the photos in this book in just three hours. Instead of trying to get each pose picture perfect, my aim was practice perfect, which is not performance. I no longer force my body into a certain shape. I now reference the classical form as a guide whereas before it was my goal.

upward bow *one leg lifted*
eka pada urdhva dhanurasana

shape prep (from upward facing bow)
- Turn left foot out slightly. Lift right foot up. Bend knee completely.
- Bring thigh vertical to floor.

shape pose
- Stay here or straighten leg.

safety (strength) prep
- Grip floor with fingertips including pinkies, thumbs. Squeeze elbows in. Move shoulders back, hollow armpits.

safety (strength) pose
- Press inner edge of bottom foot down—flare toes. Point top foot.
- Squeeze bottom thigh in slightly. Turn top leg out.
- Tighten glutes, lift tailbone, tone abdomen.
- Don't overstay your welcome in this pose.

refinement (stretch) pose
- Lift chest, stretch spine.
- Hold pose, not breath.

Repeat on the second side.

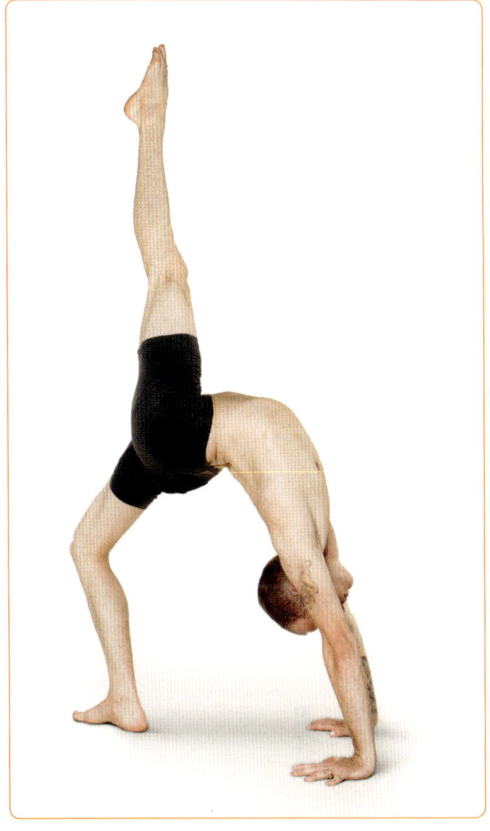

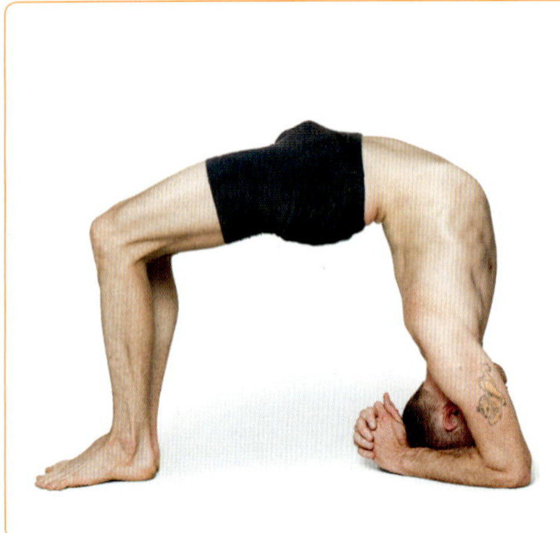

inverted staff
dwi pada viparita dandasana

shape prep (from upward facing bow)
- Place head on floor a few inches closer to feet than in upward facing bow head on floor.

shape pose
- Bring forearms to floor. Interlace fingers behind head. Place pads of thumbs against head. Point thumbs up.
- Move elbows shoulder-width apart.
- Move hips up, forward, toward head.

safety (strength) pose
- Put little to no weight on head.
- Press inner edges of feet down, flare toes.
- Tone, turn thighs down. Squeeze thighs in.
- Press wrists down.
- Tighten glutes, lift tailbone, tone abdomen, engage hamstrings.
- Move shoulders back toward feet, chest forward.

refinement (stretch) pose
- Stretch entire spine.
- Breathe evenly. Soften eyes. Relax jaw.

It is a common mistake to progress too quickly in backbends or any category of poses for that matter. I recommend not proceeding past the basic belly-down backbends and urdhva dhanurasana for the first several years of your practice. Sadhana-slow is the way to go. If you progress too fast it could turn your practice into a thing of the past.

supine twist
parivrtta supta padangusthasana prep

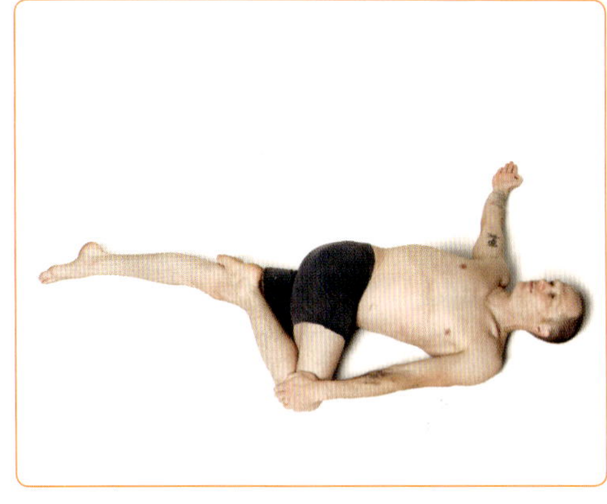

shape prep (from reclined mountain)
- Bring feet flat on floor, just in front of hips.
- Move hips four inches to left.
- Straighten right leg.
- Hook left foot under right knee.
- Extend left arm out to side, in line with shoulder. Point palm up.
- Hold left knee with right hand; straighten arm.

shape pose
- Roll onto outer right hip so that outer edge of right knee is on the floor.
- Lower left shoulder, left knee to/toward the floor.
- Look up or to left.

safety (strength) pose
- Press outer edge of right foot down, lift ankle. Press left foot, right knee together. Tone right thigh, tighten kneecap.
- Tighten glutes, press tailbone in, tone, turn abdomen to left.

refinement (stretch) pose
- Lift chest, stretch spine.

Repeat on the second side.

To enhance the calming nature of this pose move tongue away from roof of mouth. Relax jaw. Soften face and breath. Parivrtta supta padangusthasana looks like a relatively mild pose. That said, if you bring both shoulders and knee on floor it's actually quite the demanding twist. That's the nature of twists. They can be used to prepare for arm balances and backbends; they can be used as cool down.

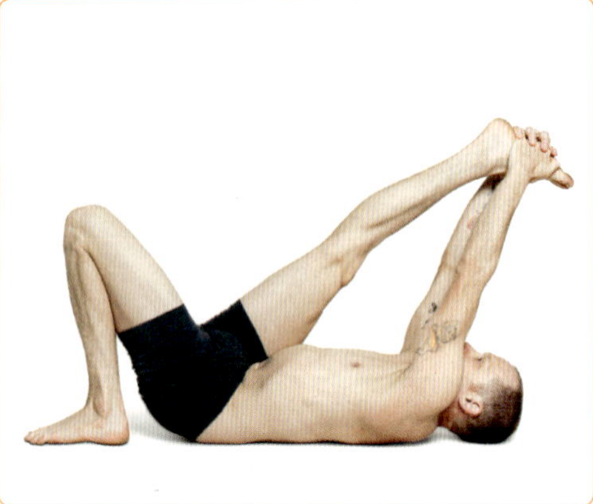

reclined bowing sage
supta dwi hasta padasana

shape prep (from reclined mountain)
- Bend left knee, place foot directly in front of left hip. Point knee up.
- Bring right thigh to torso with knee bent, shin vertical to floor.
- Hold right foot with hands. Straighten arms. Flex foot, flare toes.

shape pose
- Stay here or straighten right leg. Allow shoulders to move away from floor.

safety (strength) pose
- Tone right thigh, tighten kneecap, firm hamstrings.
- Press hands and top foot together.
- Tighten glutes, lift tailbone, tone abdomen.

Repeat on the second side.

Tibetan weaponry 1

eka pada supta virasana

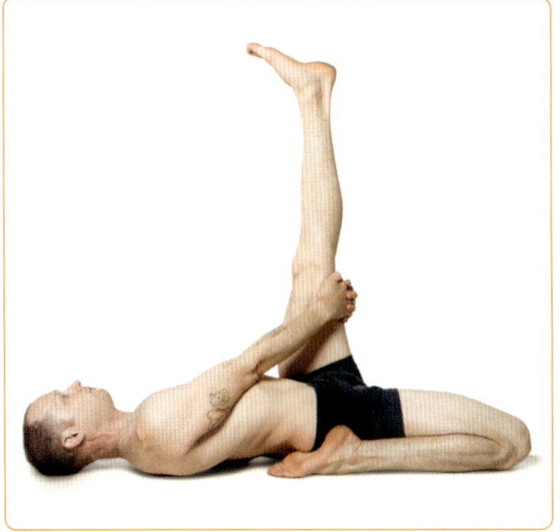

shape prep (from staff pose)

▫ Lean onto right hip. Bend left knee, catch ankle with hand. Flip top of shin to floor. Point left foot, flare toes. Bring inner edge of of left foot against outer left hip.

▫ Keeping right leg straight, lie down on back.

shape pose

▫ Bend right knee, interlace fingers behind right thigh, just below knee.

▫ Straighten arms and right leg (more doable: keep knee bent).

▫ Floint right foot—halfway between flex and point (more doable: allow left knee to lift up and out).

safety (strength) prep

▫ Press top of left foot down, squeeze left ankle in.

safety (strength) pose

▫ Tone right thigh, tighten kneecap, firm hamstrings.

▫ Press hands and leg together.

▫ Tighten glutes, lift tailbone, tone abdomen.

refinement (stretch) pose

▫ Lift chest, stretch spine.

Repeat on the second side.

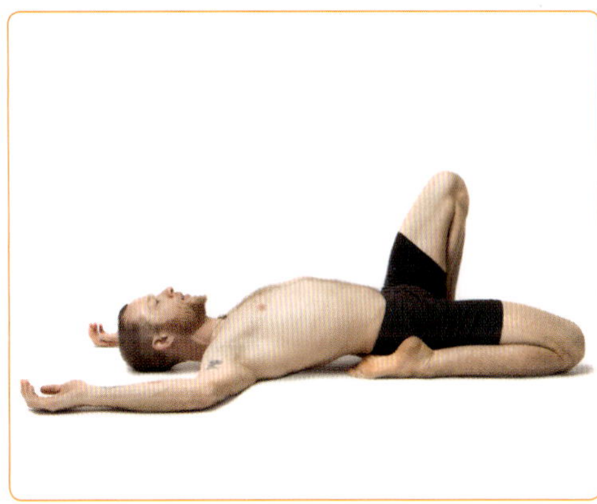

Tibetan weaponry 1 *foot on floor*

Some poses promote stress reduction. This one promotes stress destruction in the quads!

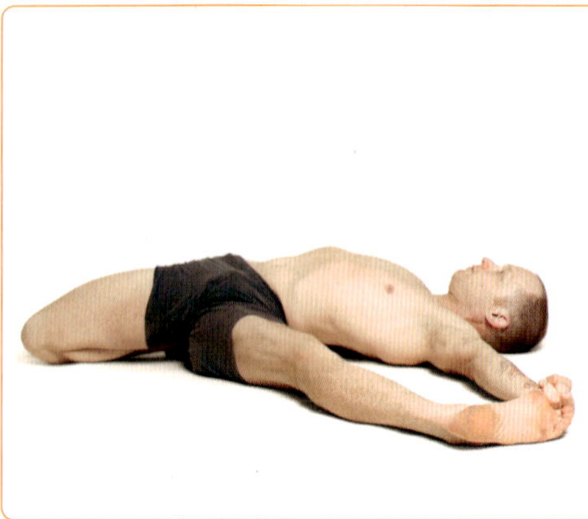

Tibetan weaponry 2
eka pada supta virasana

shape prep (from reclined mountain)
▦ Bring heels flat on floor just in front of hips. Lift right foot, hold outer ankle with right hand, arm outside leg. Bring heel to hip, point foot.
▦ Hold outer edge of left foot with left hand, arm inside leg. Flex foot.
▦ Lean onto left hip, knee.

shape pose
▦ Simultaneously straighten left leg to capacity, flip top of right foot to floor. Lower knee to capacity.

safety (strength) pose
▦ Press top of right foot down, squeeze ankle in.
▦ Tone left thigh, tighten kneecap, firm hamstrings.
▦ Press left hand, left foot together.
▦ Tighten glutes, lift tailbone, tone abdomen.
▦ Press shoulders down.

refinement (stretch) pose
▦ Lift chest, stretch.

Repeat on the second side.

Tibetan weaponry 3

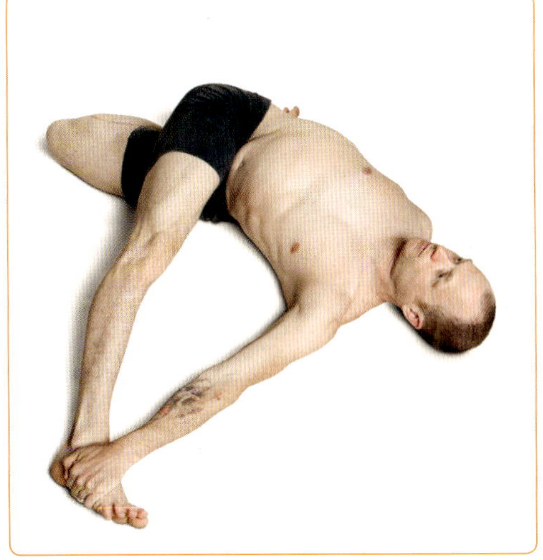

shape prep (from reclined revolved sage)
■ Bend left knee slightly.

shape pose
■ Bend right knee, catch right foot with left hand. Bring right heel to right hip.
■ Stay here, or point right knee toward top of mat.
■ Straighten left leg to capacity.

safety (strength) pose
■ Tone left thigh, tighten kneecap, firm hamstrings.
■ Press right hand, left foot together.
■ Squeeze left hip, right inner thigh together.
■ Tighten glutes, press tailbone in. Tone, turn abdomen to left.

refinement (stretch) pose
■ Lift chest, stretch spine.

Repeat on the second side.

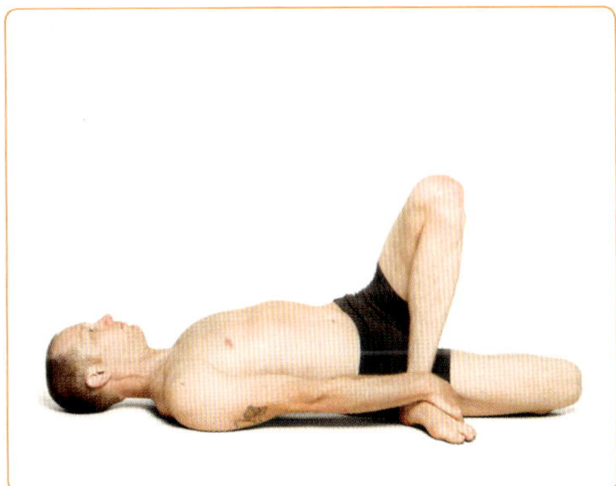

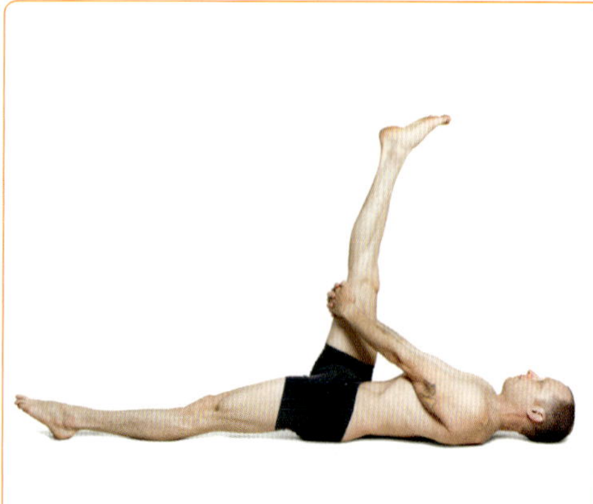

reclined big toe *hands to thigh*
supta padangusthasana 1 prep

shape prep (from reclined mountain)
- Bend right knee. Interlace fingers behind right thigh next to knee.

shape pose
- Straighten right leg. Floint foot (halfway between flex and point).
- Allow shoulders to lift off floor.

safety (strength) pose
- Tone thighs, tighten kneecaps, firm hamstrings.
- Press inner edge of left thigh down. Turn right leg out.
- Press hands and top leg together.
- Tighten glutes, lift tailbone, tone abdomen.

refinement (stretch) pose
- Lift chest, stretch spine.

Repeat on the second side.

Reclined poses are similar to twists in that they are equally good for warming up or cooling down.

reclined big toe 1
supta padangusthasana 1

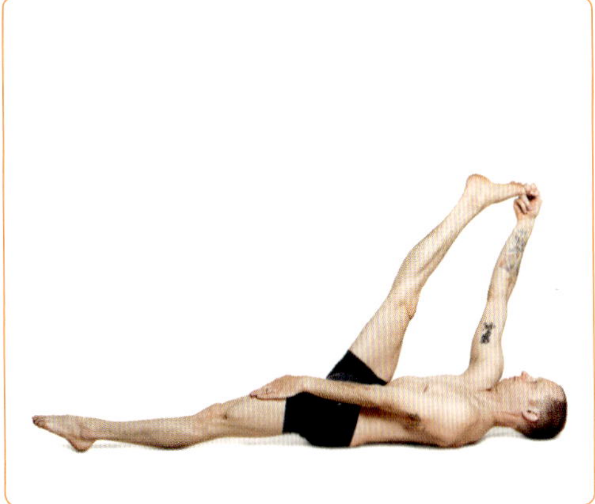

shape prep (from reclined mountain)
■ Point left foot. Place left hand on left thigh. Straighten arm, close fingers.
■ Bend right knee, hold big toe with first two fingers and thumb of right hand—arm inside leg.

shape pose
■ Straighten right leg (more doable: loop strap around foot to reach foot or lift left leg a few feet off floor). Floint top foot (halfway between flex and point).
■ Lift chin slightly. Allow both shoulders to lift off floor.

safety (strength) prep
■ Press right big toe, fingers together.

safety (strength) pose
■ Tone thighs, tighten kneecaps, firm hamstrings.
■ Tighten glutes, lift tailbone, tone abdomen.
■ Press bottom heel down, in. Extend inner edge of left leg towards floor. Turn top leg out.

refinement (stretch) pose
■ Reach toward left knee with hand.
■ Extend legs out.

Repeat on the second side.

In supine poses, students often press their chin into their throat, which can be a sign of overworking.

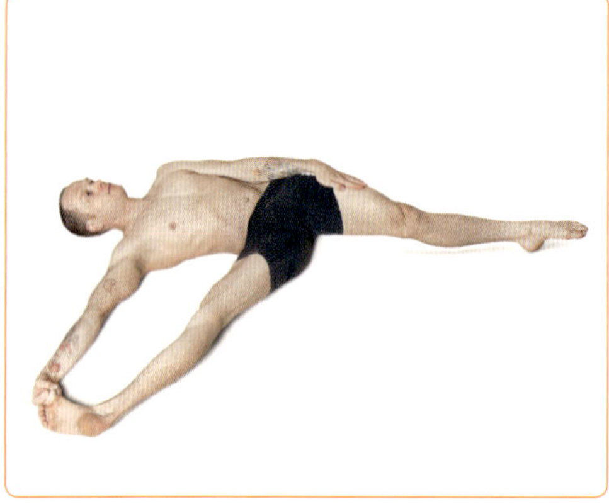

reclined big toe *leg to side*
supta padangusthasana 2

shape pose (from reclined big toe 1)
▌ Lower right leg to right—foot to/toward floor (more doable: bend and place right elbow on floor; or use a strap to hold foot).

safety (strength) prep
▌ Tone thighs, tighten kneecaps, firm hamstrings.
▌ Press right big toe and fingers together.

safety (strength) pose
▌ Tighten glutes, lift tailbone, tone abdomen.
▌ Press left heel down, in. Extend inner edge of left leg down. Turn top leg out.

refinement (stretch) pose
▌ Reach toward left knee with hand.
▌ Extend legs out.

Repeat on the second side.

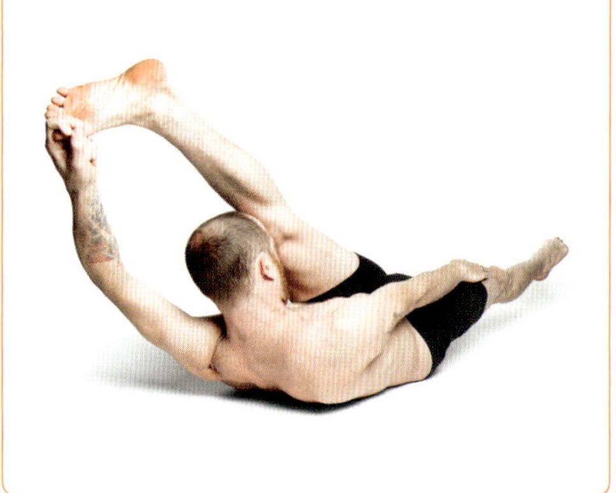

reclined big toe *forehead to knee*
supta padangusthasana 3

shape prep (from reclined big toe 1)
▌ Lift head and shoulders off floor.

shape pose
▌ Stay here or bend right elbow, bring forehead to knee/chin to shin.

safety (strength) prep
▌ Tone thighs, tighten kneecaps, firm hamstrings.
▌ Press right big toe and fingers together.
▌ Tighten glutes, lift tailbone, tone abdomen.
▌ Press left heel down, in. Extend inner edge of left leg down. Turn top leg out.

refinement (stretch) pose
▌ Reach toward left knee with hand.
▌ Extend legs out.

Repeat on the second side.

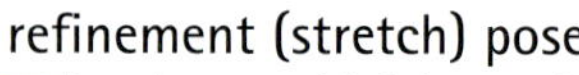

This pose strengthens the abdomen and neck as much as it stretches the hamstrings of the top leg.

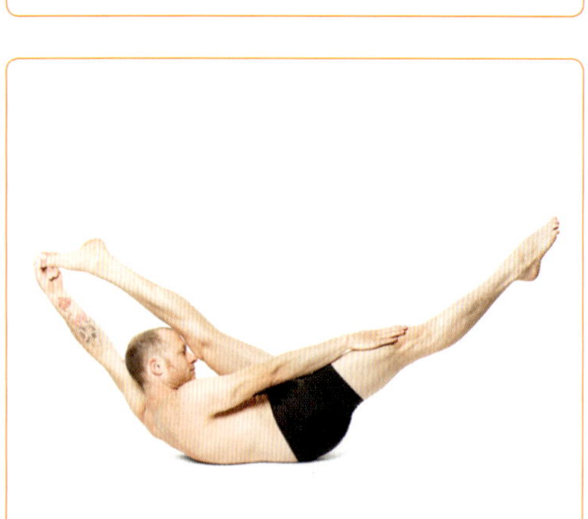

radical reclined big toe
supta padangusthasana

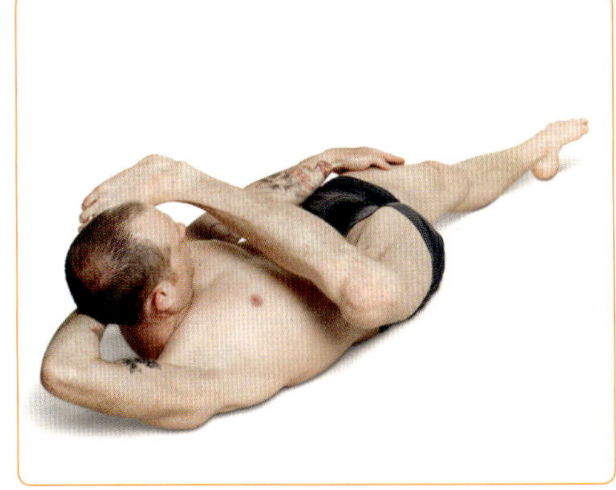

shape prep (from reclined big toe 1 prep)
- Bend right knee, bring shin across chest, point knee out.
- Sickle foot, flare toes (with control not collapse).

shape pose
- Keeping left hand on thigh, place right wrist or elbow behind head.
- Much more doable: lift left leg vertical to floor, hook right ankle with left elbow, clasp hands; or clasp right wrist with left hand.
- Lower left heel to/toward floor.

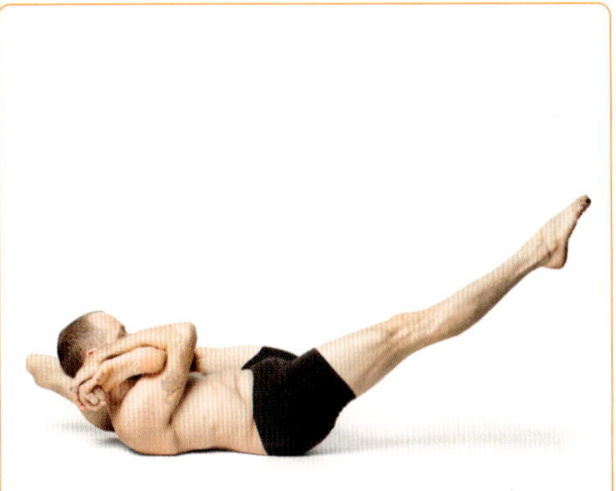

safety (strength) pose
- Straight leg: tone thigh, tighten kneecap, firm hamstrings; press inner edge of knee down.
- Bent knee: fuse ankle, press inner edge of big toe and fingers together, pull foot toward head.
- Bent arm: press head and arm together. Press shoulder down.
- Squeeze right hip and left inner thigh toward each other.
- Tone, turn abdomen to left.

refinement (stretch) pose
- Reach toward left knee with hand.

Repeat on the second side.

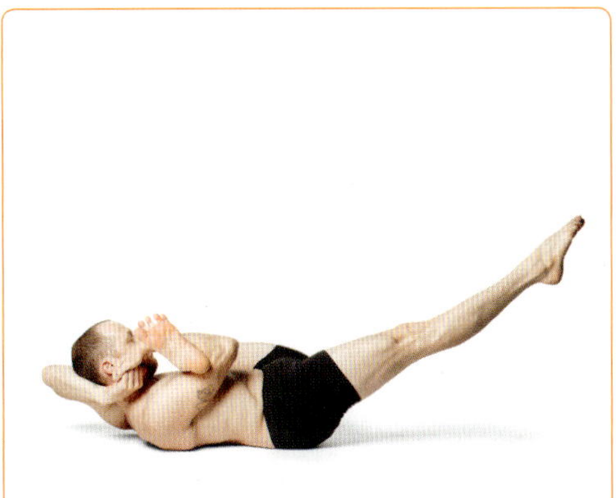

In radical reclined big toe, the sickle shape of your ankle must be strong so that it doesn't overly stretch. A collapsed ankle leads to a collapsed knee. Protect your ankle and knee by adding the action of flexing your foot without changing its shape.

A good alternate to this pose: any other pose than this one (needle's eye or reclined pigeon).

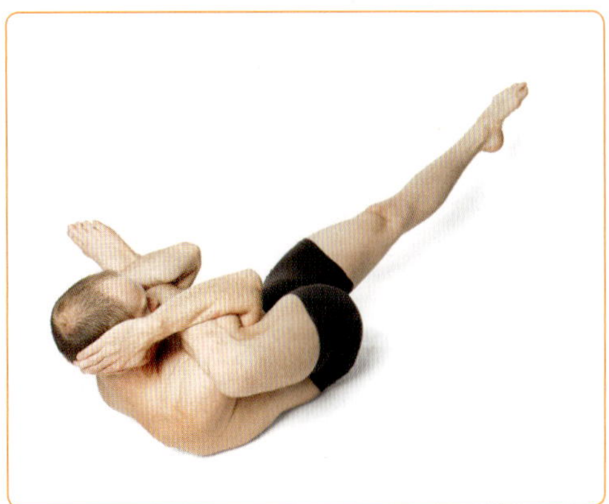

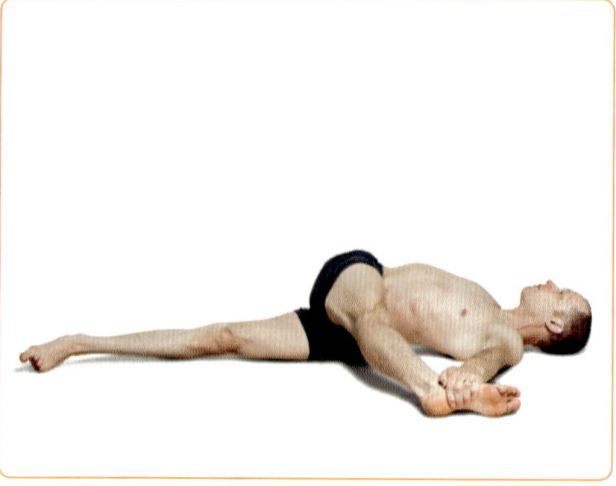

reclined revolved sage
parivrtta supta padangusthasana

shape prep (from reclined mountain)
▨ Bring left arm out to side in line with shoulder. Straighten arm, point palm up.
▨ Bend left knee into chest, hold outside of left foot with right hand. Straighten arm.
▨ Push head and right heel down, lift and slide hips four inches to the left.
▨ Roll onto outer right hip. Lower left foot to/toward floor.

shape pose
▨ Stay here or straighten left leg.
▨ Flex feet, flare toes (more difficult: place both shoulders on floor).
▨ Lift chin slightly, look up or to the left.

safety (strength) prep
▨ Press right hand, left foot together.

safety (strength) pose
▨ Press outer edge of right foot down, lift ankle.
▨ Squeeze feet towards each other.
▨ Tone thighs, tighten kneecaps, firm hamstrings.
▨ Squeeze left hip, right inner thigh together.
▨ Tighten glutes, press tailbone in. Tone, turn abdomen to left.

refinement (stretch) pose
▨ Lift chest, stretch spine.
▨ Extend legs out.

Repeat on the second side.

reclined hero
supta virasana

shape prep
- Sit on floor/block between feet—tops of feet on floor.
- Bring inner heels against hips/block.
- Point feet. Point knees straight ahead or out slightly.
- Hold knees with hands, straighten arms, look straight ahead or down.

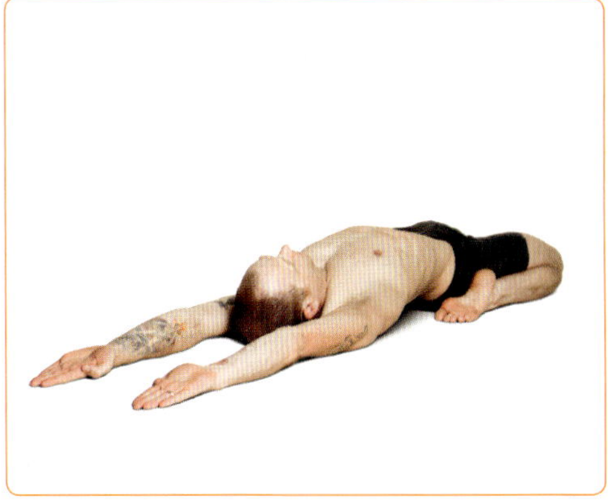

shape pose
- If seated on block, stay here. If hips firmly on floor, lie down on back.
- Stretch arms overhead. Point palms up. Close fingers, open palm (don't cup palms).

safety (strength) prep
- Press tops of feet down, squeeze ankles in.
- Tone, turn inner thighs down.

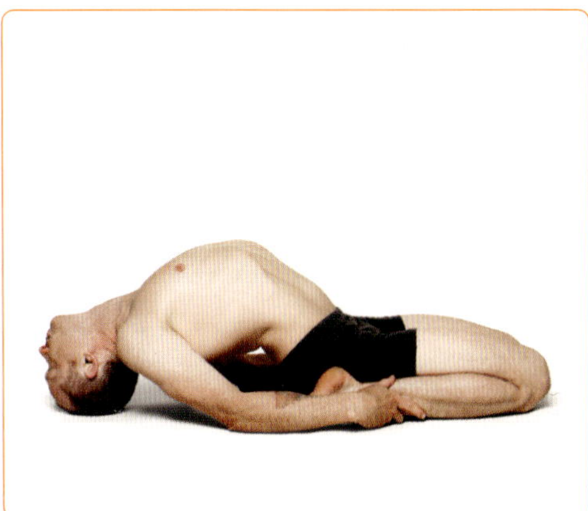

safety (strength) pose
- Tighten glutes, lift tailbone, tone abdomen.
- Press shoulders into floor.

refinement (stretch) pose
- Lift chest, stretch spine.
- Stretch arms.

How does one open, not cup, palms? The thumbs are key. Press thumbs against inner edges of hands. Keep pressing thumbs against hands as you bend them to capacity so they slide towards wrist. Try and touch floor with thumbs (kind of like moving the shoulders onto the back, move the thumbs onto the backs of the hands). Press the backs of the hands onto the floor so the hand is as flat as paper. Aside from those thumb actions, this pose is deeply calming; it promotes digestion and sleep.

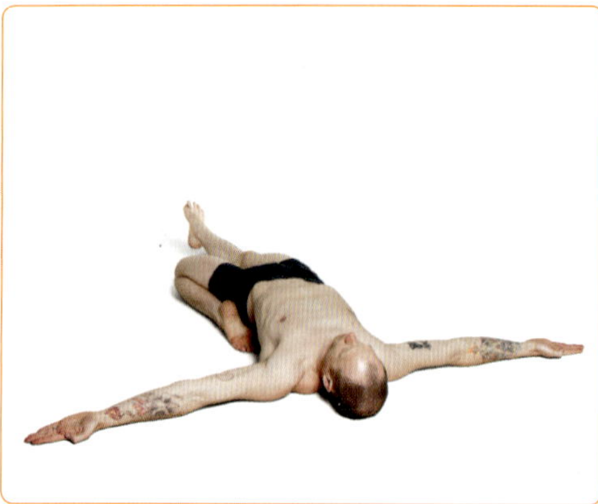

one-leg reclined hero
eka pada supta virasana

shape pose (from staff pose)
▨ Lean to left hip, bend right knee and hold right ankle with right hand. Place right heel against right hip. Point right foot and place top of right foot and shin on floor. Point right knee straight ahead (more doable: allow bent knee to move out slightly—keep inner heel against outer hip).
▨ Keeping left leg straight, lie down on back.
▨ Extend arms overhead. Straighten arms. Point palms up, close fingers.

safety (strength) pose
▨ Tighten glutes, lift tailbone, tone abdomen.
▨ Press top of right foot down, squeeze ankle in.

refinement (stretch) pose
▨ Lift chest, stretch spine. Stretch arms.

Repeat on the second side.

needle's eye
sucirandhrasana

shape prep
■ Lie down on back. Bring feet to floor in front of hips.
■ Place left ankle on right knee.

shape pose
■ Thread left arm through space between legs and interlace fingers around right shin. Straighten arms (more doable: interlace hands around right thigh).
■ Stay here or bend elbows, bring shin to/toward chest.
■ Lift chin slightly.
■ Allow low back to round.

safety (strength) prep
■ Flex left foot, flare toes. Clamp knee closed.

safety (strength) pose
■ Tone abdomen.

refinement (stretch) pose
■ Extend left knee out.

Repeat on the second side.

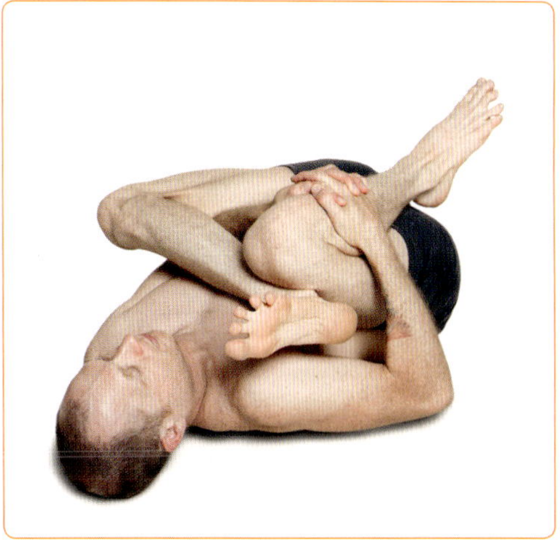

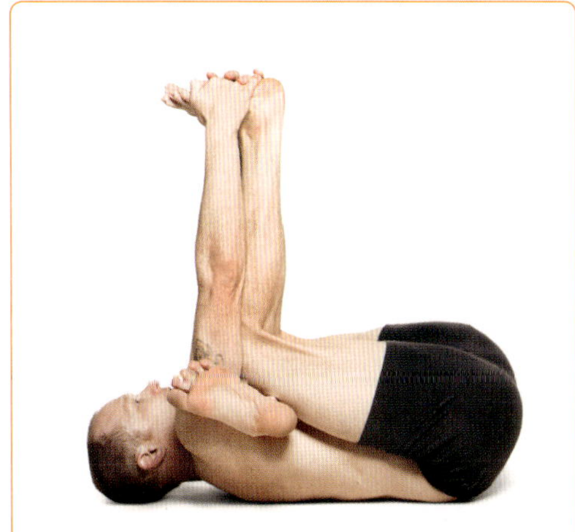

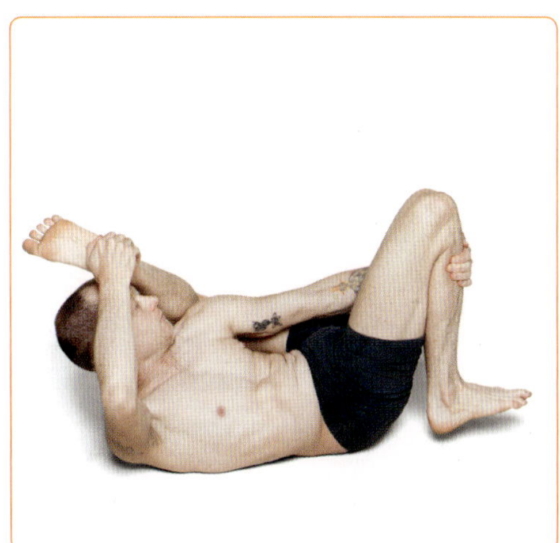

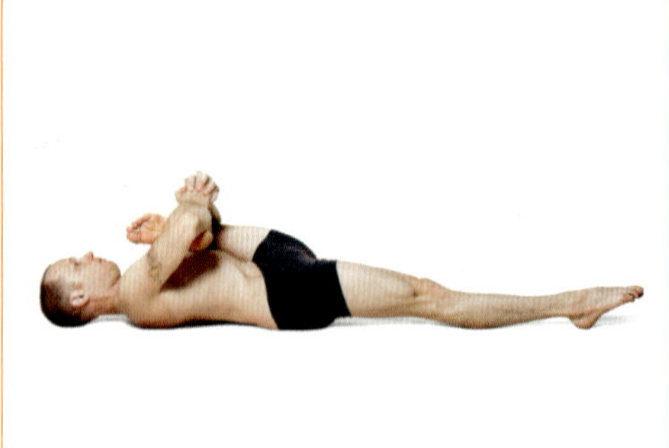

reclined pigeon
supta hindolasana

shape prep (from reclined mountain)
- Bring feet to floor in front of hips.
- Place left ankle on right knee. Flex left foot, flare toes.

shape pose
- Wrap right elbow around left foot, left elbow around left knee. Interlace fingers mid shin.
- Stay here or lift head, right foot equidistant to floor.
- Straighten right leg to capacity.

safety (strength) pose
- Squeeze elbows in.
- Clamp left knee closed.
- Extend inner right knee down.
- Tone abdomen.

refinement (stretch) pose
- Extend left thigh out with elbows.

Repeat on the second side.

This pose is an excellent prep for flying pigeon.
A good alternate to this pose is needle's eye.
Other good options: reclined eagle and reclined cow face.

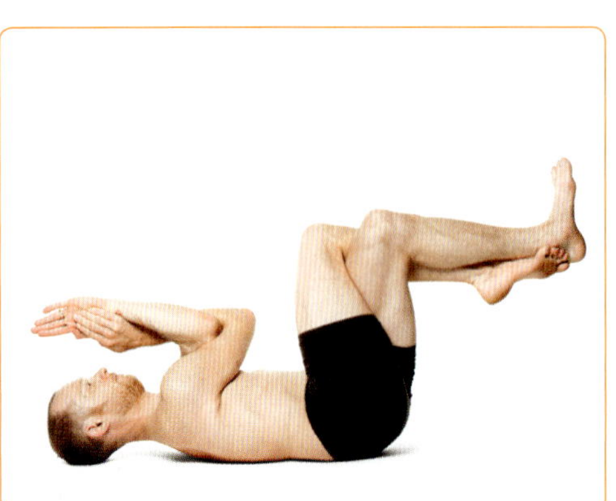

reclined eagle

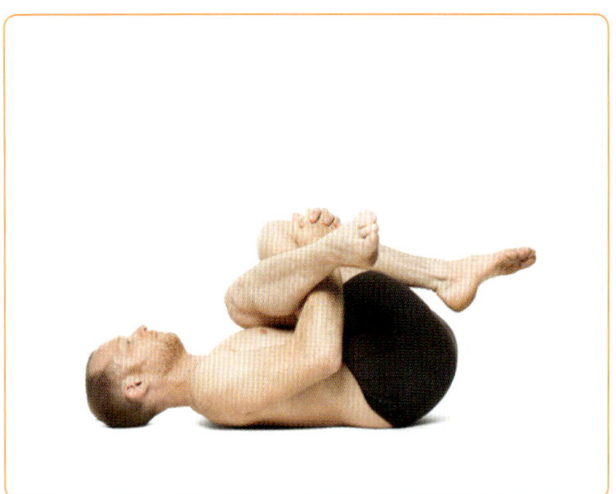

reclined cow face

firmly rotated pose
jathara parivartanasana

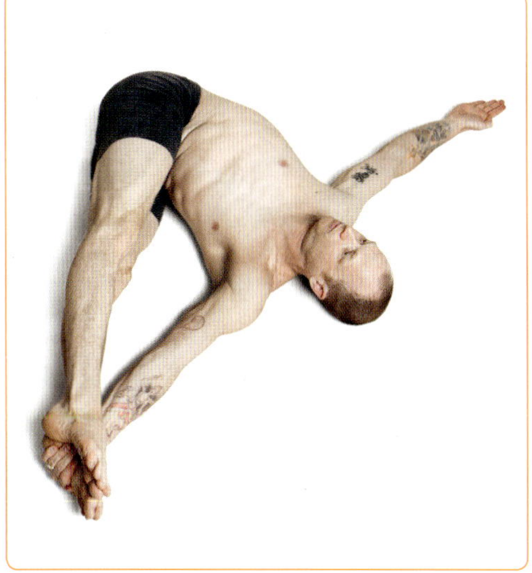

shape prep (from reclined mountain)
- Extend arms out to side in line with shoulders. Point palms up.
- Lift legs vertical to floor.
- Lift hips up and to the right four inches.

shape pose
- Stay here or lower feet to left hand (more doable: same pose with bent knees or lower left foot only; keep right leg vertical).
- Bring right shoulder to/toward floor.
- Flex feet, flare toes—feet as flush as possible.

safety (strength) prep
- Squeeze legs together.
- Tone quads, tighten kneecaps, firm hamstrings.

safety (strength) pose
- Tone, turn abdomen to right.

refinement (stretch) pose
- Lift chest, stretch spine.

Repeat on the second side.

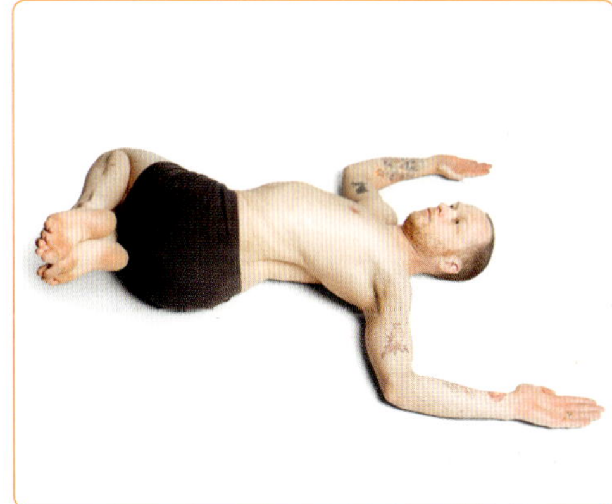

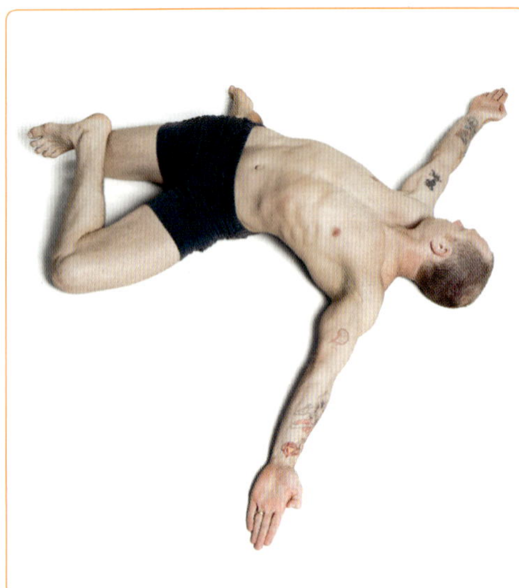

double diamond
visvavajrasana

shape prep (from reclined mountain)
▮ Extend arms out to side in line with shoulders. Point palms up.
▮ Place feet on floor directly in front of hips—feet slightly wider than hips. Lift hips up and to left four inches.

shape pose
▮ Without moving the feet, lower legs to right—left knee directly above right foot (more difficult: place right foot on top of left knee).
▮ Flex feet, flare toes.
▮ Look to left.

safety (strength) pose
▮ Squeeze feet toward hips.

refinement (stretch) pose
▮ Extend knees out.

Repeat on the second side.

This pose is inherently calming. It is like bright lights being dimmed for the nervous system. Become heavy with relaxation—a precious, and all too often scarce, resource.

reclined lunge
eka pada sukha balasana

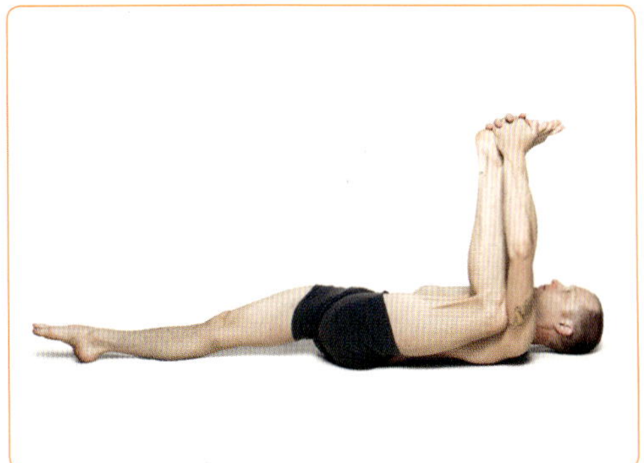

shape (from reclined mountain)
- Bend right knee. Hold right foot with hands—arms inside leg, shin vertical.
- Pull right knee to/toward floor just outside torso.
- Flex right foot, flare toes.

safety (strength) pose
- Press right foot, hands together.
- Tone abdomen.
- Tone left thigh, tighten kneecap, firm hamstrings.
- Press left heel down, in. Extend inner edge of left leg towards floor.

refinement (stretch) pose
- Lift chest, stretch spine.

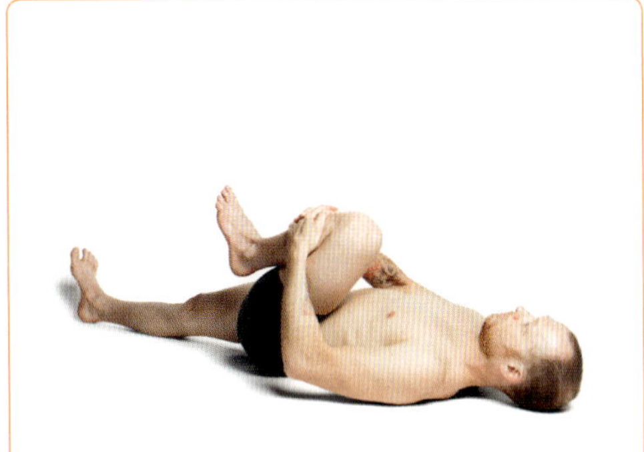

happy baby
sukha balasana

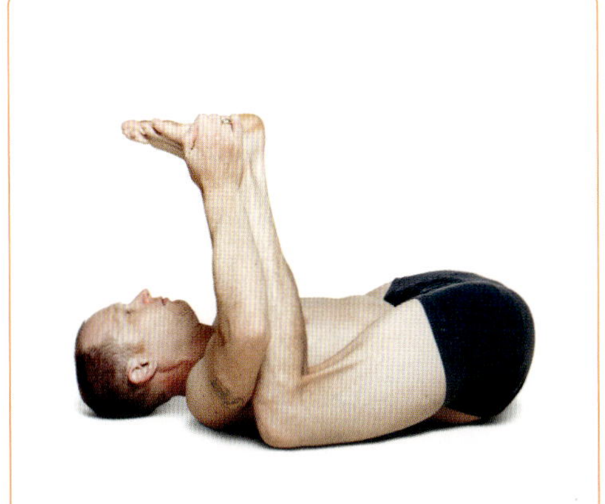

shape pose (from reclined mountain)
- Bend knees, hold outer edges of feet with hands—shins vertical.
- Pull knees to/toward floor just outside torso.
- Flex feet, flare toes.
- Allow low back to round.
- Lift chin slightly.

safety (strength) pose
- Press feet, hands together.
- Tone abdomen.

refinement (stretch) pose
- Lift chest, stretch spine.

For the low back, this pose is similar to legs-behind-the-head pose.

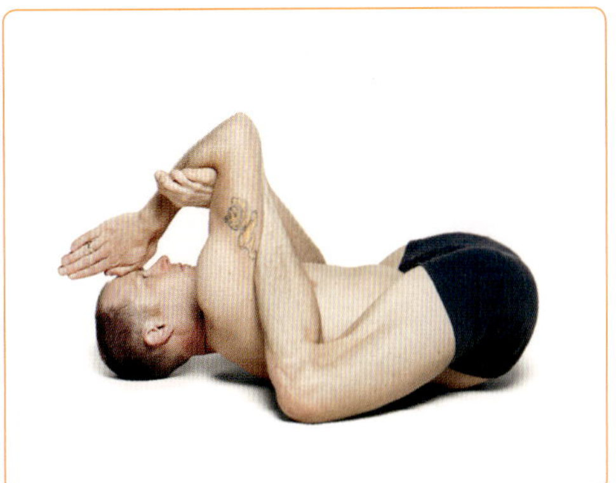

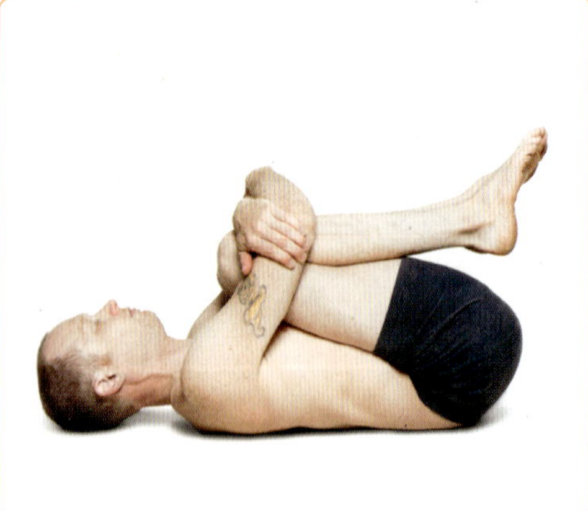

reclined child's pose
supta balasana

shape pose (from reclined mountain)
- Hug legs to chest.
- Bring inner edges of feet together.
- Lift chin slightly. Look up.

safety (strength) pose
- Tone abdomen.

refinement (stretch) pose
- Breathe. Soften face/jaw.

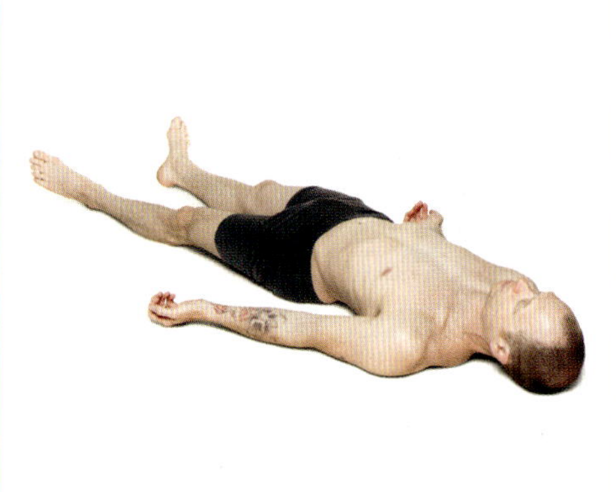

pose of repose
savasana

shape pose
- Lie down on back.
- Separate feet slightly wider than hip distance apart.
- Separate arms slightly away from torso. Point palms up.
- Close eyes.

safety (strength) pose
- Allow this time to rest.

refinement (stretch) pose
- Release breath. Receive benefits of practice.

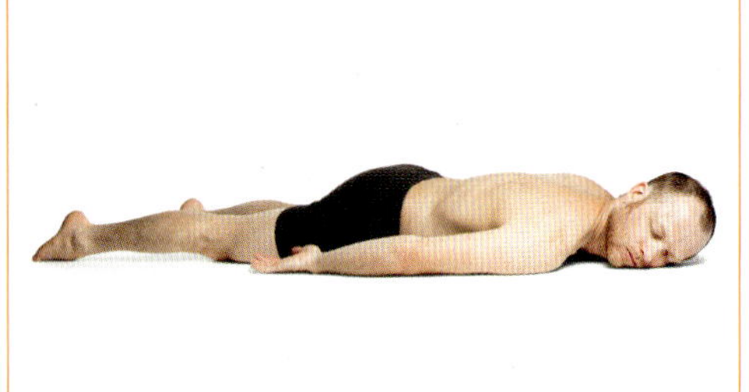

B.K.S. Iyengar says this apparently easy posture is one of the most difficult to master. The practice of remaining quiet and motionless teaches you to relax, often not an easy task.

Yoga teaches us how to both fully engage and completely relax. For many, like myself, complete relaxation is actually more difficult to attain. After stretching away stress for an hour, however, relaxation comes naturally and with ease.

A

accomplished pose · 74
adho mukha svanasana · 55
agnistambhasana · 92
akarna dhanurasana 1 · 96
akarna dhanurasana 2 · 97
anantasana · 79
anjaneyasana · 28
archer's pose 1 · 96
archer's pose 2 · 97
ardha chandrachapasana · 50
ardha chandrasana · 49
ardha hanumanasana · 81
ardha matsyendrasana 1 · 99
ardha matsyendrasana 1 prep · 96
ardha navasana · 70
arm pressure pose · 115
astangasana · 133
astavakrasana · 113

B

baby bird · 111
baddha hasta parsvakonasana · 21
baddha hasta salabhasana · 132
baddha hasta utkatasana · 38
baddha hasta vajrasana · 61
baddha konasana · 75
baddha parsvakonasana · 22
bakasana · 116
balasana · 56
bharadvajasana 1 · 93
bhekasana · 149
bhujangasana · 125
bhujangasana prep · 124, 125
bhujapidasana · 115
bitilasana · 134
boat · 69
both-big-toes pose · 67
bound angle · 75
bound side angle · 22
bow · 154
bowing sage · 41, 42
bridge · 152
building bridge · 153

C

camatkarasana · 110
camel · 158
cat · 53
cat forehead to knee · 54

chaturanga dandasana · 105
child's pose · 56
cobra elbows bent · 125
cobra torso on floor · 124
cosmic abs · 70
cow · 134
cowface 1 · 89
cowface 2 · 90
crane · 116
crescent · 8
crescent 1 wrist · 9
crescent 2 triceps · 10
crescent 3 leg lifted · 11
crocodile · 128
crooked sage · 113

D

dancing yogi · 48
dandasana · 64
dhanurasana · 154
double diamond · 178
downward facing dog · 55
down-dog lunge · 13
dwi hasta padasana · 41, 42
dwi pada koundinyasana · 120
dwi pada viparita dandasana · 162

E

eagle · 47
east stretch · 143
easy pose · 72
eight angle pose · 133
eka hasta bhujasana · 112
eka pada bakasana 2 · 118
eka pada bhekasana · 148
eka pada dhanurasana · 138, 139, 155
eka pada galavasana · 119
eka pada gomukha paschimottanasana · 88
eka pada koundinyasana 1 · 121
eka pada koundinyasana 2 · 122
eka pada rajakapotasana 1 prep · 144, 145
eka pada rajakapotasana 2 prep · 150
eka pada rajakapotasana prep · 84, 85, 86
eka pada sukha balasana · 179
eka pada supta virasana · 165, 166, 174
eka pada urdhva dhanurasana · 161
elevated bow 1 same leg and arm · 139
elevated bow 2 opposite leg and arm · 138
elevated half frog · 149
elevated locust · 33

index

elevated pigeon · 46
elevated thunderbolt · 60
endless pose · 79
extended side angle · 20

F
fallen sage · 87
fire logs · 92
firmly rotated pose · 177
flying pigeon · 119
foot to hand · 19
forward fold · 18
forward fold knees bent · 17
frog · 149

G
garland 2 · 59
garland prep · 58
garudasana · 47
gate keeper · 80
gomukhasana 1 · 89
gomukhasana 2 · 90

H
half boat · 70
half frog · 148
half lord of the fishes · 99
half lord of the fishes elbow bent · 98
half moon · 49
hand-to-big-toe · 39, 40, 43
happy baby · 179
head knee pose · 77, 78
hero · 62
heron · 95
high lunge · 29
hindolasana · 91
holy cow pose · 88

I
indudalasana · 8, 9, 10, 11
intense east stretch · 143
intense west stretch · 66
inverted locust · 131
inverted staff · 162

J
janu sirsasana · 77
jathara parivartanasana · 177

K
k sage 1 · 121
k sage 2 · 122
kapinjalasana prep · 111
king pigeon prep · 157
kneeling sage · 81
krounchasana · 95

L
lateral seated angle · 83
leg lifts · 71
levitating sage · 44
locust 1 · 127
locust 2 · 127
locust hands bound · 132
lolasana · 114
lunge · 12

M
m sage 1 · 101
m sage 3 · 102
makarasana · 128
malasana 2 · 59
malasana prep · 58
marichyasana 1 · 101
marichyasana 3 · 102
marjarasana · 53
mayurasana · 123
meditation pose · 73
mermaid 1 · 146
mermaid 2 · 147
monkey lunge · 28
monkey lunge quad stretch · 150
mountain · 6

N
naginyasana 1 · 146
naginyasana 2 · 147
natarajasana · 48
navasana · 69
needle's eye · 175
no-handed lunge · 21
noose elbow bent · 103

O

one-hand arm pose · 112
one-leg bow · 155
one-leg crane (a) · 118
one-leg crane (b) · 118
one-leg reclined hero · 174

P

padahastasana · 19
parighasana · 80
parivrtta adho mukha svanasana · 56
parivrtta ardha chandrachapasana prep · 52
parivrtta ardha chandrasana · 51
parivrtta hasta padangusthasana · 43
parivrtta janu sirsasana · 78
parivrtta marichyasana 1 · 100
parivrtta supta padangusthasana prep · 163
parivrtta supta padangusthasana · 172
parivrtta trikonasana · 25
parivrtta utkatasana · 37
parivrtta virasana · 63
parsva bakasana · 117
parsva dhanurasana · 156
parsva upavistha konasana · 83
parsvottanasana · 26, 27
parvatasana · 7
pasasana prep · 103
paschimottanasana · 65, 66
peacock · 123
pigeon prep · 84
pigeon quad stretch · 145
pigeon torso upright · 144
plank · 104
plank leg in tree · 105
pose of repose · 180
power pose · 35
power pose hands bound · 38
power pose head to knee · 36
prasarita padottanasana · 23
purvottanasana · 143
purvottanasana prep · 141, 142

R

radical reclined big toe · 171
rajakapotasana prep · 157
reclined big toe 1 · 169
reclined big toe leg to side · 170
reclined big toe forehead to knee · 170
reclined big toe hands to thigh · 168

reclined bowing sage · 164
reclined child's pose · 180
reclined hero · 173
reclined west stretch · 68
reclined lunge · 179
reclined pigeon · 176
reclined revolved sage · 172
reverse mudra · 27
reverse mudra hands on floor · 26
reverse table · 141
reverse table leg lifted · 142
reverse warrior · 32
revolved half moon · 51
revolved head knee pose · 78
revolved lunge · 15
revolved m sage 1 clasp wrist · 100
revolved sage · 43
revolved sugar cane prep · 52
revolved triangle · 25

S

salabhasana 1 · 127
salabhasana 2 · 127
seated angle · 82
seated pigeon · 91
setu bandha sarvangasana · 151
siddhasana · 74
sideways bow · 156
southpaw tiger · 135
staff · 64
standing sage · 39
standing sage leg to side · 40
star · 76
sucirandhrasana · 175
sugar cane · 50
sukha balasana · 179
sukhasana · 72
summit · 7
superhero · 129
supine twist · 163
supta balasana · 180
supta dwi hasta padasana · 164
supta hindolasana · 176
supta padangusthasana · 169, 170. 171
supta padangusthasana prep · 168
supta virasana · 173

index

T

tadasana · 6
tarasana · 76
thunderbolt arms extended · 61
thunderbolt hands bound · 61
thunderbolt quad stretch · 140
Tibetan weaponry 1 · 165
Tibetan weaponry 2 · 166
Tibetan weaponry 3 · 167
tiger opposite leg and arm · 136
tiger same leg and arm · 137
topsy-turvy superhero · 130
tree · 45
tremulous · 114
triad · 94
triang mukhaikapada paschimottanasana · 94
triangle · 24
turned crane · 117
twisted child's pose · 57
twisted down dog · 56
twisted hero · 63
twisted lunge · 16
twisted monkey · 153
twisted pigeon 1 shoulder to knee · 85
twisted pigeon 2 shoulder to arch of foot · 86
twisted power pose · 37
twisted sage · 93
two leg k sage · 120

U

ubhaya padangusthasana · 67
upavistha konasana · 82
upward bow · 160
upward bow head on floor · 159
upward bow one leg lifted · 161
upward facing dog · 126
urdhva dhanurasana · 160
urdhva dhanurasana prep · 159
urdhva eka pada bhekasana · 149
urdhva mukha paschimottanasana 2 · 68
urdhva mukha svanasana · 126
urdhva prasarita padasana · 71
ustrasana · 158
utkatasana · 35, 36
uttana mayurasana prep · 152
uttanasana · 18
utthita eka padasana · 44
utthita hasta padangusthasana 1 · 39
utthita hasta padangusthasana 2 · 40

U

utthita hindolasana · 46
utthita parsvakonasana · 20
utthita trikonasana · 24

V

v sage · 109
v sage bottom leg in tree · 108
v sage prep · 106
v sage top leg in tree · 107
vajrasana · 60, 61, 140
vasisthasana · 107, 108, 109
vasisthasana prep · 106
viparita salabhasana prep · 131
viparita virabhadrasana · 32
virabhadrasana prep · 29
virabhadrasana 1 · 30
virabhadrasana 1 prep · 29
virabhadrasana 2 · 31
virabhadrasana 3 · 34
virasana · 62
visvavajrasana · 178
vrksasana · 45
vyaghrasana · 54, 135, 136, 137

W

warrior 1 · 30
warrior 2 · 31
warrior 3 · 34
west stretch knees bent · 65
wide-leg forward fold · 23
wild thing · 110